FOURTH EDITION

4

CASES WORKBOOK FOR THE MRCGP

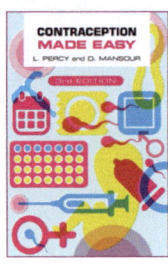
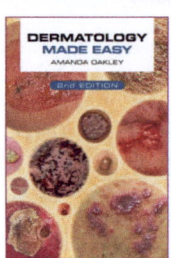
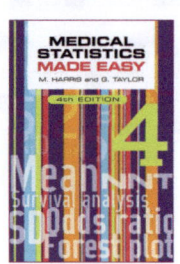
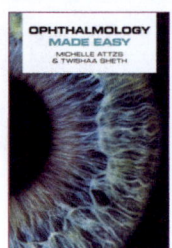
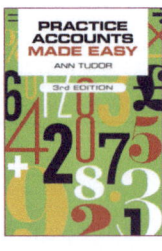
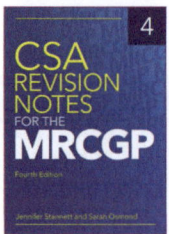
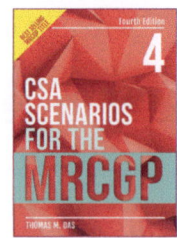
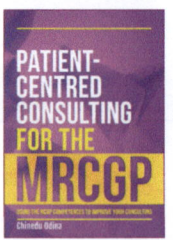
For more details see www.scionpublishing.com

Over 100 SCA cases aligned to the RCGP Blueprint areas

FOURTH EDITION

4

CASES WORKBOOK FOR THE MRCGP

Ellen Welch (MBChB, MRCGP (2013), MRCEM, BA (Hons), DTMH, DFSRH)
GP, Carlisle, Cumbria

and Jennifer Lyall (MBBS, MRCGP (2013), DRCOG, DFSRH)
GP, Workington, Cumbria

With contributions from:
Irina Zacharcenkova and George Bardsley

Scion

© **Scion Publishing Limited, 2024**

ISBN 9781914961571 (hardback ring-bound version)
ISBN 9781914961441 (loose-leaf version)

Fourth edition first published 2024
Third edition published 2019
Second edition published 2017
First edition published 2014

Scion Publishing Limited
The Old Hayloft, Vantage Business Park, Bloxham Road, Banbury OX16 9UX, UK
www.scionpublishing.com

Important Note from the Publisher
The information contained within this book was obtained by Scion Publishing Ltd from sources believed by us to be reliable. However, while every effort has been made to ensure its accuracy, no responsibility for loss or injury whatsoever occasioned to any person acting or refraining from action as a result of information contained herein can be accepted by the authors or publishers.

Readers are reminded that medicine is a constantly evolving science and while the authors and publishers have ensured that all dosages, applications and practices are based on current indications, there may be specific practices which differ between communities. You should always follow the guidelines laid down by the manufacturers of specific products and the relevant authorities in the country in which you are practising.

Although every effort has been made to ensure that all owners of copyright material have been acknowledged in this publication, we would be pleased to acknowledge in subsequent reprints or editions any omissions brought to our attention.

Registered names, trademarks, etc. used in this book, even when not marked as such, are not to be considered unprotected by law.

Typeset by Evolution Design & Digital Ltd (Kent)
Printed in the UK
Last digit is the print number: 10 9 8 7

Contents

Preface to the fourth edition

The first edition of this workbook was written in 2013 when we were all still GP Registrars preparing for the CSA ourselves. We struggled to find the resources we needed at the time to revise in a meaningful way for the exam, so decided to create our own. *Cases Workbook for the MRCGP* presents a practical and organised approach to the exam, allowing candidates to access SCA role-play scenarios aligned to the RCGP Curriculum and Blueprint areas, alongside a logical structure to exam preparation and revision.

The Workbook has been enthusiastically received and we have been delighted to read positive feedback from GP Registrars who have gone on to pass the exam using our book. We were delighted to win the Young Author Award at the BMA Book Awards, as well as being highly commended in the General Practice category. We've also taken on the criticisms – the main one being that this book doesn't provide 'the answers'. Our response to this is that every consultation in general practice is unique; what works for one clinician may not work for another. The purpose of this workbook is not to provide a script with all the answers, but to allow you to practise clinical scenarios and find your own consultation style. What we do provide is up-to-date links to the clinical information you need, and a basic structure to your revision that follows what the SCA examiners are looking for.

Our fourth edition presents over 100 remote consultation scenarios, alongside QR codes, accessible by smartphone, to help keep abreast of ever-changing guidelines. You will find the QR codes throughout the book and they take you to hyperlinked PDFs for every Curriculum area and every Blueprint area (and there's one at the start that takes you to a single PDF that covers all the weblinks in the entire book), so that during a revision session, any clinical queries can be addressed using the most up-to-date resources available.

We hope this newest edition will continue to provide a valuable resource for registrars applying to sit their SCA.

All the best – you can do it!

Ellen Welch
Jenny Lyall

Acknowledgements

Huge thanks need to go firstly to Jonathan Ray at Scion Publishing, for bringing this workbook into its 4th edition, more than 10 years after the first one came out. Thank you for sticking with us and always being patient with the deadlines being missed, and always hugely supportive of our ideas. Clare Boomer also deserves big thanks for her painstaking checking of case numbers and the finer details. The 4th edition needed a huge re-do since the structure of the exam has changed over recent years, but we did keep some of the original cases that Irina and George Bardsley wrote – thanks to you both for your time on these. Thank you to Elissa Abi-Raad for your suggestions about the structure of the book, as one of the first cohorts of registrars to sit the new exam. And thank you to Dr Sarah Jacques and Dr Lizzie Toberty for proofreading the book. Thanks to our own revision group who helped us get through our own exam, and finally to you the reader – thanks for buying this book and we hope it helps you.

Abbreviations

AAA	Abdominal aortic aneurysm	DM	Diabetes mellitus
A&E	Accident and Emergency department	DNAR	Do not attempt resuscitation
ABPI	Ankle brachial pressure index	DRE	Digital rectal examination
ACEi	ACE inhibitor	DSH	Deliberate self-harm
ACL	Anterior cruciate ligament	DVLA	Driver and Vehicle Licensing Agency
ACR	Albumin–creatinine ratio	DVT	Deep vein thrombosis
ACS	Acute coronary syndrome	ECG	Electrocardiogram
ADHD	Attention deficit hyperactivity disorder	eGFR	Estimated glomerular filtration rate
ADL	Activities of daily living	ENT	Ear, nose and throat
AF	Atrial fibrillation		(Otorhinolaryngology)
AiT	Associate in training	ESR	Erythrocyte sedimentation rate
AKT	Applied knowledge test	ET	Exercise tolerance
ALP	Alkaline phosphatase	FBC	Full blood count
ALT	Alanine aminotransferase	FEV_1	Forced expiratory volume in 1 second
AS	Ankylosing spondylitis	FGM	Female genital mutilation
ASD	Atrial septal defect	FSH	Follicle-stimulating hormone
BCC	Basal cell carcinoma	FVC	Forced vital capacity
BMD	Bone mineral density	GCS	Glasgow Coma Scale
BMI	Body mass index	GFR	Glomerular filtration rate
BMJ	*British Medical Journal*	GGT	Gamma-glutamyl transferase
BNF	*British National Formulary*	GI	Gastro-intestinal
BNP	Brain natriuretic peptide	GMC	General Medical Council
BP	Blood pressure	GORD	Gastro-oesophageal reflux disease
BS	Bowel sounds	GTN	Glyceryl trinitrate
BTS	British Thoracic Society	GUM	Genito-urinary medicine
CAMHS	Child and Adolescent Mental Health	Hb	Haemoglobin
	Services	HbA1c	Glycated haemoglobin
CBT	Cognitive behavioural therapy	HIV	Human immunodeficiency virus
CCF	Congestive cardiac failure	HOCM	Hypertrophic cardiomyopathy
CCT	Certificate of completion of training	HPV	Human papillomavirus
CFU	Colony-forming units	HR	Heart rate
CHD	Chronic heart disease	HRT	Hormone replacement therapy
CI	Contraindication	HS	Heart sounds
COCP	Combined oral contraceptive pill (or COC)	HTN	Hypertension
COPD	Chronic obstructive pulmonary disease	I&D	Incision and drainage
COT	Consultation observation tools	IBD	Inflammatory bowel disease
CKD	Chronic kidney disease	IBS	Irritable bowel syndrome
Cr	Creatinine	ICE	Ideas, concerns and expectations
CRF	Chronic renal failure	ICP	Intracranial pressure
CRP	C-reactive protein	IELTS	International English Language Testing
CSA	Clinical Skills Assessment		System
CVD	Cardiovascular disease	IM	Intramuscular
CVS	Chorionic villus sampling	IMB	Inter-menstrual bleeding
CXR	Chest X-ray	IMG	International medical graduates
DEXA	Dual-energy X-ray absorptiometry	IUD	Intrauterine device (e.g. copper coil)
DH	Drug history	IUS	Intrauterine system (e.g. Mirena)

IVDU	Intravenous drug user	PO	*Per orum* (orally)
K	Potassium	POP	Progesterone-only contraceptive pill
LARC	Long-acting reversible contraception	PPI	Proton pump inhibitor
LD	Learning disability	PR	Per rectum (examination)
LFTs	Liver function tests	prn	Pro re nata (as needed)
LGV	Lymphogranuloma venereum	PSA	Prostate-specific antigen
LMP	Last menstrual period	PTSD	Post-traumatic stress disorder
LOC	Loss of consciousness	PVD	Peripheral vascular disease
LRTI	Lower respiratory tract infection	RA	Rheumatoid arthritis
LTOT	Long-term oxygen therapy	RCA	Recorded Consultation Assessment
LUTS	Lower urinary tract symptoms	RCGP	Royal College of General Practitioners
MCS	Microscopy, culture and sensitivities	RCOG	Royal College of Obstetricians and Gynaecologists
MCV	Mean corpuscular volume		
MDT	Multi-disciplinary team	RhF	Rheumatoid factor
ME/CFS	Myalgic encephalomyelitis / chronic fatigue syndrome	RICE	Rest, ice, compression, elevation
		RR	Respiratory rate
MI	Myocardial infarction	Rx	Treatment
MMR	Measles, mumps, rubella vaccination	SCA	Simulated Consultation Assessment
MRCGP	Member of the Royal College of General Practitioners	SCBU	Special care baby unit
		SCC	Squamous cell carcinoma
MS	Multiple sclerosis	SI	Sacroiliac
MSU	Mid-stream urine	SIGN	Scottish Intercollegiate Guidelines Network
Na	Sodium		
NAD	Nothing abnormal detected	SLE	Systemic lupus erythematosus
NAI	Non-accidental injury	SOB	Shortness of breath
NHS	National Health Service	SpO$_2$	Pulse oximetry measurement
NICE	National Institute for Health and Care Excellence	SSRI	Selective serotonin reuptake inhibitor
		ST3	Specialist trainee year 3
NIV	Non-invasive ventilation	STD	Sexually transmitted disease
NRT	Nicotine replacement therapy	STI	Sexually transmitted infection
NSAID	Non-steroidal anti-inflammatory drug	SVC	Superior vena cava
NTDs	Neural tube defects	SVT	Supraventricular tachycardia
NVD	Normal vaginal delivery	T	Temperature
OCP	Ova, cysts and parasites	T2DM	Type 2 diabetes mellitus
OE	On examination	TATT	Tired all the time
OOH	Out of hours	TB	Tuberculosis
OSA	Obstructive sleep apnoea	TCA	Tricyclic antidepressant
OSCE	Objective structured clinical examination	TFTs	Thyroid function tests
		TIA	Transient ischaemic attack
OTC	Over-the-counter	TSH	Thyroid-stimulating hormone
PCB	Post-coital bleeding	U&Es	Urea and electrolytes
PCOS	Polycystic ovary syndrome	UPSI	Unprotected sexual intercourse
PE	Pulmonary embolism	Ur	Urea
PEFR	Peak expiratory flow rate	URTI	Upper respiratory tract infection
PERL	Pupils equal and reactive to light	USS	Ultrasound scan
PID	Pelvic inflammatory disease	UTI	Urinary tract infection
PIL	Patient information leaflet	VA	Visual acuity
PLAB	Professional and linguistic assessment board exam	VTE	Venous thromboembolism
		WCC	White cell count
Plt	Platelets	WPBA	Workplace-based assessments
PND	Paroxysmal nocturnal dyspnoea		

PART I: THE SCA

Chapter 1: An introduction to the MRCGP

The College of General Practitioners was founded back in 1952 as an academic body to improve standards and establish general practice as a discipline. Prior to this, GPs were widely regarded as second-rate compared to those pursuing hospital careers. GPs had no specific training, no body of scientific knowledge and no journals or college of their own. The membership exam (MRCGP) was set up in 1965, the same year the College called for vocational training for general practice. It was granted its Royal Charter in 1972, becoming the Royal College of General Practitioners (RCGP). The MRCGP exam was an optional qualification until 2007, when it became an integrated training and assessment system to prepare doctors for NHS general practice. Known initially as the nMRCGP ('new MRCGP') it was introduced as an evidence-based assessment of professional competency based on modern educational theory.

The format of the MRCGP has been tweaked over the years and the Simulated Consultation Assessment (SCA) emerged as the latest incarnation of the Clinical Skills Assessment (CSA) at the end of 2023. This replaced the temporary Recorded Consultation Assessment (RCA) brought in during the Covid-19 pandemic, which allowed GP registrars to complete their training within the restrictions caused by the pandemic.

The three separate components of the MRCGP exam currently include:
* Applied Knowledge Test (AKT) – a computer-based 200-question multiple choice exam, taken after reaching the ST2 stage of training; tests the knowledge base behind NHS general practice. It takes place four times a year at Pearson VUE test centres across the UK, taking 3 hours 10 minutes to complete.
* Simulated Consultation Assessment (SCA) – a practical examination taken during the ST3 training year and conducted remotely in a local GP surgery. It assesses a doctor's ability to integrate and apply clinical, professional, communication and practical skills appropriate for general practice via an evaluation of 12 simulated consultations.
* Workplace-Based Assessments (WPBA) – evaluate day-to-day practice by completion of specific assessments and reports, documentation of naturally occurring evidence and mandatory training (such as Basic Life Support and Child Safeguarding) – carried out throughout GP training.

Completion of all three parts of the MRCGP is required before trainees are issued a certificate of completion of training (CCT). The RCGP website provides further information on the necessary requirements and should be checked prior to the examination for any updates (www.rcgp.org.uk/training-exams/mrcgp-exams-overview.aspx).

1.1 Overview of the SCA exam

The SCA is a practical OSCE-style online exam, sat during the ST3 year, which aims to simulate a busy day at work in an NHS GP surgery. The college created the SCA to reflect real-life general practice and to recognise the different types of consultation that now occur in primary care.

The exam consists of 12 remote consultations, a mix of both video and telephone, each lasting 12 minutes, with a 3-minute gap between each case. It is carried out remotely at a local GP surgery via an online IT platform. Ideally this will be in the candidate's usual training practice, and the college is working to ensure as many practices as possible meet the necessary IT requirements.

The patients in each case are performed by professional role-players, trained and standardised to provide the same standard of case for each trainee, but with the ability to respond to the approach of each individual doctor. Each case is based on a remote consultation – in some, the simulated patient will be visible, others will be audio only. Cases may involve the patient themselves, their carer / parent or other health and social care workers. Notably, physical examinations are not assessed as part of the SCA and are instead covered within WPBA.

1.2 When to sit the SCA

At present the SCA can only be taken during the ST3 stage of GP specialty training. There are 9 sittings throughout the year which you can book 12 months in advance via a link on the trainee e-portfolio. The current fee for the exam is £1180 and you can book and pay 7 weeks ahead of your exam date. Reserving a slot does not constitute a booking (although you must reserve to be eligible to book). This does mean, however, that you can adjust your reservation date at any time up to 7 weeks prior to your examination date. This is all done via your trainee e-portfolio.

1.3 Marking scheme

The RCGP has produced guidance on the passing grade (the standard) used by the examiners.

Each case will be marked in three domains:

1. Data gathering and diagnosis
2. Clinical management and medical complexity
3. Relating to others

These domains all link to the capabilities used in WPBA which are available here: www.rcgp.org.uk/getmedia/073d0d80-a8fb-42ae-a23d-a8be6aa12572/WPBA-capabilities-with-IPUs-detailed-descriptors.pdf

Each domain will be graded as follows:
- CP (clear pass) – this domain is clearly demonstrated above the standard of a newly qualified, independent GP
- P (pass): this domain is sufficiently demonstrated at the standard of a newly qualified, independent GP
- F (fail): this domain is insufficiently demonstrated at the standard of a newly qualified, independent GP
- CF (clear fail): this domain is clearly demonstrated below the standard of a newly qualified, independent GP

The trainee's mark is determined by their performance across the whole assessment, and they will not be required to pass a certain number of stations. Examiners will mark the three domains, and will also judge the candidate's general performance on each case. The pass mark for each case will be based on this assessment through a standard setting process typical for OSCE-type exams (called borderline regression). This means there is no fixed pass mark for each case.

The standard descriptors are detailed below, but the RCGP clearly emphasises that they are not 'tick boxes' for passing the examination, and each behaviour listed does not need to be demonstrated by candidates in every case. They are used to guide judgements for examiners and to enhance consistency. An examiner marks the same case all day. The three domains in each case may be weighted, meaning that the domains contribute to the overall mark for the case in different ways (e.g. clinical management may carry more weight in one case). Examiners are not aware of this weighting to avoid it influencing their marking.

Data gathering and diagnosis (passing level)

- Systematically gathers and organises relevant and targeted information to address the needs of the patient and their problem(s).
- Adopts a structured and informed approach to problem-solving, generating an appropriate differential diagnosis or relying on first principles where the presentation is undifferentiated, uncertain or complex.

Data gathering
- Systematically gathers information, using questions targeted to the problem, ensuring patient safety.
- Makes effective use of existing information about the problem and the wider context.
- Establishes the presence or absence of red flags.
- Elicits relevant psychological and social information to place the patient's problem(s) in context.

Making a diagnosis
- Uses a structured and evidence-based approach to diagnostic reasoning.
- Uses an understanding of probability based on prevalence, incidence and natural history to aid decision-making.
- Revises hypotheses as necessary in the light of additional information.
- Addresses problems that present early and/or in an undifferentiated way by integrating all the available information to help generate a reasonable working hypothesis.

Clinical management and medical complexity (passing level)

- Demonstrates the ability to formulate safe and appropriate management options which includes effective prioritisation, continuity and time and self-management.
- Demonstrates commitment to providing optimum care in the short and long term, whilst acknowledging the challenges.

Clinical management
- Considers a "wait and see" approach where appropriate.
- Encourages patient understanding with suggestions for self-care or lifestyle modification.
- Applies local and/or national guidelines, including for drug and non-drug therapies.
- Demonstrates principles of safe prescribing.
- Refers when required, being mindful of available resources.
- Suggests safe and sensible follow-up arrangements, as well as continuity of care.

- Ensures care is coordinated within the practice team and/or with other services, where necessary.
- Varies management options responsively according to the circumstances, priorities and preferences of all those involved.
- Makes safe, evidence-based decisions that are defensible even when difficult.
- Thinks flexibly around problems, generating functional solutions.

Medical complexity

- Concurrently manages all health conditions, both short- and long-term, acute and chronic, and multimorbidity.
- Prioritises management options based on an understanding of risk.
- Manages uncertainty, including that experienced by the patient.
- Adjusts care as necessary in the management of multiple problems, recognising the implications of multimorbidity and polypharmacy.
- Manages health improvement, rehabilitation, prevention and health promotion.

Practising holistically, promoting health and safeguarding

- Engages support agencies targeted to the needs of the patient and/or their family and carers.
- Recognises and responds to adult and child safeguarding concerns, including ensuring information is shared and referrals are made when required.

Relating to others (passing level)

- Demonstrates ethical awareness.
- Shows ability to communicate in a person-centred way.
- Demonstrates initiative and flexibility in using various consultation approaches in order to overcome any communication barriers and to reach a shared understanding with the patient.

Fitness to practise

- Shows respect for patients, treating them fairly and without discrimination.
- Takes ownership of decisions and with confidence, whilst being aware of own limitations.

Maintaining an ethical approach

- Recognises cultural and personal differences in patients and/or colleagues.
- Recognises that everyone has their own values and beliefs.
- Acts non-judgmentally with equity and fairness.
- Recognises and respects patient autonomy.
- Acts with beneficence, and in the patient's best interests.
- Shows awareness of medico-legal concepts, such as informed consent, mental capacity and best interests of the patient.

Communication and consultation skills

- Explores and clarifies the patient's agenda, health beliefs and preferences.
- Employs a range of communication skills, both verbal and non-verbal, including active listening skills.
- Responds to important, significant cues (verbal and non-verbal). Uses language that is understandable and takes into consideration the needs and characteristics of the patient.
- Uses a variety of communication techniques and materials to adapt explanations to the patient.
- Uses the patient's understanding, agenda, health beliefs and preferences to help tailor any explanation offered.

- Works in partnership with the patient, negotiating a mutually acceptable plan which is clear and understandable.
- Checks the patient's understanding of the consultation including any agreed plans.
- Demonstrates an empathetic approach, including a willingness to help and care for the patient.

Working with colleagues
- Works collaboratively, understanding the context within which different team members work, respecting their role, and valuing their opinions.
- Shows respect for colleagues, treating them fairly and without discrimination.

Practising holistically, promoting health, and safeguarding
- Recognises and acknowledges the impact of the problem on the patient, their family and/or carers.
- Challenges assertively unhelpful health beliefs or behaviours, whilst remaining respectful and maintaining a continuing and productive relationship.
- Recognises what matters to the patient and works collaboratively to enhance patient care.

1.4 SCA practicalities

Because the SCA is carried out remotely, trainees need to ensure their surgery is set up with the appropriate IT requirements to be SCA-ready, and the college has created a comprehensive surgery preparation guide which we advise checking in case of updates (www.rcgp.org.uk/mrcgp-exams/simulated-consultation-assessment/trainee-surgery-guide).

☐ **Book a room**
Office space in GP surgeries is a precious resource, and it is important to liaise with your trainer and wider team to ensure you can book a suitable space where you can undertake the exam without being disturbed. The morning exam sessions run between 08:45 and 13:25, and the afternoon sessions between 13:20 and 18:05. Trainees will be informed of their allocated examination date and session at least one month before the exam.

☐ **Room set-up**
To make the space SCA-ready, the allocated examination room needs to ensure:
- Only one computer monitor is used; all others in the room should be unplugged
- Any landline telephones in the room are disconnected
- The room should be free from noise
- Clinical guidance documents and medical posters on the wall should be covered or removed
- An 'examination in progress' sign is placed outside the door.

☐ **IT set-up**
The exam is conducted via a program called Osler Online, which is an online application that can run through your web browser, requiring no download or installation. Candidates are not required to purchase any additional equipment to sit the SCA. The following technical requirements are needed for the platform to work, however:
- A laptop or PC (Osler Online does not currently run on tablets or mobile devices)
- Minimum screen resolution of 1024×768
- Windows or Mac operating systems only (Windows 10 or newer, Sierra 10.12 or newer)
- A built-in camera on a laptop or monitor or an external webcam attached to a monitor. If the webcam is bolted on or embedded in the monitor, the invigilator will ask you to perform an environment check using a combination of your webcam and the camera on your mobile phone

- A built-in microphone and speaker, or external wired headphones and microphone. Bluetooth headsets are not permitted.
- The minimum recommended bandwidth for Osler Online is 10 Mbps download and 4 Mbps upload. You can check your internet speed from the device and room you intend to use for your examination via Speed Test: www.speedtest.net.

Osler Online is only compatible with Google Chrome and Microsoft Edge. It's advisable to update your browser ahead of examination day (do this by opening the browser, click 'more' at the top right, click 'update' then 'relaunch').

Platform onboarding

As part of the examination process, you are required to book an onboarding session, which needs to be done on the same device and in the same location you will use on your examination day. This session will guide you through logging in, followed by a platform check (connection, webcam and sound check) and ensuring you understand how the program works, alongside basic troubleshooting.

What to bring on the day

- Your mobile phone, placed out of arm's reach and on silent.
- A paper copy of the *BNF* and children's *BNF* (optional).
- A blank whiteboard and pen on your desk to take notes (optional). There is a function within the platform to take notes. Paper or a notepad is not allowed into the examination.
- A drink bottle or glass of water (optional).

Please do not bring:

- Personal electronic devices such as tablets, iPads, cameras or recording devices
- Any preparation materials or notes
- Food or hot drinks.

If any additional necessary items are required such as medications, this needs to be stipulated as a reasonable adjustment which can be applied for via the RCGP website. Find out more about reasonable adjustments here: www.rcgp.org.uk/mrcgp-exams/mrcgp-important-info/reasonable-adjustments.

1.5 Resources available

Despite this exam being brand new, resources are already available to help registrars to prepare. Practising cases with peers is probably the most useful way to get into exam mode, and any material originally designed to guide candidates through the old-style CSA exam is still useful for the SCA. Specific SCA revision courses are appearing online. The RCGP has put together several webinars for both trainers and trainees, along with an SCA consultation toolkit: www.rcgp.org.uk/mrcgp-exams/simulated-consultation-assessment/toolkit.

Chapter 2: How to use this book

2.1 Introduction

We based this workbook around our own preparation for the CSA and have adapted it to work for the SCA. For us, regularly practising different case scenarios and trying out different phrasing or consultation styles was essential exam preparation.

Our approach was to form a revision group and meet on a weekly basis to rehearse case scenarios together and give each other feedback. You can do this in person or remotely. To make each session productive, we suggest choosing a different RCGP curriculum area to focus cases on each week and reading up on the guidelines specific to that topic area. This allows the group sessions to focus on practising consultation skills and role-playing the cases.

The workbook is designed to be used by revision groups as follows:
- The case scenarios we provide (in *Chapter 4*) are divided into the **12 RCGP Blueprint areas of Clinical Experience Groups**. The college has developed a 'Blueprint' to ensure the spread of each assessment is representative and not focused on any one area of practice. These Blueprint areas may already be familiar as they are similar to those used in WPBA. The first 5 Blueprint areas are likely to come up in every diet of the exam.
- The **RCGP Curriculum topic guides** are listed in *Chapter 3*. The topic guides are split into Clinical topic guides, Life stage topic guides and Professional topic guides. Being up-to-date with guidelines and ensuring good medical knowledge is essential for the SCA and the cases can test any area of the curriculum. We suggest revising guidelines and cases following the clinical areas, which are more focused and specific than the Blueprint areas.

How to use the RCGP Curriculum resources (*Chapter 3*)

Each curriculum area comprises a list of useful resources relevant to that topic including:
- *cases provided in this Workbook* – to guide you to the cases relevant to that clinical topic area for your revision sessions
- *possible cases* – those cases most likely to come up in the SCA
- *revision notes* – key clinical guidelines, along with other helpful references and websites, that the whole revision group can read ahead of your practice sessions
- *material for patient* – a list of resources that you could usefully guide the patient towards in the consultation
- *practice explanations* – topics, tests and procedures that you should be able to describe to the patient in a couple of minutes
- *practice examinations* – procedures that you should be able to undertake confidently (although you will not be expected to undertake examinations in the SCA, we think it is still important that you are confident in them for your GP work in the real world).

QR codes
We have used QR codes to give quick access to the weblinks in this book.
- If you scan the QR code on the left using your mobile device, you will be taken to a page on our website where all the weblinks detailed in the book are available as clickable links. Alternatively you can access that page at https://scionpublishing.com/casesworkbook – then click on the Resources tab to reach the clickable weblinks.
- The QR code at the start of each curriculum area takes you to a hyperlinked pdf just for that section.

How to use the cases (*Chapter 4*)

Each case comprises several pages:

- **information for the doctor** – this page provides the doctor with a brief summary of their patient and should be given to the person in your revision group acting as the doctor in the next revision session
- **information for the patient** – this page provides all the background information (including ICE, information divulged freely and information only divulged if specifically asked about) to allow a person in your group to act as the patient, including any results and examination findings that you can provide to the doctor if they ask for it appropriately (we have kept these to basic readings that many patients may be able to provide from home: BP, heart rate, oxygen sats; for some video consultations, we have also provided images of skin lesions)
- **marking scheme for the observer** – this page provides the observer in your group with a simple checklist of descriptors in each of the three domains (data gathering and diagnosis, clinical management and medical complexity, and relating to others) and allows the 'observer' to rank the 'doctor' as pass, borderline, or fail for each descriptor.

This design allows the 'doctor', 'patient' and 'observer' to take out just the pages they need ahead of the next revision session, making the practice consultations as exam-like as possible.

Cases provided in this Workbook

Each curriculum topic area in *Chapter 3* starts by listing the cases in the Workbook that are relevant to that clinical topic area. Note that some of the cases appear more than once because, as in real life, they are relevant to more than one clinical area.

Possible cases

Each topic area also lists possible cases that could potentially come up in the exam – this is a list we have brainstormed together and is not exhaustive, so feel free to think of more of your own. Thinking about potential cases gave us a structure for improving our clinical knowledge, and ensuring we were familiar with current guidelines in the management of common conditions. This is useful not just for the exam, but for life as a GP afterwards, ensuring patients are managed appropriately. The RCGP GP Curriculum provides an overview of the knowledge and skills needed for each topic area, and is available online (www.rcgp.org.uk/mrcgp-exams/gp-curriculum).

Revision notes

The breadth of knowledge needed to be a GP is quite daunting, and we found that dealing with one or two topic areas in each session made the revision process more manageable. Our approach was to try to read around each topic area before meeting up with our revision group, to become familiar with the up-to-date management of common conditions. This allowed us to fill in gaps in our knowledge, and feel more confident that we were prepared at least clinically, even if our communication skills needed some work. We felt strongly that the focus of our revision groups should be to practise the role-playing we all felt nervous about, so doing the clinical preparation in our own time ahead of this meant we could concentrate on the area we didn't get to practise often elsewhere.

To help you with this part of the revision process, we decided to list helpful resources and guidelines relevant to each topic area, along with some patient resources it is useful to be able to signpost to in the exam and beyond.

Smartphone links

In addition to the revision notes, cases have useful weblinks provided – use the QR code next to them to be taken to hyperlinked pages on the resources section of the website that supports the book (https://scionpublishing.com/casesworkbook). These weblinks can be found at the top of every marking scheme and are usually links to clinical information relevant to each case for the observer to access on their smartphone. When the role-playing ends, any questions regarding the current management of the condition in the case can be quickly reviewed using these links. We have also included links to videos of examination techniques, which although not tested in the SCA, is still essential knowledge as a GP.

Explaining and examining

This is something you can do as part of a group or by yourself. Explaining common conditions and treatments to patients in jargon-free language can sometimes be challenging. At the end of our revision group sessions, we would often take turns trying to explain common conditions to each other in two minutes, which made us realise that even if we thought we understood certain conditions well ourselves, our explanations were often not very eloquent. For each topic area we have listed a selection of topics and tests we think it is useful to be well versed in, and which you should practise explaining. We have also listed examination techniques, even if these skills will not be tested in the SCA, because they remain an important part of general practice and you will need to be able to demonstrate them as part of your WPBA.

2.2 Setting up a study group

We still believe that forming a study group together was one of the most important factors in our exam preparation. The beauty of being part of a GP training scheme is that you are likely to already be part of a year group of other GP trainees, all facing the same exam. We would suggest you form a group together. A minimum of three per group is ideal so that there is always a 'doctor', 'patient' and 'observer'. If it's difficult for you to join a group, you can practise cases with just two people, and the person playing the 'patient' can also give feedback as an observer. Ten years ago we didn't have Zoom or Teams, but these platforms now allow you to set up remote study groups with trainees around the country, meaning it should be easy to find people to practise with.

Start revision early and make a commitment to meet on a weekly basis. We recommend meeting up for roughly 3 hours each week, starting 4–6 months before the exam, which should leave plenty of time to cover all the topic areas and approach the exam feeling prepared.

To make the most of your meetings, try to organise each session so that one person takes the lead in organising the cases you will practise. The group leader should be responsible for deciding who will play the 'patient', and providing them with their 'script' in advance, so that your sessions aren't wasted reading through the cases on the day. The leader can rotate each week so that everyone gets a chance to be the 'doctor'.

Decide on the topic you are going to cover each week and agree that everyone in the group will make an effort to read through the main guidelines in that subject area. This will be even more useful if you are also planning on sitting the AKT around the same time as the SCA. If you manage to read a little each week, by the time the exam comes around, you will feel more confident about your clinical knowledge as well as your communication skills.

Remember, all of this practice is on top of the GP registrar year, where you will be seeing patients every day in surgery anyway. Read up on the cases you are unsure about, and even the ones you are confident with – check the guidelines to ensure you are up to date. Ask your trainer to watch videos of your consultations and do joint surgeries together so you can get constructive feedback.

Chapter 3: RCGP curriculum topic guides

3.1 Introduction to the topic guides

The cases in this book are ordered by Blueprint area in line with the SCA exam structure. However, we felt these areas did not lend themselves to revision as easily as the RCGP curriculum topic guides did, so we have listed the revision resources under the following headings in line with the RCGP curriculum:

3.2 Structure of revision help provided

Case provided in the Workbook

If you prefer to practise cases by RCGP curriculum areas rather than by Blueprint areas, then simply work through the cases listed in this section for each curriculum area.

Possible cases

Each curriculum topic guide section begins with a list of possible cases which may come up in the exam, including 'emergency cases'. We advise you to become familiar with 'red flags' and the emergency management of common conditions. The exam is also likely to feature 'special cases' where you will encounter scenarios such as an angry patient, a patient refusing hospital admission, or a situation where you have to break bad news. We have tried to incorporate these 'special cases' into the scenarios we have written, but we have also listed potential special areas to think about at the start of each topic section to enable you to cover these during your revision.

Revision notes

To make your weekly preparation easier, we have listed relevant guidelines and useful websites to read, to improve your clinical knowledge. The following websites contain resources for almost every curriculum area, and we found them consistently useful so we list them here to avoid repetition:

Patient.info provides detailed information suitable for both patients and professionals: www.patient.info

GPnotebook is a popular encyclopaedia of medical knowledge: www.gpnotebook.com

The RCGP online learning environment provides evidence-based CPD modules: elearning.rcgp.org.uk

BMJ Learning site: new-learning.bmj.com

Clinical Knowledge Summaries provides a good source of evidence-based information on common primary care conditions: cks.nice.org.uk

Red Whale knowledge (requires payment): www.redwhale.co.uk

E-learning for health is available to all NHS doctors: www.e-lfh.org.uk

Doctors.net provides educational resources for doctors including textbooks and e-learning modules: www.doctors.net.uk

Practise explanations and examinations

At the end of each revision session we suggest you take turns practising how you explain common conditions and medical information, to think about how you communicate this information to patients. To start you off, we have provided a list to work from, but feel free to make your own.

We have listed clinical examinations relevant to each topic area. Even though the SCA does not formally test this, it remains useful and important as a GP to have strong examination skills and if you have time you can also practise these in your revision sessions.

C1 Allergy and immunology

Cases provided in *Workbook*: B1.4, B3.6, B9.17, B10.2

Possible cases
- Allergy testing request
- Anaphylaxis
- Angioedema
- Atopy – asthma, eczema, hay fever
- Autoimmune conditions
- Chickenpox in pregnancy
- Drug reactions / allergies
- Food allergies
- Gastrointestinal symptoms of allergy
- Immune deficiency states (inherited and acquired, e.g. HIV, chemotherapy)
- Immunisation
- Needlestick injury and bloodborne disease
- Occupational allergies (contact allergies – latex / hair dye / metals / plants)
- Pollen food syndrome
- Transplantation patients in primary care
- Urticaria and rashes

Emergency cases
- Acute management of anaphylaxis
- Emergency treatment of venom allergy

Special cases
- Discussing allergy tests – skin patch plus specific IgE testing
- Discussing indications / contraindications to routine immunisation in an immunosuppressed child

Revision notes

Applicable guidelines and useful resources

Relevant NICE guidelines and pathways:
- cks.nice.org.uk/specialities/allergies
- cks.nice.org.uk/specialities/immunizations

The British Society for Allergy & Clinical Immunology: www.bsaci.org

British Society for Immunology: www.immunology.org

British HIV Association: www.bhiva.org

British Transplantation Society: bts.org.uk

Resuscitation Council UK – emergency treatment of anaphylaxis: www.resus.org.uk/library/additional-guidance/guidance-anaphylaxis

RCEM Learning – management of needlestick injury: www.rcemlearning.co.uk/reference/needlestick-injury

Vaccine Knowledge (University of Oxford): vaccineknowledge.ox.ac.uk/home
UK immunisation schedule: www.gov.uk/government/publications/the-complete-routine-immunisation-schedule
Guidance on allergy and specific IgE testing: www.coventryrugbygpgateway.nhs.uk/pages/guidance-on-allergy-and-specific-ige-testing

Material for patient

Allergy UK: www.allergyuk.org
ASCIA info leaflets: www.allergy.org.au/patients
Immunodeficiency UK: www.immunodeficiencyuk.org
Patient leaflets from BSACI: www.bsaci.org/professional-resources/patient-information-leaflets-2
Transplant patient information: www.nhsbt.nhs.uk/organ-transplantation
UK PIPS (Primary immune deficiency patient support): ukpips.org.uk

Practise explaining

Practise explaining the following to a patient in less than 2 minutes:
- Exclusion and reintroduction in non-IgE disease
- How to effectively administer nasal steroids
- Signposting patients to pharmacy for over-the-counter hay fever treatments
- Benefits and risks of different vaccinations (try: MMR; influenza for a 2-year old and for a 65-year old)
- The role of immunotherapy for chronic allergic disorders

Practise examining

Ensure that you can undertake the following procedures confidently and efficiently:
- How to administer adrenaline

C2 Cardiovascular health

Cases provided in *Workbook*: B3.1, B3.2, B6.3, B9.2, B9.3, B9.5, B10.1, B11.4, B11.5, B12.10

Possible cases
- Aneurysms
- Arrhythmias
- Cardiomyopathy
- Cerebrovascular disease
- Congenital heart disease
- Heart failure
- Hypertension
- Infections (viral myocarditis / pericarditis, infective endocarditis, rheumatic fever and complications)
- Ischaemic heart disease (angina, MI)
- Lipids and statins
- NOACs (apixaban, dabigatran and rivaroxaban)
- Peripheral vascular disease
- Prevention of cardiovascular disease (risk factor modification)
- Syncope, dizziness and collapse
- Varicose veins
- Venous thromboembolism

Emergency cases
- Acute coronary syndrome
- Arrhythmias
- Cardiac arrest
- Heart failure
- Limb ischaemia
- Stroke

Special cases
- Complications / malfunctions of pacemakers
- Discussion of post-MI treatment such as return to work / sex / driving
- Reassuring patients concerned about musculoskeletal chest pain

Revision notes

Applicable guidelines and useful resources

Relevant NICE guidelines and pathways: www.nice.org.uk/guidance/conditions-and-diseases/cardiovascular-conditions
SIGN guidelines for cardiovascular disease: www.sign.ac.uk/search-results?q=cardiovascular&LibGo=Search
AAA screening programme: www.nhs.uk/conditions/abdominal-aortic-aneurysm-screening

British Society for Heart Failure guidelines: www.bsh.org.uk/patient-information
The British and Irish Hypertension Society provides up-to-date guidance: bihsoc.org/guidelines
The King's Thrombosis Centre guidelines on anticoagulation: www.kingsthrombosiscentre.org.uk/index.php/anticoagulation/anticoagulation-guidelines
Life in the Fast Lane is an emergency medicine site which provides a useful collection of ECGs as well as many explanations of common emergency conditions: litfl.com/ecg-library
Resuscitation Council UK guidance: www.resus.org.uk/professional-resources
British Cardiovascular Society guidelines: www.britishcardiovascularsociety.org/resources
Stroke Association guidance: www.stroke.org.uk/professionals/resources-professionals/national-clinical-guideline-stroke

Material for patient

British Heart Foundation: www.bhf.org.uk
Patient.info resources: patient.info/search?searchterm=cardiovascular%2520disease

Practise explaining

Practise explaining the following to a patient in less than 2 minutes:

- Angina
- Why anticoagulation is needed in AF
- Calculating cardiovascular risk (using a tool such as QRISK2)
- Coronary artery calcium scoring

Practise examining

Ensure that you can undertake the following procedures confidently and efficiently:

- Cardiovascular system
- ECG – be able to interpret and perform
- Ankle brachial pressure index (ABPI) – interpret and perform

---

Cardiovascular examination: youtu.be/eBnzjerIHj0
Peripheral vascular examination: youtu.be/6beOTEKx1ek

C3 Dermatology

Cases provided in *Workbook:* B1.4, B2.6, B3.6, B3.7, B9.19, B10.5, B10.10

Possible cases
- Acne and rosacea
- Actinic keratosis
- Balanitis
- Contact dermatitis / eczema
- Corns and calluses
- Discoid lupus
- Erythema nodosum
- Haemangioma
- Hair and nail disorders (alopecia, ingrown toenail)
- Hidradenitis suppurativa
- Hypopigmentation and hyperpigmentation presentations
- Infestations (lice / scabies)
- Lichen planus / sclerosus
- Light-sensitive disorders (polymorphic light eruption, porphyria, drug reactions)
- Lupus
- Lymphoedema
- Molluscum contagiosum
- Nappy rash
- Pemphigus and pemphigoid
- Pityriasis rosea / versicolor
- Pressure sores
- Psoriasis
- Seborrhoeic dermatitis
- Skin infections (bacterial, viral, fungal)
- Skin tumours (benign and malignant: melanoma, BCC, SCC, dermatofibroma)
- Ulcers
- Urticaria
- Vasculitis
- Vitiligo
- Warts and benign skin lesions (seborrhoeic keratosis / sebaceous cysts)
- Wound management

Emergency cases
- Angioedema and anaphylaxis
- Disseminated herpes simplex
- Erythroderma
- Meningococcal sepsis
- Necrotising fasciitis
- Stevens–Johnson syndrome
- Toxic epidermal necrolysis

Special cases
- Complications following minor surgery (anaphylaxis / infection)
- Discussing why certain cosmetic procedures and certain investigations are restricted on the NHS (e.g. patch testing / access to phototherapy / skin tag removal) – and explaining this to a patient
- Drug eruptions – discussing potential skin side-effects with a patient recently started on methotrexate / amiodarone / lithium
- Skin manifestations of psychiatric conditions (dermatitis artefacta, trichotillomania)

Revision notes

Applicable guidelines and useful resources

Relevant NICE guidelines and pathways:
www.nice.org.uk/guidance/conditions-and-diseases/skin-conditions
RCGP Dermatology toolkit: elearning.rcgp.org.uk/mod/book/view.php?id=12891
British Association of Dermatologists provides clinical guidelines and standards for dermatologists: www.bad.org.uk
Primary Care Dermatology Society has a wealth of resources for GPs: www.pcds.org.uk
Examining black and brown skin:
- Black & Brown Skin: www.blackandbrownskin.co.uk/our-vision
- BAD training: www.bad.org.uk/education-training/skin-of-colour-in-dermatology-education

Skin patterns associated with Covid-19: covidskinsigns.com
Collections of skin images:
- DermNet NZ: www.dermnetnz.org
- DermIS: www.dermis.net

Material for patient

The British Association of Dermatologists has produced a range of PILs: www.bad.org.uk/patient-information-leaflets
Allergy UK: www.allergyuk.org
Alopecia UK: www.alopecia.org.uk
Anaphylaxis UK: www.anaphylaxis.org.uk
Lupus UK: www.lupusuk.org.uk
National Eczema Society: www.eczema.org
National Psoriasis Foundation: www.psoriasis.org
National Rosacea Society: www.rosacea.org
Skin Cancer Foundation: www.skincancer.org/melanoma

Practise explaining

Practise explaining the following to a patient in less than 2 minutes:
- Shingles
- Psoriasis
- Urticaria
- Molluscum contagiosum
- Impetigo
- Suspicious lesion – atypical mole / possible malignant melanoma / BCC / SCC

Practise examining

- Be prepared to carry out an appropriate examination of the skin, hair and nails. This might sometimes require a chaperone.
- Skin lesions: assess distribution, morphology, size and colour, symmetry, shape.
- Various images are available via www.dermnetnz.org. Choose an image, then practise describing different skin lesions within your study groups to improve your dermatological examination skills and knowledge.

C4 Ear, nose and throat, speech and hearing

Cases provided in *Workbook:* B3.4, B3.5, B9.8, B9.9, B9.14

Possible cases
- Bell's palsy
- Cholesteatoma
- Chronic cough
- Croup
- Dental problems
- Dizziness
- Epistaxis
- Facial pain
- Head and neck cancers
- Hearing impairment
- Hoarseness
- Mouth ulcers
- Nasal polyps
- Neck lumps
- Obstructive sleep apnoea
- Otitis media / externa and otalgia
- Ramsay Hunt syndrome
- Rhinosinusitis
- Salivary gland disorders (infection, mumps, stones, Sjögren's syndrome, tumours)
- Septal haematoma
- Snoring
- Sore throat – tonsillitis, quinsy, glandular fever, GORD
- Speech delay
- Tinnitus
- Trigeminal neuralgia
- Vertigo

Emergency cases
- Epistaxis
- Foreign bodies
- Mastoiditis
- Peritonsillar abscess
- Septal haematoma
- Tracheotomy indications

Special cases
- Communicating with patients who are hearing impaired
- Discussing hearing aids, cochlear implants and tinnitus maskers

Revision notes

Applicable guidelines and useful resources

NICE pathways and guidelines:
* ENT conditions: cks.nice.org.uk/specialities/ear-nose-throat
* Oral health: cks.nice.org.uk/specialities/oral-health
* Head and neck cancers: www.nice.org.uk/guidance/ng12/chapter/Recommendations-organised-by-site-of-cancer#head-and-neck-cancers

The RCGP TARGET Antibiotic stewardship tools: elearning.rcgp.org.uk/mod/book/view.php?id=12649&chapterid=793

RCGP Deafness and hearing loss toolkit: elearning.rcgp.org.uk/mod/book/view.php?id=12532

ENT UK provides resources for professionals and patient leaflets: www.entuk.org

As does

British Association of Oral and Maxillofacial Surgeons (BAOMS): www.baoms.org.uk

Paediatric screening for hearing loss: www.nhs.uk/conditions/hearing-tests-children

Material for patient

British Snoring & Sleep Apnoea Association: www.britishsnoring.co.uk

The British Tinnitus Association: www.tinnitus.org.uk

Royal National Institute for Deaf People: rnid.org.uk

Practise explaining

In less than 2 minutes, how would you explain the following to a patient:
* Ménière's disease
* Benign paroxysmal positional vertigo and the Epley manoeuvre
* Reasons for not prescribing antibiotics to a child with otitis media
* Glue ear

Practise examining

Ensure that you can undertake the following procedures confidently and efficiently:
* Otoscopy
* Tuning fork tests
* Neck examination
* Dix–Hallpike test

Neck lump examination: youtu.be/oVhKjmOrzwM

C5 Eyes and vision

Cases provided in *Workbook:* B1.6, B8.3, B9.10

Possible cases
- Age-related macular degeneration
- Altered vision (floaters, halos, flashes)
- Colour blindness
- Congenital problems – congenital cataract, vitamin A deficiency
- Conjunctivitis
- Contact lens problems – acanthamoeba, corneal damage
- Corneal ulcers
- Diabetic and hypertensive eye disease
- Diplopia, squint, amblyopia
- Dry eye syndrome
- Epiphora
- Episcleritis / scleritis
- Foreign body / corneal abrasion
- Glaucoma
- Iritis / uveitis (association with systemic disease, e.g. ankylosing spondylitis, Reiter's syndrome)
- Lid disorders (blepharitis, chalazion, ectropion, BCC, nasolacrimal obstruction)
- Malignancy (retinoblastoma, lymphoma, melanoma)
- Migraine
- Refractive disorders (cataract, astigmatism)
- Temporal arteritis
- Thyroid eye disease
- Vitreo-retinal disorders (retinal / vitreous detachment, retinoblastoma**)**

Emergency cases
- Acute red eye
- Arc eye
- Eye trauma
- Herpes zoster ophthalmicus
- Orbital cellulitis
- Raised intracranial pressure causing papilloedema
- Retinal detachment
- Sudden loss of vision
- TIA

Special cases
- A blind patient asks you how to get a guide dog
- Discussing eye complications with a newly diagnosed diabetic
- Discussing fitness to drive with a patient with severe visual impairment

Revision notes

Applicable guidelines and useful resources

NICE pathways for eye conditions: cks.nice.org.uk/specialities/eyes

Moorfields Eye Hospital has resources for primary care providers: www.moorfields.nhs.uk/for-health-professionals/for-primary-care-providers

The British Undergraduate Ophthalmology Society has produced concise factsheets on a range of eye conditions: buos.co.uk/learning/notes

Material for patient

Moorfields Eye Hospital hosts a patient information library: www.moorfields.nhs.uk/content/patient-leaflets

RNIB: www.rnib.org.uk

Vision Express provides useful condition leaflets for patients: www.visionexpress.com/eye-health/eye-conditions

Practise explaining

Practise explaining the following to a patient in less than 2 minutes:

- Acute conjunctivitis
- Bell's palsy
- Temporal arteritis
- Age-related macular degeneration
- Cataract

Practise examining

Ensure that you can undertake the following procedures confidently and efficiently:

- Visual acuity – be familiar with how to use a Snellen chart
- Fundoscopy
- Targeted eye examination – pupils, eyelids, eye movements
- Visual fields examination

Examination of eyes and vision: youtu.be/IwBEjEbU-Yw

C6 Gastroenterology

Cases provided in *Workbook:* B1.1, B3.3, B4.3, B9.4, B9.7, B11.10

Possible cases
- Abnormal liver function tests
- Acute abdomen
- B12 deficiency
- Coeliac disease / malabsorption
- Constipation
- Diarrhoea
- Diverticular disease
- Dyspepsia, gastritis, peptic ulcer
- Dysphagia
- 'Embarrassing' complaints (flatulence, hiccups)
- Gallstones / gallbladder disease
- Gastroenteritis
- GI cancers and their red flags
- *H. pylori* eradication
- Hernias
- Inflammatory bowel (Crohn's / colitis)
- Irritable bowel syndrome
- Jaundice
- Liver disease
- Nutrition (impact on health, obesity, vitamin deficiency)
- Pancreatic disease
- Perianal disease (abscess, anal fissure, haemorrhoids, pruritis ani)
- Post-operative complications
- Stoma management
- Weight loss surgery

Emergency cases
- Acute abdomen
- Haematemesis / melaena
- Strangulated hernia

Special cases
- Breaking bad news (GI cancer diagnosis)
- Talking through lifestyle with the family of a morbidly obese toddler
- Travellers' diarrhoea

Revision notes

Applicable guidelines and useful resources

Relevant NICE guidelines and pathways: cks.nice.org.uk/specialities/gastrointestinal

The Primary Care Society for Gastroenterology: www.pcsg.org.uk
British Society of Gastroenterology: www.bsg.org.uk
British Society of Lifestyle Medicine: bslm.org.uk
RCGP toolkits:
- Inflammatory bowel disease: elearning.rcgp.org.uk/course/view.php?id=702
- Liver disease: elearning.rcgp.org.uk/mod/book/view.php?id=13042

FIT (faecal immunochemical testing): www.faecal-immunochemical-test.co.uk/about-faecal-immunochemical-testing
NHS Bowel Cancer Screening: cks.nice.org.uk/bowel-screening

Material for patient

British Liver Trust: www.britishlivertrust.org.uk
Coeliac UK: www.coeliac.org.uk
Colostomy UK: www.colostomyuk.org
Crohn's & Colitis UK: www.crohnsandcolitis.org.uk
IBS network: www.theibsnetwork.org
Weight loss resources: www.claphamparkgp.com/weight-loss-resources

Practise explaining

Practise explaining the following to a patient in less than 2 minutes:
- Fatty liver disease
- *Helicobacter pylori* infection
- Hiccups
- IBS
- FIT testing

Practise examining

Ensure that you can undertake the following procedures confidently and efficiently:
- Abdominal examination
- DRE if required (on a model)

Abdominal examination: youtu.be/XOefpxm38bc
Rectal examination: youtu.be/bK1GTLpL_F8

C7 Genomic medicine

Cases provided in *Workbook*: B2.2, B2.3, B3.1, B11.2, B11.3, B12.10

Possible cases
- Autosomal dominant disorders
  - Ehlers–Danlos syndrome
  - Familial adenomatous polyposis
  - Hereditary haemorrhagic telangiectasia
  - HOCM
  - Huntington's disease
  - Hypercholesterolaemia
  - Marfan syndrome
  - Neurofibromatosis
  - Polycystic kidney disease
  - Prader–Willi syndrome
  - von Willebrand disease
- Autosomal recessive disorders
  - Cystic fibrosis
  - Haemochromatosis
  - Haemoglobinopathies (sickle cell / thalassaemia)
  - Wilson's disease
- Chromosomal disorders
  - Down's syndrome
  - Klinefelter's syndrome
  - Turner's syndrome
- Conditions with a genetic component
  - Alzheimer's disease
  - Bipolar disorder
  - Cardiovascular disease
  - Diabetes
- Familial cancers (bowel, breast)
- X-linked disorders
  - Fragile X
  - Haemophilia
  - Muscular dystrophies

Revision notes

RCGP feedback has highlighted that candidates score poorly in this curriculum area, since cases on genetics often involve rare conditions. One approach to revision is to be able to recognise basic patterns of inheritance and draw a family tree to illustrate this. If you are not sure about certain conditions, often being able to discuss further referral for genetic counselling and testing, and discussing the implications of this, may be more important than a detailed knowledge of the condition itself.

Applicable guidelines and useful resources

Relevant NICE guidelines and pathways:
- cks.nice.org.uk/topics/pre-conception-advice-management/management/genetic-risk-assessment
- www.nice.org.uk/guidance/ng201

Royal College of Obstetricians & Gynaecologists – Prenatal testing: www.rcog.org.uk/guidance/browse-all-guidance/other-guidelines-and-reports/supporting-women-and-their-partners-through-prenatal-screening-for-downs-syndrome-edwards-syndrome-and-pataus-syndrome

Information on sickle cell and thalassaemia screening across the UK: www.gov.uk/guidance/sickle-cell-and-thalassaemia-screening-programme-overview

Newborn screening: www.gov.uk/government/publications/handbook-for-sickle-cell-and-thalassaemia-screening/newborn-screening

British Society for Genetic Medicine: bsgm.org.uk

Primary Care Genetics Society: www.primarycaregenetics.org/?page_id=109&lang=en

The NHS Genomics Education Programme provides e-learning resources on taking a family history and drawing genetic diagrams: www.genomicseducation.hee.nhs.uk

RCGP Genomics toolkit: elearning.rcgp.org.uk/mod/book/view.php?id=12892

Material for patient

Down's Syndrome Association: www.downs-syndrome.org.uk/about-downs-syndrome/pregnancy-and-baby

Genetic Alliance UK: geneticalliance.org.uk

National Hereditary Breast Cancer Helpline: www.breastcancergenetics.co.uk

NHS Genomic Medicine Service: www.england.nhs.uk/genomics

Practise explaining

Practise explaining the following to a patient in less than 2 minutes:
- Cystic fibrosis
- Antenatal screening
- Thalassaemia
- A family tree diagram for a condition that might have a:
    1. dominant
    2. recessive
    3. sex-linked inheritance

C8 Gynaecology and breast

Cases provided in *Workbook:* B1.5, B2.3, B2.4, B2.5, B2.6, B2.10, B2.11, B2.12, B5.2, B6.1, B7.2, B8.2, B10.3, B12.1

Possible cases
- Abnormal smear results
- Breast pain / lumps / nipple discharge / cancer / screening
- Breastfeeding and common problems
- Contraception
- Gynaecological malignancies
- Infertility
- Menopause, perimenopause and HRT
- Menstrual disorders (amenorrhoea, dysmenorrhoea, menorrhagia, intermenstrual bleeding, premenstrual syndrome, premenstrual dysphoric disorder, post-coital bleeding)
- Mental health problems in pregnancy
- Ovarian cancer
- Pelvic infection
- Polycystic ovarian syndrome
- Post-menopausal bleeding
- Pregnancy (see resources in L3)
- Premature ovarian insufficiency (premature menopause)
- Prolapse
- Recurrent miscarriage
- Sexual dysfunction
- Urinary incontinence
- Vaginal discharge / infections (e.g. Bartholin's abscess, bacterial vaginosis)
- Vulval symptoms (FGM, malignancy (vulval intraepithelial neoplasia, VIN)), skin disorders (lichen sclerosus, psoriasis, intertrigo, warts), atrophy, Bartholin's problems

Emergency cases
- Ectopic pregnancy

Special cases
- Cases of potential sexual abuse / child protection concerns
- Discussing medication with an epileptic patient wishing to conceive
- Please also see the following resources closely related to this topic area:
    - C11 Kidney and urology (p. 35)
    - C18 Sexual health (p. 50)
    - L3 Maternity and reproductive health (p. 62)

Revision notes

Applicable guidelines and useful resources

Relevant NICE guidelines and pathways:

* cks.nice.org.uk/specialities/womens-health
* cks.nice.org.uk/specialities/pregnancy

SIGN guidelines for the following conditions are available at www.sign.ac.uk:

* 134 Treatment of primary breast cancer
* 135 Management of epithelial ovarian cancer
* 169 Perinatal mental health disorders

RCGP Women's health toolkit: elearning.rcgp.org.uk/mod/book/view.php?id=12534

Primary Care Women's Health Forum resources: pcwhf.co.uk/resources/?_sft_source=pcwhf-resource

Green top guidelines specific to women's health are available on the RCOG website: www.rcog.org.uk/guidelines

British Menopause Society: www.thebms.org.uk

International Menopause Society training: www.imsociety.org/education/impart-registration

The Faculty of Sexual & Reproductive Healthcare: www.fsrh.org/home

Medication use in pregnancy:

* uktis.org
* www.medicinesinpregnancy.org

Medication use in breastfeeding:

* lacted.org/iable-breastfeeding-education-handouts/breastfeeding-and-medications
* gpifn.org.uk

Material for patient

Breast Cancer Research Foundation: www.bcrf.org

Endometriosis UK: www.endometriosis-uk.org

Female Cancer Foundation: www.femalecancerfoundation.org

International Association for Premenstrual Disorders (support and resources for women with PMDD and PME): iapmd.org

Lichen sclerosus and vulval cancer awareness: www.lsvcukawareness.co.uk

Menopause resources:

* www.menopausematters.co.uk
* www.balance-menopause.com
* rockmymenopause.com

National Association for Premenstrual Syndromes (information and support for PMS sufferers): www.pms.org.uk

National fertility awareness service: www.fertilityuk.org

Ovarian Cancer Action: www.ovarian.org.uk

PCOS Awareness Association: www.pcosaa.org

Support through miscarriage: www.miscarriageassociation.org.uk

Supporting women with premature ovarian insufficiency: www.daisynetwork.org/about-us/what-we-do

The UK's gynaecological cancer research charity: www.eveappeal.org.uk

The Vulval Pain Society: vulvalpainsociety.org

Women's health resources:

- www.womens-health-concern.org
- www.womens-health.co.uk

Practise explaining

Practise explaining the following to a patient in less than 2 minutes:

- Polycystic ovarian syndrome
- Premenstrual dysphoric disorder
- Bacterial vaginosis
- Menopause

Practise examining

Ensure that you can undertake the following procedures confidently and efficiently:

- Pelvic examination including speculum and digital bimanual on a model
- Breast examination

Breast examination: youtu.be/76g_tNWMhCE
Vaginal examination: youtu.be/Z-O_JYtyQqE

C9 Haematology

Cases provided in *Workbook*: B4.3, B11.2

Possible cases

- Anaemia and its causes (iron, folate, B12 deficiency; haemolytic, sideroblastic, chronic disease)
- Anticoagulants
- Bleeding, bruising, petechiae and purpura
- Blood film abnormalities (macrocytosis, microcytosis, spherocytosis, neutrophilia)
- Bone pain and pathological fractures
- Clotting disorders (haemophilia, von Willebrand's disease, DIC, septicaemia)
- Fatigue
- Haematological malignancies: acute / chronic leukaemias, lymphomas, multiple myeloma
- Haemochromatosis
- Haemoglobinopathies (thalassaemia, sickle cell disease)
- Haemolytic diseases
- Lymphadenopathy / splenomegaly
- Lymphoedema
- Management of a single enlarged lymph node
- Myelodysplasia
- Myeloproliferative disorders (polycythaemia rubra vera, thrombocytosis)
- Neutropenia
- Pancytopenia
- Thrombocytosis and thrombocytopenia
- Venous thromboembolism
- Emergency cases
- Acute promyelocytic leukaemia (APML)
- Disseminated intravascular coagulation (DIC)
- Hypercalcaemia in haematological malignancy
- Neutropenic sepsis
- Sickle cell crisis
- Spinal cord compression in multiple myeloma
- Thrombotic thrombocytopenic purpura

Special cases

- Patient with a splenectomy discussing the implications

Revision notes

Applicable guidelines and useful resources

Relevant NICE guidelines and pathways: cks.nice.org.uk/specialities/haematology
British Society for Haematology: b-s-h.org.uk
RCEM Haematology resources: www.rcemlearning.co.uk/haematology
Thrombosis UK: thrombosisuk.org

British Society for Haemostasis and Thrombosis: bsht.org.uk/related-organisations-useful-links/
Haematological Malignancy Research Network: hmrn.org

Material for patient

Blood Cancer UK: bloodcancer.org.uk
Haemochromatosis UK: www.haemochromatosis.org.uk
Haemophilia Society: haemophilia.org.uk/bleeding-disorders/haemophilia-a-and-b
Leukaemia Care: www.leukaemiacare.org.uk
Lymphoma Action: lymphoma-action.org.uk
Sickle Cell Society: www.sicklecellsociety.org

Practise explaining

Practise explaining the following to a patient in less than 2 minutes:
- Different anticoagulant therapies
- Sickle cell disease

Practise examining

Ensure that you can undertake the following procedures confidently and efficiently:
- Examination of lymph nodes in the neck
- Examining / recognising a purpuric rash

C10 Infectious disease and travel health

Cases provided in *Workbook*: B2.1, B8.1, B9.17, B10.2, B10.6

Possible cases

- Bone, joint and soft tissue infections (septic arthritis, osteomyelitis)
- Cardiovascular infections (endocarditis, pericarditis, rheumatic fever)
- Childhood infections (viral, bacterial, fungal)
- ENT infections
- Fever in the returning traveller (e.g. malaria, dengue, typhoid, paratyphoid, viral haemorrhagic fevers)
- GI infections (amoebiasis, amoebic dysentery, food poisoning, giardiasis, hydatid disease, traveller's diarrhoea, typhoid)
- GU infections (UTI, STIs)
- Healthcare-associated infections (MRSA, *Clostridioides difficile*)
- Helminth infections (hookworm, schistosomiasis, strongyloides, threadworm)
- Hepatitis
- HIV/AIDS (prevention, prophylaxis, testing, transmission and associated diseases)
- Malaria
- Neurological infections (encephalitis, meningitis)
- Occupational infections (e.g. needlestick infections)
- Ocular infections (conjunctivitis, ophthalmia neonatorum)
- Pandemics (Covid-19, influenza)
- Post-operative infections
- Respiratory infections (Legionnaire's disease, influenza)
- Skin infections (bed bugs, flea bites, ringworm, scabies, leishmaniasis, orf)
- Tick-borne diseases (Lyme disease)
- Trauma (injuries, animal bites, wounds)
- Travel-related conditions (altitude sickness, motion sickness, sun exposure, hypothermia, water activities / drowning, VTE)
- Tuberculosis
- Vaccine-preventable communicable diseases
- Zoonotic diseases (leptospirosis, brucellosis)

Emergency cases

- Necrotising fasciitis
- Sepsis

Special cases

Discussing a 'fitness to fly' letter request with a patient (discuss as a group any practice policy, what falls within the work of the GP contract, who would/would not write one and why?)

Revision notes

Applicable guidelines and useful resources

Relevant NICE guidelines and pathways:
- cks.nice.org.uk/specialities/infections-infestations
- cks.nice.org.uk/specialities/preventative-medicine

RCGP toolkits:
- TARGET antibiotics: elearning.rcgp.org.uk/course/view.php?id=553
- Lyme disease: elearning.rcgp.org.uk/mod/book/view.php?id=12535
- Sepsis: elearning.rcgp.org.uk/mod/book/view.php?id=12896

British Infection Association: www.britishinfection.org

Royal Society of Tropical Medicine & Hygiene: www.rstmh.org

UK Health Security Agency: www.gov.uk/government/organisations/uk-health-security-agency

The UK Sepsis Trust: sepsistrust.org

Antibiotic Guardian resources: antibioticguardian.com/healthcare-professionals/

Antimicrobial stewardship: www.gov.uk/government/publications/antimicrobial-stewardship-start-smart-then-focus

Travel advice:
- nathnac.net
- travelhealthpro.org.uk
- cdc.gov/travel

Disease outbreak news: www.who.int/emergencies/disease-outbreak-news

Current outbreaks: www.who.int/publications/journals/weekly-epidemiological-record

Material for patient

Fitness to fly information: www.caa.co.uk/passengers/before-you-fly/am-i-fit-to-fly

Travel advice: www.fitfortravel.nhs.uk/home

Well Travelled Clinics: www.welltravelledclinics.co.uk

Practise explaining

Practise explaining the following to a patient in less than 2 minutes:
- NHS travel health provision and the role of the private sector
- Pre-exposure prophylaxis in HIV

Practise examining

Ensure that you can undertake the following procedures confidently and efficiently:
- Recognising red and amber flags for sepsis

C11 Kidney and urology

Cases provided in *Workbook*: B1.2, B1.3, B2.8, B2.9, B11.1, B11.7

Possible cases
- Acute kidney injury (AKI)
- Balanitis / balanoposthitis
- Benign prostatic hyperplasia
- Cancers: bladder, kidney, penile, prostate, testicular, ureteric
- Chronic kidney disease (CKD)
- Congenital abnormalities of the urinary tract
- Epididymo-orchitis
- Haematospermia
- Haematuria
- Inherited kidney disease (polycystic kidney disease, Alport syndrome)
- Intrinsic renal disease (glomerulonephritis)
- Mumps orchitis
- Overactive bladder
- Penile warts and ulcers (trauma; cancer; syphilis; herpes covered in C18)
- Peyronie's disease
- Prostatism (LUTS)
- Proteinuria
- PSA testing
- Renovascular disease (renal artery stenosis)
- Scrotal pain / swellings / lumps (testicular cancer; hernias; hydrocele; varicocele; cysts)
- Systemic causes of kidney disease (diabetes, hypertension, connective tissue disease, nephrotic syndrome, myeloma)
- Undescended testicles
- Urethral discharge / urethritis (STIs)
- Urinary incontinence in men and women
- Urinary tract obstruction
- Urolithiasis
- UTI in children and adults

Emergency cases
- Acute urinary retention
- Phimosis / paraphimosis
- Priapism
- Testicular torsion

Special cases
- Prostate cancer (breaking bad news)
- Request for NHS circumcision for religious reasons
- Request for NHS prescription for Caverject
- Sterilisation request

Revision notes

Applicable guidelines and useful resources

Relevant NICE guidelines and pathways:
* cks.nice.org.uk/specialities/kidney-disease-urology
* cks.nice.org.uk/specialities/mens-health

RCGP Acute Kidney Injury Toolkit: elearning.rcgp.org.uk/mod/book/view.php?id=12897

The UK Kidney Association: ukkidney.org

UK eCKD Guide: ukkidney.org/health-professionals/information-resources/uk-eckd-guide#sthash.aR3HaMDP.dpbs

The British Association of Urological Surgeons: www.baus.org.uk

The International Society for Men's Health & Gender (ISMH): www.jomh.org

PSA testing guide for GPs: www.gov.uk/government/publications/prostate-specific-antigen-testing-explanation-and-implementation

RCEM urology resources: www.rcemlearning.co.uk/foamed/male-urological-issues-in-the-ed/

Prostate Cancer UK: prostatecanceruk.org/for-health-professionals/guidelines?category=

GP Gateway Renal Medicine: www.coventryrugbygpgateway.nhs.uk/category/medical/renal-medicine/?post_type=gpage

Material for patient

Kidney Care UK: kidneycareuk.org

Kidney Research UK: www.kidneyresearchuk.org

The Men's Health Forum website: www.menshealthforum.org.uk

Prostate Cancer UK: www.prostatecanceruk.org

The Urology Foundation: www.theurologyfoundation.org

Practise explaining

Practise explaining the following to a patient in less than 2 minutes:
* PSA test
* Benign prostatic hyperplasia
* Phimosis
* Peyronie's disease
* Dialysis

Practise examining

Ensure that you can undertake the following procedures confidently and efficiently:
* Examination of the genitalia and digital rectal examination on a model
* Differentiating scrotal lumps on examination

C12 Mental health

Cases provided in *Workbook*: B5.1, B5.2, B5.3, B5.4, B5.5, B5.6, B5.7, B5.8, B5.9

Possible cases
- Addictive and dependent behaviour
- Affective disorders (depression, mania, bipolar disorder)
- Anxiety disorders
- Attention deficit hyperactivity disorder (ADHD) (also see C15)
- Behaviour problems (ADHD, enuresis, encopresis, school refusal)
- Bereavement reactions
- Eating disorders (anorexia, bulimia, body dysmorphia, morbid obesity)
- Mental health and physical health (e.g. steroid-induced psychosis, Parkinson's disease and depression)
- Obsessive–compulsive behaviours
- Organic reactions (e.g. delirium)
- Perinatal mental health
- Personality disorders (borderline, antisocial, narcissistic)
- Post-traumatic stress disorder
- Pregnancy-related disorders (perinatal depression, puerperal psychosis)
- Schizophrenia
- Self-harm
- Sleep disorders
- Somatisation disorder
- Trauma

Emergency cases
- Attempted suicide
- Delirium
- Panic attack
- Psychosis

Special cases
- Abuse (child / elder, domestic, emotional, physical, sexual)
- Application of the Mental Health Act
- Violent patients

Revision notes

Applicable guidelines and useful resources

Relevant NICE guidelines and pathways: cks.nice.org.uk/specialities/mental-health
The Royal College of Psychiatrists: www.rcpsych.ac.uk
The RCGP toolkits:
- Mental health and perinatal mental health: elearning.rcgp.org.uk/mod/book/view. php?id=13115

- Gambling Harms Hub: elearning.rcgp.org.uk/course/view.php?id=734
- Veterans' Health Hub: elearning.rcgp.org.uk/course/view.php?id=803

The Academy for Eating Disorders resources: www.aedweb.org/resources/professional-resources

BMA Mental Capacity Act England and Wales Toolkit: www.bma.org.uk/advice-and-support/ethics/adults-who-lack-capacity/mental-capacity-act-toolkit

Deprivation of Liberty Safeguards (DOLS): www.lawsociety.org.uk/support-services/advice/articles/deprivation-of-liberty

Medication guidance

Prescribing in psychiatry: Maudsley Guidelines available via Athens:

- www.knowledge.scot.nhs.uk/library-resources/medicines-information
- www.maudsley-prescribing-guidelines.co.uk

Material for patient

ADHD Psychiatry-UK: psychiatry-uk.com/adhd

The National Attention Deficit Disorder information and support service: www.addiss.co.uk

Royal College of Psychiatrists support leaflets: www.rcpsych.ac.uk/mental-health/treatments-and-wellbeing

Support for UK Armed Forces: www.gov.uk/guidance/mental-health-support-for-the-uk-armed-forces

Women's Aid (charity to end domestic abuse): www.womensaid.org.uk

'You Okay Doc?' have a directory of resources: youokaydoc.org.uk/resources

Practise explaining

Practise explaining the following to a patient in less than 2 minutes:

- Starting an antidepressant (answering questions on side-effects, duration of treatment, monitoring progress)
- Schizophrenia

Practise examining

Ensure you can undertake the following confidently and efficiently:

- Assessing risk of suicide in a depressed patient
- Assessing severity of depression
- Capacity assessment
- Mental State Examination

C13 Metabolic problems and endocrinology

Cases provided in Workbook: B3.1, B4.2, B6.5, B8.4, B9.11, B10.1, B11.5, B11.6, B11.8

Possible cases

- Adrenal disease (Addison's disease, Cushing's syndrome, phaeochromocytoma, hyperaldosteronism, malignancy)
- Carcinoid syndrome
- Diabetes:
    - type 1, type 2, maturity onset diabetes of the young, latent autoimmune diabetes in adults
    - pre-diabetes, impaired glucose tolerance, insulin resistance, gestational diabetes
    - micro- and macrovascular complications, medication and lifestyle modification
- Disorders of calcium metabolism (hypoparathyroidism, hyperparathyroidism and osteomalacia, CKD, myeloma, bony metastases)
- Haemochromatosis and disorders of iron metabolism
- Hirsutism
- Hyperlipidaemia
- Hyperprolactinaemia
- Hyperuricaemia
- Hypogonadism
- Inherited metabolic diseases (phenylketonuria, glycogen storage diseases, porphyrias)
- Metabolic effects of prescribed medication (e.g. hypokalaemia with diuretics)
- Metabolic syndrome
- Non-alcoholic fatty liver disease
- Obesity and overweight
- Osteoporosis
- Parathyroid disease
- Pituitary disorders (acromegaly, diabetes insipidus, prolactinoma)
- Poisoning (deliberate or unintentional)
- Polycystic ovary syndrome (see C8)
- Psychogenic polydipsia
- Replacement and therapeutic steroid therapy
- Sex hormone problems (hirsutism, virilism, gynaecomastia, impotence, androgen deficiency, androgen insensitivity syndrome)
- Thyroid problems
- Vitamin D and bone health

Emergency cases

- Addisonian crisis
- Diabetic ketoacidosis
- Hyperglycaemic hyperosmolar non-ketotic coma
- Hypoglycaemic coma
- Thyroid crisis

Special cases
- Explaining newly diagnosed diabetes to an uninterested teenager
- Fitness to drive case with diabetic having frequent hypos

Revision notes

Applicable guidelines and useful resources

NICE pathways and guidelines:
- cks.nice.org.uk/specialities/endocrine-metabolic
- cks.nice.org.uk/specialities/poisoning

RCGP Acute Kidney Injury toolkit: elearning.rcgp.org.uk/mod/book/view.php?id=12897

RCGP Physical Activity Hub: elearning.rcgp.org.uk/course/view.php?id=536

Rethink Obesity: www.rethinkobesity.global/au/en/resources/obesity-resources-for-physicians-and-patients.html

National Osteoporosis Guideline Group: www.nogg.org.uk

TOXBASE – National Poisons Information Service: www.toxbase.org/login/?ReturnUrl=

Resources from the London Endocrine Centre: www.londonendocrinecentre.co.uk/pituitary-disorders.html

Material for patient

Addison's Disease Self-Help Group: www.addisonsdisease.org.uk

British Inherited Metabolic Diseases Group: www.bimdg.org.uk/site/index.asp

British Thyroid Foundation: www.btf-thyroid.org

Diabetes UK: www.diabetes.org.uk

Metabolic Support UK: metabolicsupportuk.org

Pituitary Foundation: www.pituitary.org.uk

RCPCH Clinical guideline directory: www.rcpch.ac.uk/resources/clinical-guideline-directory

Royal Osteoporosis Society: theros.org.uk

UK National Kidney Federation: www.kidney.org.uk

Practise explaining

Practise explaining the following in less than 2 minutes:
- 'Sick day rules' in adrenal insufficiency
- How statins work
- Cardiovascular risk reduction to a diabetic (lipids / BP / aspirin)
- Addisonian crisis and how to avoid it

Practise examining

Ensure that you can undertake the following procedures confidently and efficiently:
- Neck examination
- Diabetic foot examination

Thyroid status examination: youtu.be/ziaYBkgEZNU
Diabetic foot examination: youtu.be/vwIyuIPnXcg

C14 Musculoskeletal health

Cases provided in *Workbook*: B4.2, B6.5, B8.5, B9.6, B9.18

Possible cases

- Acute / chronic arthropathies
- Avascular necrosis
- Bone cancers (metastatic disease, Ewing's and soft tissue sarcoma)
- Cervical spine disorders (spondylosis, torticollis and 'whiplash' injuries, vertebral fracture)
- Chronic pain management (complex regional pain syndrome)
- Common injuries
- Congenital / inherited diseases (osteogenesis imperfecta, Marfan's syndrome, Ehlers–Danlos syndrome, Gaucher's disease, hypermobility syndromes)
- Fibromyalgia
- Fracture and dislocation management
- Gout
- Hallux valgus
- Hand disorders (trigger finger, Dupuytren's contracture, carpal tunnel syndrome, ulnar nerve compression)
- Infections (septic arthritis and osteomyelitis)
- Inflammatory arthritis and connective tissue disease (rheumatoid arthritis, sero-negative arthritis, reactive arthritis, scleroderma, systemic sclerosis)
- Knee pain
- Lymphoedema
- Muscular dystrophies and myasthenia gravis
- Osteoarthritis and joint replacement surgery
- Osteoporosis (see C13)
- Plantar fasciitis
- Polymyalgia rheumatica and giant cell arteritis
- Polymyositis
- Shoulder disorders
- Sjögren's syndrome
- Skeletal problems including disorders of calcium homeostasis (osteomalacia, rickets, Paget's disease) (see C13)
- Soft tissue disorders (Achilles tendon problems, bursitis, synovitis, tendonitis)
- Spinal disorders (mechanical back pain, disc lesions, malignancy, infection, spinal stenosis, developmental disorders, trauma, red flag recognition)
- Systemic lupus erythematosus (SLE)

Emergency cases

- Burns
- Cauda equina
- Head injury
- Septic arthritis / osteomyelitis
- Trauma management

Special cases
- Appropriate use of steroid injections
- Dealing with uncertainty – patient with rarer rheumatological disease you may not know much about
- Inappropriate imaging requests
- Recognising injuries in children as non-accidental injury

Revision notes

Applicable guidelines and useful resources

Relevant NICE guidelines and pathways: cks.nice.org.uk/specialities/musculoskeletal
RCGP Physical Activity Hub: elearning.rcgp.org.uk/course/view.php?id=536
British Institute of Musculoskeletal Medicine: www.bimm.org.uk
British Orthopaedic Association: www.boa.ac.uk
The Primary Care Rheumatology and Musculoskeletal Medicine Society: www.pcrsmm.org.uk
British Lymphology Society: www.thebls.com
Versus Arthritis: versusarthritis.org
British Association of Sport & Exercise Medicine: www.basem.co.uk
Royal Osteoporosis Society: theros.org.uk
Advanced Trauma Life Support: www.facs.org/quality-programs/trauma/education/advanced-trauma-life-support/
RCGP Inflammatory Arthritis Toolkit: https://elearning.rcgp.org.uk/mod/book/view.php?id=13455&chapterid=777
UK Spine Societies: www.ukssb.com/improving-spinal-care-project

Material for patient

BackCare: www.backcare.org.uk
British Sjögren's Syndrome Association: www.bssa.uk.net
Children's Chronic Arthritis Association: www.ccaa.org.uk
Living Made Easy – independent living for people with disabilities: livingmadeeasy.org.uk
Lupus UK: lupusuk.org.uk
Lymphoedema Support Network: www.lymphoedema.org
Muscular Dystrophy UK: www.musculardystrophyuk.org
National Ankylosing Spondylitis Society (Act on Axial SpA): www.actonaxialspa.com
National Rheumatoid Arthritis Society: nras.org.uk
Polymyalgia Rheumatica and Giant Cell Arteritis Scotland: pmrgcascotland.com
Repetitive Strain Injury charity: www.rsiaction.org.uk
Scleroderma & Reynaud's UK: www.sruk.co.uk
Sheffield Aches & Pains: sheffieldachesandpains.com
Versus Arthritis: versusarthritis.org

Practise explaining

Practise explaining the following to a patient in less than 2 minutes:
- Ankylosing spondylitis
- The role of an osteopath / chiropractor / physiotherapist / podiatrist
- Fibromyalgia
- Medication used for musculoskeletal problems: methotrexate, steroids
- The Ottawa ankle rules for imaging ankles (to a medical student)

Practise examining

- Knee exam to exclude ACL rupture
- Assessment of carpal tunnel syndrome (Phalen and Tinel's tests / awareness of median nerve distribution)
- The elbow of a patient you suspect has golfer's elbow (medial epicondylitis)
- Evaluation of the rotator cuff (choose the provocation tests you are most comfortable / familiar with)

Shoulder examination: youtu.be/TDs1IOFYnMo
Hip joint examination: youtu.be/KAgRJTsXHrU
Knee examination: youtu.be/B76oGAFKb28
Spine examination: youtu.be/CJVGpciEMol
Hand examination: youtu.be/xKNBflxRlCs
GALS (gait / arms / legs / spine) examination: youtu.be/g8-dMuzWal4

C15 Neurodevelopmental disorders, intellectual and social disability

Cases provided in *Workbook:* B2.2, B4.4, B7.2, B7.3, B7.4, B7.5, B7.6, B7.7

Possible cases

- Annual health checks for patient with learning disability
- Autism and autism spectrum disorder
- Behaviour change in patients with severe learning difficulties
- Carer strain
- Cerebral palsy (child presenting with delayed developmental milestones)
- Dyspraxia
- Genetic causes of intellectual disability (Fragile X, Williams, Prader–Willi, Rett's, Down's and Sturge–Weber syndromes, phenylketonuria, neurofibromatosis, tuberous sclerosis)
- Health promotion (using easy to understand explanations)
- Mental health problems in patients with intellectual disability (Alzheimer's disease, anxiety and depression, bereavement reactions, bipolar affective disorder, schizophrenia)
- Non-genetic causes of intellectual disability (fetal alcohol syndrome, brain injury, neglect)
- Physical health problems in patients with intellectual disability (aspiration pneumonia, cardiovascular disease, epilepsy / seizures, MSK problems / joint contractures, obesity, sleep disorders, visual / speech / hearing / mobility problems)
- Screening tools for autism / ADHD in adulthood
- Emergency cases
- Safeguarding adults – dealing with an adult with intellectual disability at risk of abuse / neglect

Special cases

- Third party consultations / telephone consultations with carers

Revision notes

Applicable guidelines and useful resources

Relevant NICE guidelines and pathways:
- cks.nice.org.uk/topics/learning-disabilities
- cks.nice.org.uk/topics/attention-deficit-hyperactivity-disorder
- cks.nice.org.uk/topics/autism-in-adults
- cks.nice.org.uk/topics/autism-in-children

The RCGP Toolkits are available:
- Resources for secure environments: elearning.rcgp.org.uk/mod/book/view.php?id=13151&chapterid=625
- Autism and ADHD: elearning.rcgp.org.uk/mod/book/view.php?id=13115&chapterid=608
- Adult safeguarding: elearning.rcgp.org.uk/mod/book/view.php?id=12530
- Child safeguarding: elearning.rcgp.org.uk/mod/book/view.php?id=12531

Intellectual disability and health resource from the University of Hertfordshire: www.intellectualdisability.info

Material for patient

ADHD Psychiatry-UK: psychiatry-uk.com/adhd

Down's Syndrome Association: www.downs-syndrome.org.uk

Intellectual disability charities and support groups: www.intellectualdisability.info/links

Mencap (support for people with intellectual disability): www.mencap.org.uk

The National Attention Deficit Disorder information and support service: www.addiss.co.uk

Royal College of Psychiatrists support leaflets: www.rcpsych.ac.uk/mental-health/treatments-and-wellbeing

Scope (support for disabled people and their families): www.scope.org.uk

Practise explaining

Practise explaining the following to a patient in less than 2 minutes:

- Autism spectrum disorder
- Cervical screening to a patient with intellectual disability (www.gov.uk/government/publications/cervical-screening-easy-read-guide)
- Testicle self-examination to a patient with intellectual disability (www.intellectualdisability.info/how-to-guides/articles/how-to-look-after-my-balls)
- ADHD diagnosis and current NHS waiting times, self-help strategies / resources

Practise examining

Ensure you can undertake the following confidently and efficiently:

- Cognitive screening
- Consider how you would approach a breast examination in a patient with intellectual disability

C16 Neurology

Cases provided in *Workbook*: B4.8, B9.1, B9.12, B9.13, B9.14, B9.15, B10.8, B11.3

Possible cases

- Cerebellar disorders (tumours, demyelination)
- Cerebral palsy
- Myalgic encephalomyelitis / chronic fatigue syndrome (ME/CFS)
- Complex regional pain syndrome
- Cranial nerve disorders (Bell's palsy, trigeminal neuralgia, bulbar palsy)
- Delirium / acute confusional state
- Dementia (Alzheimer's, vascular, Lewy body, Pick's disease (behavioural variant frontotemporal dementia), normal pressure hydrocephalus)
- Epilepsy (generalised / focal seizures, febrile convulsions, medical causes of seizures)
- Essential tremor
- Head injury
- Headache (tension, cluster, migraine, sinusitis, dental pain, medication overuse headache, tumours, subarachnoid haemorrhage, temporal arteritis)
- Infections (meningitis, encephalitis, arachnoiditis)
- Inherited neurological disease (Huntington's disease, Charcot–Marie–Tooth, myotonic dystrophy, neurofibromatosis)
- Motor neurone disease
- Movement disorders (tremor and gait problems: athetosis, chorea, tardive dyskinesia, dystonia, tics. Underlying causes such as Sydenham's chorea, Huntington's disease, drug-induced parkinsonism)
- Multiple sclerosis and demyelinating disorders
- Muscle disorders (muscular dystrophy, myasthenia gravis)
- Nerve entrapment (carpal tunnel)
- Neuropathies
- Parkinson's disease and progressive degenerative disorders (progressive supranuclear palsy, multisystem atrophy)
- Recurrent falls
- Sensory and motor disturbances (peripheral nerve problems, mono- / polyneuropathies such as nerve compression and palsies, Guillain–Barré syndrome)
- Spinal injuries causing paralysis, care of tetra- / paraplegic patients
- Stroke and TIA
- Tumours of the brain and peripheral nervous system (meningioma, glioblastomas, astrocytomas, neurofibromatosis, secondary metastases)

Emergency cases

- Collapse
- Head injury / loss of consciousness
- Intracranial haemorrhage (subarachnoid, subdural, extradural, thrombosis, congenital aneurysms)

- Meningococcal septicaemia
- Raised intracranial pressure
- Seizures
- Stroke

Special cases
- Discussing fitness to drive with a patient with epilepsy
- Discussing prognosis with patients with progressive / disabling neurological conditions

Revision notes

Applicable guidelines and useful resources

Relevant NICE guidance and pathways: cks.nice.org.uk/specialities/neurological
National Stroke Association Resource Library: www.stroke.org/category/resource
DVLA guidance assessing fitness to drive: www.gov.uk/government/publications/assessing-fitness-to-drive-a-guide-for-medical-professionals

Material for patient

Epilepsy Society: epilepsysociety.org.uk
Meningitis Research Foundation: www.meningitis.org
www.migraine.org.uk
Motor Neurone Disease Association: www.mndassociation.org
Multiple Sclerosis Society: www.mssociety.org.uk
Parkinson's UK: www.parkinsons.org.uk
The Stroke Association: www.stroke.org.uk

Practise explaining

Practise explaining the following to a patient in less than 2 minutes:
- Parkinson's disease
- Medication overuse headache
- Restless legs
- Carpal tunnel syndrome

Practise examining

Ensure that you can undertake the following procedures confidently and efficiently:
- 'Targeted' neurological exam – peripheral and cranial nerves (particularly visual fields)
- Tests to exclude carpal tunnel – Tinel's / Phalen's
- Fundoscopy
- Visual acuity – be familiar with how to use a Snellen chart

Upper limb neurological examination: youtu.be/4uAAjYzi7SY
Lower limb neurological examination: youtu.be/IdmQSVZN05I
Cranial nerve examination: youtu.be/yZ5kV7dJoZw

C17 Respiratory health

Cases provided in *Workbook:* B9.16, B10.9, B11.9, B12.4

Possible cases
- Asthma (new diagnosis; annual review)
- Bronchiectasis
- Connective tissue disease affecting the lungs (RA, SLE, sarcoidosis)
- COPD
- Cough (infection; reflux; post-nasal drip; medications; asthma; psychogenic)
- CXR result (lung cancer; pleural plaques; pleural effusion; heart failure)
- Cystic fibrosis
- Emphysema including alpha1-antitrypsin deficiency
- Haemoptysis
- Hay fever and allergy
- Immunosuppression affecting the respiratory system (TB, fungal, parasitic, atypical pneumonias including Legionnaire's disease, sepsis)
- Influenza
- Lower respiratory tract infections
- Occupational respiratory diseases (pneumoconiosis, asthma, extrinsic allergic alveolitis and asbestos-related disease)
- Pleural effusion and its causes
- Pulmonary embolism
- Respiratory failure
- Respiratory malignances (laryngeal, bronchial, pleural, paraneoplastic syndromes)
- Smoking cessation
- Spirometry results (obstructive / restrictive pattern)
- Upper respiratory tract infections
- Ventilation methods including CPAP for sleep apnoea
- Whooping cough

Emergency cases
- Acute exacerbation of asthma / COPD
- Anaphylaxis
- Inhaled foreign body
- Pneumothorax
- Pulmonary embolism

Special cases
- Discussing rescue medication with a COPD patient having frequent ED admissions
- Request for antibiotics for self-limiting illness

Revision notes

Applicable guidelines and useful resources

Relevant NICE guidelines and pathways: cks.nice.org.uk/specialities/respiratory

BTS guidelines relevant to primary care (among others) are available at:
www.brit-thoracic.org.uk/quality-improvement
British Infection Association guidelines: www.britishinfection.org/guidance/published-guidelines
Thrombosis UK VTE guidelines: thrombosisuk.org/guidelines.php
The RCGP TARGET antibiotic toolkit: elearning.rcgp.org.uk/course/view.php?id=553
International Primary Care Respiratory Group: www.ipcrg.org
Primary Care Respiratory Society: www.pcrs-uk.org
The National Centre for Smoking Cessation and Training: www.ncsct.co.uk
The British Society for Allergy & Clinical Immunology: www.bsaci.org
Occupational diseases info: www.hse.gov.uk/statistics/causdis/
Death certification reforms: www.gov.uk/government/publications/changes-to-the-death-certification-process/an-overview-of-the-death-certification-reforms (relevant to occupational lung disease)

Material for patient

Asthma + Lung UK: www.asthmaandlung.org.uk
Cystic Fibrosis Trust: www.cysticfibrosis.org.uk
How to read your chest X-ray report: www.radiologyinfo.org/en/info/article-chest-xray-report
Physio for COPD: www.csp.org.uk/conditions/copd
Smoking cessation help: www.smokefreeaction.org.uk
Support for people with asbestos diseases: hasag.co.uk
TB Alert: www.tbalert.org
Thrombosis UK: www.thrombosisuk.org

Practise explaining

Practise explaining the following to a patient in less than 2 minutes:
- Inhaler technique including use of spacer and cleaning advice
- Asthma diagnosis and difference between 'preventer' and 'reliever' inhalers
- Difference between viral and bacterial infection
- Smoking cessation – lifestyle measures; nicotine replacement therapies

Practise examining

Ensure that you can undertake the following procedures confidently and efficiently:
- Respiratory examination
- Instruct patient to perform peak flow measurements
- Interpretation of spirometry results (the BTS has a useful document on spirometry at www.brit-thoracic.org.uk/media/70454/spirometry_e-guide_2013.pdf

> Respiratory examination: youtu.be/gRWSyqatWQQ
> Peak expiratory flow rate (PEFR) demonstration: youtu.be/jdA8KU_D9JU

C18 Sexual health

Cases provided in *Workbook:* B1.5, B2.7, B2.9, B2.10, B2.12, B7.2, B8.1, B8.2, B10.3, B10.4, B10.6, B12.1

Possible cases
- Asymptomatic sexual screening
- Bacterial vaginosis
- Candida
- Cervical screening / cancer
- Conjunctivitis (e.g. caused by chlamydia / gonorrhoea)
- Contraception – knowledge of methods available, efficacy, risks / benefits / side-effects
- Dysuria
- Erectile dysfunction and premature ejaculation
- Female sexual dysfunction (anorgasmia, dyspareunia, hypo-oestrogenism, loss of libido, vaginismus)
- Gender identity, dysphoria and reassignment
- Genito-urinary skin disorders (lichen sclerosus, balanitis)
- HIV – testing, counselling and pre-exposure prophylaxis; possible presentations (*Pneumocystis* pneumonia, candidiasis, Kaposi's sarcoma, TB, toxoplasmosis)
- HPV vaccination
- Infestations (pubic lice, scabies)
- Pelvic inflammatory disease
- Reiter's syndrome
- STIs – chlamydia, gonorrhoea, hepatitis B and C, herpes, HPV, LGV, syphilis, trichomonas, genital warts
- Termination of pregnancy (variation in services between the four UK nations)
- Transgender health issues including access to Gender Identity clinics
- Vaginal bleeding – intermenstrual, post-coital, infection- / contraception-related

Emergency cases
- Emergency contraception
- Post-exposure prophylaxis in HIV prevention
- Sexual assault

Special cases
- Discussing contraceptive options with a patient under the age of 16 (Fraser guidelines)
- Discussing partner notification with a patient diagnosed with an STI
- Female genital mutilation
- Screening for domestic and intimate partner violence
- Sexual abuse (adult and child)

There may be cross-over with other topic areas.

Revision notes

Applicable guidelines and useful resources

Relevant NICE guidelines and pathways: cks.nice.org.uk/specialities/sexual-health

British Association for Sexual Health and HIV: www.bashh.org/resources/guidelines

The Faculty of Sexual & Reproductive Healthcare (FSRH): www.fsrh.org

- UK Medical Eligibility criteria for contraceptive use: www.fsrh.org/standards-and-guidance/uk-medical-eligibility-criteria-for-contraceptive-use-ukmec
- Sexual and reproductive health e-learning: www.e-lfh.org.uk/programmes/sexual-and-reproductive-healthcare

The Royal College of Obstetricians and Gynaecologists: www.rcog.org.uk

RCEM Sexual assault aftercare in the emergency department: www.rcemlearning.co.uk/reference/sexual-assault-aftercare-in-the-emergency-department/#1658839414645-60c6b10d-148b

A directory of hormonal contraceptives from around the world can be found at www.ippf.org/sites/default/files/dohc.pdf which may be useful when patients present with unfamiliar brands from overseas

Drugs that interact with antiretroviral therapy: www.hiv-druginteractions.org

National FGM centre: nationalfgmcentre.org.uk/fgm/fgm-resources

The Gender Identity Clinic provides resources and referral advice for GPs including a telephone advice line for queries regarding hormonal treatment: gic.nhs.uk/gp-support

GMC ethical hub: Trans healthcare: www.gmc-uk.org/professional-standards/ethical-hub/trans-healthcare

College of Sexual and Relationship Therapists offers advice on psychosexual problems for both clinicians and patients: www.cosrt.org.uk

The RCGP toolkits are available:

- Adult safeguarding: elearning.rcgp.org.uk/mod/book/view.php?id=12530
- Child safeguarding: elearning.rcgp.org.uk/mod/book/view.php?id=12531

Material for patient

56 Dean Street is an NHS sexual health clinic in central London providing STI/HIV care, PEP/PrEP, Chemsex support, psychosexual counselling and Trans and non-binary services: www.dean.st

British Pregnancy Advisory Service: www.bpas.org

Brook clinics provide advice on STIs, contraception and pregnancy: www.brook.org.uk

Family Planning Association (FPA): www.fpa.org.uk

Gender identity resources:

- Young Minds: www.youngminds.org.uk/parent/parents-a-z-mental-health-guide/gender-identity
- Stonewall: www.stonewall.org.uk
- Mermaids: mermaidsuk.org.uk
- Marie Stopes (abortion and vasectomy care): www.msichoices.org.uk

HIV resources:

- HIV peer support: www.positivelyuk.org/Project-100
- HIV treatment info and advocacy: i-base.info
- Reliable HIV information: www.aidsmap.com
- Terrence Higgins Trust (HIV, AIDS and sexual health): www.tht.org.uk

Relate is a charity offering advice, relationship counselling and sex therapy: www.relate.org.uk

Practise explaining

Practise explaining the following to a patient in less than 2 minutes:

- Intrauterine methods of contraception
- Missed pill rules (COC/POP)
- Pre-exposure prophylaxis for HIV
- Emergency contraception options
- Waiting times for transgender patients for specialist care and support available in the interim

Practise examining

Ensure that you can undertake the following procedures confidently and efficiently:

- Pelvic examination (digital and speculum)
- Swab taking (male / female; anogenital areas)

C19 Smoking, alcohol and substance misuse

Cases provided in *Workbook*: B5.3, B5.4, B5.6, B5.7, B5.8, B5.9, B10.8, B10.11

Possible cases
- Alcohol excess and its complications (accidents, anaemia, AF, dyspepsia, erectile dysfunction, fetal alcohol syndrome, GI bleeding, liver damage, mental health problems, neurological damage, obesity, peripheral neuropathy, seizures, violence, Wernicke–Korsakoff syndrome, withdrawal)
- Anabolic steroid use
- Cannabis use and mental health problems
- Chronic liver disease
- Cocaine use and cardiac problems
- Drug use: awareness of the main problem drugs, e.g. anabolic steroids, new psychoactive substances, opiates, solvents, stimulants
- Medical complications of substance misuse (local and systemic infections, malnutrition, nasal / respiratory symptoms, cardiac complications, venous thromboembolic disease)
- Methadone request
- Misuse of over-the-counter medications
- Pregnancy complicated by alcohol / substance misuse (including fetal alcohol spectrum disorder, growth retardation, neonatal withdrawal, pre-term delivery)
- Relative concerned about patient with drug / alcohol problems
- Request for alcohol detoxification
- Request for benzodiazepines or gabapentinoids
- Request for sleeping tablets
- Smoking (types of tobacco, health impacts, passive smoking, nicotine addiction and treatment, vaping)
- Social consequences of substance misuse (contact with the criminal justice system, domestic violence, homelessness, poor school / work attendance, relationship issues, safeguarding concerns, unemployment)

Emergency cases
- Alcohol withdrawal / emergencies (delirium, psychosis, seizures, head injury)
- Drug-related emergencies (overdose, arrhythmias, cocaine-induced chest pain, psychosis)

Special cases
- Child protection case – parents who misuse drugs / alcohol
- Sick note for patient who is not engaging with drug and alcohol team
- Substance misuse in pregnancy

Revision notes

Applicable guidelines and useful resources
Relevant NICE guidelines and pathways:

- cks.nice.org.uk/topics/alcohol-problem-drinking
- www.nice.org.uk/guidance/ng64

RCGP Mental health toolkit substance misuse:
- elearning.rcgp.org.uk/mod/book/view.php?id=13115&chapterid=609
- elearning.rcgp.org.uk/mod/book/view.php?id=13151&chapterid=626

Alcohol Health Alliance: ahauk.org

British Society of Gastroenterology: www.bsg.org.uk

National Centre for Smoking Cessation and Training: www.ncsct.co.uk

RCEM – Drug misuse and the Emergency Department: rcem.ac.uk/wp-content/uploads/2021/10/RCEM_BPC_DrugMisuse_FINAL2019.pdf

NHS guidelines on management of drug misuse and dependence: www.gov.uk/government/collections/alcohol-and-drug-misuse-prevention-and-treatment-guidance

Chemsex resources: www.dean.st/chemsex/what-is-chemsex

Material for patient

Action on Smoking and Health: www.ash.org.uk

Alcohol and the brain: www.rcpsych.ac.uk/mental-health/mental-illnesses-and-mental-health-problems/alcohol-mental-health-and-the-brain

Alcoholics Anonymous: www.alcoholics-anonymous.org.uk

FRANK – honest information about drugs: www.talktofrank.com

Narcotics Anonymous (UK): ukna.org

RCPSYCH young people:
- Cannabis and mental health: www.rcpsych.ac.uk/mental-health/parents-and-young-people/cannabis-and-mental-health-information-for-young-people
- Drugs and alcohol: www.rcpsych.ac.uk/mental-health/parents-and-young-people/drugs-and-alcohol-for-young-people

Support with drugs, alcohol and mental health: www.wearewithyou.org.uk

Practise explaining

Practise explaining the following to a patient or colleague in less than 2 minutes:
- Alcohol withdrawal – physical effects
- Risks of sharing needles for drug use
- Chemsex – what it is and the risks it poses

Practise examining

Ensure that you can undertake the following procedures confidently and efficiently:
- Examining for signs of liver failure, e.g. liver flap, hepatomegaly, hepatic encephalopathy
- Using a screening tool for alcohol abuse (AUDIT / CAGE)

C20 Urgent and unscheduled care

Cases provided in *Workbook:* B4.6, B6.1, B6.2, B6.3, B6.4, B6.5, B9.1, B9.2, B9.3, B9.5

Possible cases
- Acute abdomen and its causes
- Anaphylaxis
- Aneurysms
- Arrhythmias – AF, SVT, bradyarrhythmias
- Cancer presenting with hypercalcaemia, neutropenic sepsis, spinal cord compression, superior vena cava obstruction
- Choking
- Critical limb ischaemia
- Diabetic ketoacidosis
- Ectopic pregnancy / antenatal emergencies
- Intestinal obstruction or perforation
- Limb ischaemia
- Loss of consciousness
- Malignant hypertension
- Meningitis
- Mental health crisis (suicide, psychosis, mania)
- Myocardial infarction / acute coronary syndrome
- Pre-eclampsia
- Pulmonary embolus
- Sepsis
- Status epilepticus
- Stroke
- Subarachnoid haemorrhage
- Suicidal ideation
- Visual loss (glaucoma, retinal detachment)

See also Emergency cases in each curriculum area

Special cases
- Cardiorespiratory arrest
- Death (expected / unexpected, assessment, confirmation, legal requirements)
- Identifying an unwell patient on a telephone consultation and/or a third-party consultation
- Identifying how quickly a patient needs admission (999 ambulance or own transport)
- Refusal of hospital admission

Revision notes

Applicable guidelines and useful resources

The Royal College of Emergency Medicine clinical guidance: rcem.ac.uk/clinical-guidelines

The British Thoracic Society guidelines: www.brit-thoracic.org.uk/quality-improvement/guidelines
Life in the Fast Lane educational resources for emergency physicians: litfl.com
RCGP Toolkits:
* elearning.rcgp.org.uk/mod/book/view.php?id=12896
* elearning.rcgp.org.uk/course/view.php?id=553
Royal College of Obstetricians & Gynaecologists: www.rcog.org.uk/guidelines
Resuscitation Council UK guidance: www.resus.org.uk/professional-resources
* Including basic and advanced life support for adults, paediatrics and the newborn; anaphylaxis, choking and DNACPR decisions
Surviving Sepsis campaign: www.sccm.org/SurvivingSepsisCampaign

Material for patient

British Heart Foundation: www.bhf.org.uk
Royal Society for the Prevention of Accidents: www.rospa.com

Practise explaining

Practise explaining the following to a patient in less than 2 minutes:
* Myocardial infarction
* Pre-eclampsia
* Stroke
* Subarachnoid haemorrhage

Practise examining

Ensure that you can undertake the following procedures confidently and efficiently:
* Assessment of an unwell child (awareness of normal parameters for vital signs in different age groups)
* ECG interpretation
* Calculating GCS in a confused patient

L1 Children and young people

Cases provided in *Workbook*: B1.1, B1.2, B1.3, B1.4, B1.5, B1.6, B7.1

Possible cases

- Asthma
- Autism
- Bronchiolitis
- Child abuse and safeguarding (non-accidental injury)
- Childhood cancers (leukaemias, lymphoma, brain tumours, retinoblastoma, neuroblastoma, nephroblastoma, sarcoma) (see C9)
- Childhood infections (e.g. mumps, measles, rubella, chickenpox) (see C10)
- Chromosomal disorders (e.g. Down's syndrome, fragile X, Klinefelter's syndrome, trisomy 18, Turner's syndrome) (see C7)
- Chronic disease in children (diabetes, asthma, arthritis, LD)
- Congenital abnormalities (e.g. congenital heart disease, hypothyroidism, musculoskeletal, neurological abnormalities, sensory impairment)
- Constipation
- Croup
- Dermatological disorders in childhood (seborrhoeic dermatitis, atopic eczema, impetigo, fungal infections, vitiligo, infantile haemangiomas) (see C3)
- Developmental milestones and variants
- Diabetes
- Diarrhoea and vomiting / gastroenteritis
- Eating disorders
- Failure to thrive
- Febrile convulsion / epilepsy
- GI conditions in childhood (appendicitis, Meckel's diverticulum, intussusception, malabsorption, CMPA, inflammatory bowel disease) (see C6)
- GORD / colic
- Head lice / threadworms
- Immunisations
- Infectious mononucleosis
- Kawasaki's disease
- Learning disabilities in children (see C15)
- Limping child
- Management approach to rarer conditions you may not know much about
- Mental health (see C12)
- Musculoskeletal problems in children (inflammatory arthritides, osteochondritis, Osgood–Schlatter's, Perthes' disease, slipped epiphysis, greenstick fractures, pulled elbow (see C14)
- Neonatal problems (birthmarks; feeding problems; sticky eye; jaundice; heart murmur; poor weight gain)
- Poisoning
- Psychological problems – enuresis, encopresis, school refusal, bullying, behavioural disorders, tantrums, sleep disorders

- Recognising the range of normality (developmental milestones / growth / puberty / behaviour) (this may present as a case of parental concern with the role of the GP to reassure)
- Renal disease (UTI, structural anomalies, posterior urethral valves, renal pelvic dilatation, haemolytic uraemic syndrome, nephrotic syndrome, glomerulonephritis) (see C11)
- Teenage contraception (see C18)
- Tonsillitis
- Urticaria
- Viral exanthems

Emergency cases
- Acute appendicitis
- Acute asthma attack
- Epiglottitis
- Head injury / loss of consciousness
- Meningococcal septicaemia
- Non-accidental injury
- Recognition of 'Red Flags' for serious illness in children
- Seizures
- Testicular torsion

Specific paediatric themes
- Adolescents and young people aged 10–25 as a distinct group regarding brain development
- Behavioural problems
- Developmental problems
- Faltering growth (and possible causes – ineffective intake, chronic disease, infection, abuse or neglect)
- Gender identity issues
- Gillick / Fraser competency
- Mental health problems
- Prevention and safety (prenatal diagnosis, infant feeding / breastfeeding, healthy diet, immunisation, smoking / alcohol / drugs)
- The acutely unwell child

Revision notes

Applicable guidelines and useful resources

Relevant NICE guidance and pathways: cks.nice.org.uk/specialities/child-health
Royal College of Paediatrics and Child Health (RCPCH) Clinical guideline directory: www.rcpch.ac.uk/resources/clinical-guideline-directory
Resuscitation Council UK Paediatric basic life support guidelines: www.resus.org.uk/library/2021-resuscitation-guidelines/paediatric-basic-life-support-guidelines
Great Ormond Street Hospital guidelines on many childhood conditions: www.gosh.nhs.uk/wards-and-departments/departments/clinical-specialties/thames-paediatric-anaesthetists-group-information-health-professionals/clinical-guidelines
Paediatric Pearls Primary care guidelines: paediatricpearls.co.uk/primary-care-guidelines
Childhood surveillance tools via the Health for all Children website: www.healthforallchildren.com
Sepsis screening tools for both adults and children (specifically under 5s and children 5–11): sepsistrust.org/professionalresources/clinical-tools
International Children's Palliative Care Network: icpcn.org

Safeguarding resources

RCGP Toolkits: Child safeguarding: elearning.rcgp.org.uk/mod/book/view.php?id=12531
The Victoria Climbié inquiry: www.gov.uk/government/publications/the-victoria-climbie-inquiry-report-of-an-inquiry-by-lord-laming
Safeguarding resources: www.safecic.co.uk
E-learning Resources Safeguarding Children and Young People Level 3: www.e-lfh.org.uk/programmes/safeguarding-children
National Working Group for Sexually Exploited Children: nwgnetwork.org

Material for patient

Jumo (medical information written in a child-friendly fashion): jumohealth.com
Teenage-friendly advice: www.healthforteens.co.uk
Vaccine Knowledge (University of Oxford): vaccineknowledge.ox.ac.uk
When Should I Worry? (information for parents on management of respiratory infection): www.what0-18.nhs.uk/parentscarers/worried-your-child-unwell
Young Minds: www.youngminds.org.uk

Practise explaining

Practise explaining the following to a patient in less than 2 minutes:
- Basics about childhood immunisation and schedule
- ADHD
- Allergy testing
- Enuresis
- Hand, foot and mouth disease
- Febrile convulsions

Practise examining

- A child with a fever – familiarise yourself with the 'Traffic light system for identifying risk of serious illness' www.paediatricpearls.co.uk/wp-content/uploads/Attachment-1-Remote-Assess-fever-assessment-Luton.pdf
- A child who doesn't want to be examined – share different techniques that have worked for you in practice
- Practise third party consultations within your study group
- Calculating drug doses in children

L2 People with long term conditions including cancer

Cases provided in *Workbook:* B3.1, B3.2, B3.3, B3.4, B3.5, B3.6, B3.7, B4.1, B4.2, B4.4, B4.6, B10.1, B11.3, B12.4

Possible cases
- Cancer
  - financial impact (loss of job, costs of care / unfunded treatments)
  - physical effects (chemo- / radiotherapy, hormone treatment, surgery)
  - psychological effects
  - social (loss of role, relationship breakdowns)
- Communicable diseases
  - HIV/AIDS
  - post-Covid-19 syndrome
- Mental health disorders
- Non-communicable diseases
  - cardiovascular conditions (hypertension, angina, heart failure)
  - ME/CFS
  - chronic pain
  - diabetes
  - irritable bowel syndrome
  - neurological conditions (MS)
  - respiratory conditions (asthma, COPD)
- Ongoing defined impairments
  - blindness
  - hearing impairment
  - musculoskeletal disorders

Applicable guidelines and useful resources

RCGP Toolkits: Primary care cancer: elearning.rcgp.org.uk/mod/book/view.php?id=12890
Relevant NICE guidelines and pathways
- www.nice.org.uk/guidance/conditions-and-diseases/cancer
- www.nice.org.uk/guidance/ng12
NIHR – Researching long Covid: evidence.nihr.ac.uk/themedreview/researching-long-covid-addressing a new global health challenge
Long term conditions in children: stateofchildhealth.rcpch.ac.uk/evidence/long-term-conditions
Long term conditions and medically unexplained symptoms (NHSE):
www.england.nhs.uk/mental-health/adults/nhs-talking-therapies/mus
Suspected cancer referral guidelines:
- Macmillan cancer support: www.macmillan.org.uk/healthcare-professionals/cancer-pathways/prevention-and-diagnosis/rapid-referral-guidelines
- Cancer Research UK: www.cancerresearchuk.org/health-professional/diagnosis/suspected-cancer-referral-best-practice/nice-cancer-referral-guidelines

Disability rights: www.gov.uk/rights-disabled-person

Material for patient

Cancer Research UK: www.cancerresearchuk.org

Disability Rights UK: www.disabilityrightsuk.org

Living Well Consortium UK: livingwellconsortium.com/psychological-therapies/long-term-conditions

Long COVID SOS: www.longcovidsos.org/resources

Long-term physical conditions and mental health: www.mentalhealth.org.uk/explore-mental-health/a-z-topics/long-term-physical-conditions-and-mental-health

Macmillan cancer information and support: www.macmillan.org.uk/cancer-information-and-support

OUTpatients – LGBTIQ+ cancer charity: outpatients.org.uk

The Patients Association – Long term conditions: www.patients-association.org.uk/long-term-conditions

Practise explaining

Practise explaining the following to a patient in less than 2 minutes:

- Cancer screening discussion with non-binary patient: www.cancerresearchuk.org/about-cancer/cancer-symptoms/spot-cancer-early/screening/trans-and-non-binary-cancer-screening
- Long Covid and available clinics local to your area of practice
- What is involved in the work capability assessment: www.disabilityrightsuk.org/resources/work-capability-assessment#What

Practise examining

Ensure that you can undertake the following procedures confidently and efficiently:

- Testing for possible fibromyalgia (www.arthritis.org/diseases/more-about/fibromyalgia-tests)
- What is involved in a diabetic foot check

L3 Maternity and reproductive health

Cases provided in *Workbook:* B1.5, B2.1, B2.2, B2.3, B2.5, B2.11, B2.12, B5.2, B6.1, B7.2, B8.2, B10.3, B12.1

Possible cases
- Contraception (postnatal) (see resources in C18)
- Infertility
- Maternity rights (benefits, paperwork – MatB1, exemption from prescription charges / dental treatment)
- Pregnancy
  - antenatal care and screening
  - bleeding in pregnancy
  - breastfeeding problems
  - common complaints (hyperemesis, reflux, back pain, symphysis pubis dysfunction, haemorrhoids, varicose veins)
  - ectopic pregnancy / molar pregnancy
  - gestational diabetes
  - mental health issues in pregnancy
  - miscarriage
  - normal pregnancy and labour
  - obstetric cholestasis
  - postnatal care and problems
  - pre-conception care / health promotion advice
  - pre-eclampsia
  - prescribing in pregnancy
  - rhesus status
  - unwanted pregnancy
  - VTE

Emergency cases
- Bleeding in pregnancy
- Ectopic pregnancy
- Pre-eclampsia

Special cases
- Discussing medication with an epileptic patient wishing to conceive
- Domestic violence in pregnancy

Revision notes

Applicable guidelines and useful resources
Relevant NICE guidelines and pathways:
- cks.nice.org.uk/specialities/womens-health

- cks.nice.org.uk/specialities/pregnancy

RCGP Women's health toolkit: elearning.rcgp.org.uk/mod/book/view.php?id=12534

Primary Care Women's Health Forum resources: pcwhf.co.uk/resources/?_sft_source=pcwhf-resource

Green top guidelines specific to women's health are available on the RCOG website: www.rcog.org.uk/guidelines

Medication use in pregnancy:

- uktis.org
- www.medicinesinpregnancy.org

Medication use in breastfeeding:

- lacted.org/iable-breastfeeding-education-handouts/breastfeeding-and-medications
- gpifn.org.uk
- www.sps.nhs.uk/home/guidance/safety-in-pregnancy/#:~:text=lactation

Material for patient

Breastfeeding resources:

- The Breastfeeding Network: www.breastfeedingnetwork.org.uk
- La Leche League: laleche.org.uk
- Lactation consultants of Great Britain: lcgb.org

UNICEF Baby friendly initiative: www.unicef.org.uk/babyfriendly

Practise explaining

Practise explaining the following to a patient in less than 2 minutes:

- Ectopic pregnancy
- Pre-eclampsia

Practise examining

Ensure that you can undertake the following procedures confidently and efficiently:

- Antenatal examination (abdominal palpation, symphysial fundal height, fetal heart rate)
- Discuss the postnatal assessment

L4 Older adults

Cases provided in *Workbook:* B2.4, B2.6, B4.1, B4.2, B4.3, B4.4, B4.5, B9.1

Possible cases
- Advance care planning
- Carer strain
- Chronic disease management
- Confusion
- Dementia
- Falls
- Incontinence
- Malnutrition
- Medication issues – hazards of polypharmacy, iatrogenic disease, medication errors, non-compliance
- Multimorbidity
- Osteoporosis
- Parkinson's disease
- Social isolation
- Stroke
- Unintentional weight loss

Emergency cases
- Complications of anticoagulants
- Delirium
- Injuries post fall

Special cases
- Third party consultations – confidentiality and capacity issues for patients in a care home
- Approaching patients with visual / hearing impairment or communication problems
- Elder abuse

Revision notes

Applicable guidelines and useful resources

Relevant NICE guidelines and pathways:
- www.nice.org.uk/guidance/population-groups/older-people
- www.nice.org.uk/guidance/conditions-and-diseases/multiple-long-term-conditions

The *BNF* has a section on prescribing in the elderly: bnf.nice.org.uk/medicines-guidance/prescribing-in-the-elderly

The British Geriatrics Society Comprehensive geriatric assessment toolkit for primary care practitioners: www.bgs.org.uk/sites/default/files/content/resources/files/2019-02-08/BGS%20Toolkit%20-%20FINAL%20FOR%20WEB_0.pdf

RCGP Toolkits: Adult safeguarding: elearning.rcgp.org.uk/mod/book/view.php?id=12530

Delirium training Resources – British Geriatrics Society: www.bgs.org.uk/resources/delirium-hub-education-and-training

The Royal College of Physicians has produced National Clinical guidelines for Stroke: www.rcp.ac.uk/improving-care/resources/stroke-guidelines-2016

Osteoporosis resources for primary care by the Royal Osteoporosis Society: theros.org.uk/healthcare-professionals/clinical-quality-hub/clinical-quality-toolkits

Polypharmacy in older people: awttc.nhs.wales/files/guidelines-and-pils/polypharmacy-in-older-people-a-guide-for-healthcare-professionalspdf

Material for patient

Age UK: www.ageuk.org.uk

Alzheimer's Society: www.alzheimers.org.uk

Carers UK: www.carersuk.org

Dementia United: dementia-united.org.uk

Parkinson's UK: www.parkinsons.org.uk

Royal Osteoporosis Society: theros.org.uk

Stroke Association: www.stroke.org.uk

World Delirium Awareness Day: www.deliriumday.com/links-to-info-on-delirium

Practise explaining

Practise explaining the following in less than 2 minutes:

- Capacity assessment to a medical student
- Reasons for conflicting advice when managing co-morbidity (e.g. diabetic patient advised by falls clinic to stop antihypertension, when diabetic nurses have always emphasised their importance in reducing CVD risk)
- Vertebro-basilar insufficiency
- Possible triggers for delirium in patients with dementia

Practise examining

Ensure that you can undertake the following procedures confidently and efficiently:

- Assessment of tremor
- Mini-mental state examination

L5 End of life

Cases provided in *Workbook:* B4.6, B4.7, B10.7, B12.2, B12.3

Possible cases
- 'Red flags' for diagnosing cancer ('2-week rule' referrals)
- Advance care planning
- Bereavement
- Breaking bad news
- Depression and anxiety in palliative patients
- DNAR / palliative discussion
- Gastrointestinal symptoms (nausea, vomiting, oral ulceration, constipation, diarrhoea, ascites, hiccuping)
- Pain management
- Starting syringe drivers
- Symptom control in palliative care

Emergency cases
- Haemorrhage
- Hypercalcaemia
- Neutropenic sepsis / pancytopenia
- Pathological fracture
- Raised ICP
- Spinal cord compression
- SVC obstruction
- Venous thromboembolic events

Special cases
- Discussion of the social benefits / services available to a palliative patient
- Third party consultations around DNAR / end-of-life care

Revision notes

Applicable guidelines and useful resources

Relevant NICE guidelines and pathways:
- www.nice.org.uk/guidance/ng12
- cks.nice.org.uk/specialities/palliative-care

Suspected cancer referral guidelines:
- Macmillan cancer support: www.macmillan.org.uk/healthcare-professionals/cancer-pathways/prevention-and-diagnosis/rapid-referral-guidelines
- Cancer Research UK: www.cancerresearchuk.org/health-professional/diagnosis/suspected-cancer-referral-best-practice/nice-cancer-referral-guidelines

The Gold Standards Framework: goldstandardsframework.org.uk

Scottish Palliative Care Guidelines: rightdecisions.scot.nhs.uk/scottish-palliative-care-guidelines

RCGP end of life and palliative care toolkit: elearning.rcgp.org.uk/mod/book/view.php?id=12529

UK Acute Oncology Society Guidelines: www.ukacuteoncology.co.uk/information-hub/ao-guidelines

UK Cancer Genetics Group: www.ukcgg.org/information-education/national-and-international-guidelines

International Children's Palliative Care Network: icpcn.org

End of life care for adults in the Emergency department: rcem.ac.uk/wp-content/uploads/2021/10/RCEM_End_of_Life_Care_Toolkit_December_2020_v2.pdf

Resuscitation Council UK: DNACPR and CPR decision making: www.resus.org.uk/library/additional-guidance/guidance-dnacpr-and-cpr-decisions

Material for patient

Cancer support groups:
- www.cancerresearchuk.org
- www.macmillan.org.uk
- www.mariecurie.org.uk

Compassion in Dying: compassionindying.org.uk

Dying Matters resources: www.dyingmatters.org/overview/resources

Hospice UK: www.hospiceuk.org

Practise explaining

Practise explaining the following to a patient in less than 2 minutes:
- DNAR
- Power of attorney
- Advance directives

Practise examining

Ensure that you can undertake the following procedures confidently and efficiently:
- Lower limb examination assessing for spinal cord compression
- Describe the signs you would examine for in a patient with SVC obstruction
- Confirming death in a patient

PT1 Professional topics

This section comprises aspects of everyday general practice and should be considered in conjunction with other topic guides. The RCGP curriculum explores these areas as part of *Being a General Practitioner*, dividing them into the following areas:

- Consulting in general practice
- Equality, diversity and inclusion
- Evidence-based practice, research and sharing knowledge
- Improving quality, safety and prescribing
- Leadership and management
- Population and planetary health

Cases provided in *Workbook*: B12.4, B12.5, B12.6, B12.7, B12.8, B12.9, B12.10

Possible cases
- Agenda setting (patients with a list of problems)
- Angry patient
- Breaking bad news
- Capacity assessment
- Complaints
- Communicating with patients speaking different languages or communication problems
- Confidentiality issues
- Dealing with colleagues
- Death certification
- Driving regulations
- Inappropriate requests
- Information security / data protection issues
- Probity issues – a patient gives you an expensive gift
- Private certificate requests
- Speaking with a poorly performing medical student
- Third party consulting
- Removing a patient from your practice – zero tolerance discussion
- Request from a patient to register as visually impaired
- "Sick / Fit notes"
- Sustainable clinical practice (e.g. low carbon alternatives when prescribing inhalers)

Revision notes

Applicable guidelines and useful resources

RCGP Toolkits:
- Continuity of care: elearning.rcgp.org.uk/mod/book/view.php?id=12895
- GP online services: elearning.rcgp.org.uk/mod/book/view.php?id=13455
- Multidisciplinary team working: elearning.rcgp.org.uk/mod/book/view.php?id=12898
- Patient safety: elearning.rcgp.org.uk/mod/book/view.php?id=12537

- Person-centred care: elearning.rcgp.org.uk/mod/book/view.php?id=12953

GMC Professional standards for doctors: www.gmc-uk.org/ethical-guidance

GMC Raising and acting on concerns about patient safety: www.gmc-uk.org/guidance/ethical_guidance/raising_concerns.asp

BMA core ethics guidance: www.bma.org.uk/advice-and-support/ethics/core-ethics/core-ethics-guidance?_gl=1*1h6ei81*_up*MQ..*_ga*MTIzMTYxMjM4MS4xNzE4NjQzODg5*_ga_F8G3Q36DDR*MTcxODY0Mzg4OC4xLjAuMTcxODY0Mzg4OC4wLjAuMA

eGPlearning – technology-enhanced primary care and learning: egplearning.co.uk

You are Not a Frog podcast:

- Managing your time in a system which sucks: youarenotafrog.com/episodes/74
- How to have crucial conversations: youarenotafrog.com/episodes/85

Dealing with an angry patient: www.hpso.com/risk-education/individuals/articles/Handling-the-Angry-Patient

Material for patient

Choosing wisely (promotes conversation around unnecessary medical tests and procedures): www.choosingwisely.org

Citizens Advice: www.citizensadvice.org.uk

How to complain in the NHS: www.nhs.uk/using-the-nhs/about-the-nhs/how-to-complain-to-the-nhs

Practise explaining

Discuss with your group how you would deal with the following scenarios:

- A colleague with an alcohol problem
- A social media request from a patient
- An aggressive patient
- A request from a patient's spouse for medical records
- What is social prescribing?

PART II: CASE SCENARIOS

Chapter 4: Case scenarios by RCGP Blueprint areas

Introduction to the cases

We have divided the cases into sections corresponding with the RCGP Blueprint areas:
1. Patient less than 19 years old
2. Gender, reproductive and sexual health, including women's, men's, LGBTQ+, gynaecology and breast
3. Long-term conditions, including cancer, multi-morbidity and disability
4. Older adults, including frailty and people at the end of life
5. Mental health, including addiction, smoking, and alcohol and substance misuse
6. Urgent and unscheduled care
7. Health disadvantages and vulnerabilities, including veterans, mental capacity, safeguarding, and communication difficulties
8. Ethnicity, culture, diversity and inclusivity
9. New presentation of undifferentiated disease
10. Prescribing
11. Investigations / results
12. Professional conversation / professional dilemma

Each case is made up of:
- **information for the doctor** – this page provides the doctor with a brief summary of their patient and should be given to the person in your revision group acting as the doctor in the next revision session
- **information for the patient** – this page provides all the background information (including ICE, information divulged freely and information only divulged if specifically asked about) to allow a person in your group to act as the patient, including any results and examination findings that you can provide to the doctor if they ask for it appropriately (we have kept these to basic readings that many patients may be able to provide from home: BP, heart rate, oxygen sats; for some video consultations, we have also provided images of skin lesions)
- **marking scheme for the observer** – this page provides the observer in your group with a simple checklist of descriptors in each of the three domains (data gathering and diagnosis, clinical management and medical complexity, and relating to others) and allows the 'observer' to rank the 'doctor' as pass, borderline, or fail for each descriptor.

This design allows the 'doctor', 'patient' and 'observer' to take out just the pages they need ahead of the next revision session, making the practice consultations as exam-like as possible. See p. 9 for our tips on setting up a study group and using the cases.

Structuring the consultations

Communication skills are essential in general practice and a knowledge of the common consultation models (*Table 4.1*) can help you to develop your own consultation style.

The RCGP runs several courses on consulting, and offers an extensive reading list on consultation models and 'being a GP': www.rcgp.org.uk/mrcgp-exams/gp-curriculum/being-general-practitioner

Having a structure to the consultation is important but remember to have some flexibility, to avoid coming across as too formulaic. The general model we used in our study groups was something like this:

- Greeting the patient
- Starting with an open question to allow the patient to tell their story
- Keeping quiet and allowing the patient to talk (the 'golden minute')
- Data gathering – ICE and psychosocial aspects first, then focused questions and excluding red flags
- Examination if appropriate
- Summarising

Table 4.1   Well-known consultation models

Calgary–Cambridge Model 1996 (Stages of a consultation)	Neighbour 1987 (Five checkpoint model)	Tuckett *et al.* 1985 (Meeting of two experts)
1. Initiating the session 2. Gathering information 3. Building the relationship 4. Explanation and planning 5. Closing the session	1. Connecting 2. Summarising 3. Handover 4. Safety-netting 5. Housekeeping	The consultation is a meeting between two experts (doctors in medicine, patients in their own illness) Shared understanding is the aim Doctors should seek to understand the patient's beliefs and address explanations in terms of this belief system
Pendleton *et al.* 1984, 2003 (Seven tasks model)	**Stewart *et al.* 1995, 2003 (Patient-centred clinical method)**	**Stott and David 1979 (Exceptional potential in each consultation)**
1. Define reasons for the patient's attendance (ideas, concerns and expectations) 2. Consider other problems 3. Choose appropriate action 4. Share understanding with the patient 5. Involve the patient in management decisions 6. Use time and resources well 7. Establish and maintain the doctor–patient relationship	1. Exploring both the disease and the illness experience 2. Understanding the whole person 3. Finding common ground 4. Incorporating prevention and health promotion 5. Enhancing the patient–doctor relationship 6. Being realistic (with time and resources)	1. Managing the presenting complaint 2. Managing ongoing problems 3. Opportunistic health promotion 4. Modifying health-seeking behaviour

- Explaining and sharing management options
- Checking understanding / safety-netting.

This structure may change depending on the style of the consultation – and may need to be adapted for an angry patient or a breaking bad news scenario.

Telephone and video consultations

Remote consultations are part of general practice now, and the SCA has adapted to recognise this. Consulting via telephone or video can prove to be challenging as the non-verbal clues are removed, and often the contact is made by a third party, which introduces extra issues of consent and confidentiality. Some tips to remember:

- Check the identity of the person you are speaking to (it is good practice to confirm their number / current location in case you get cut off) and ensure you can speak to the patient themselves, or if this is impossible, that the patient has consented to a relative speaking on their behalf.
- Listen actively and take a systematic history, excluding red flags, in the same way as you would face to face. Listen to how the patient sounds – are they breathless? Can they complete sentences? Do they sound distressed / in pain?
- In a third party consultation (for example with a child) ask what the child is doing right now – a flat, non-responsive child will require more urgent action than one who is happily playing.
- Safety-netting on the telephone requires specific instructions on what to look out for and when to seek face-to-face review in case of deterioration. Ensure you can justify your management and if the patient needs to be examined, arrange for a face-to-face review.
- Consider what you would do with a failed contact – how many calls would you make? What voice message would you leave? When would you consider asking the police to carry out a welfare check?

Third party consultations

Third party encounters are common in paediatric cases where patients may present with parents or carers. Ensure in these consultations that you acknowledge all members of the party, and clarify who everyone is and their relationship to each other. Aim to elicit as much history as you can from the patient themselves, using language that they will be able to understand. Be aware of any potential conflicts of interest or confidentiality; for example, if a parent accompanies a more mature child under 16, it may hinder an open discussion of certain topics such as sexual health / contraception. In certain circumstances it may be appropriate to ask to speak to the patient on their own.

Further reading

Pygall, S-A. (2023) *Telephone Assessment in Primary Care*. Scion Publishing Ltd.

Males, T. (2015) Risks of telephone consultations. *Practice Matters*, **3(1)**: 12–14. Available at: www.medicalprotection.org/uk/articles/risks-of-telephone-consultations

Case B1.1   Information for the doctor

In this case you are a doctor in surgery taking telephone consultations.	
Name:	Emma Brown
Age:	2 years old
Past medical history:	NVD with no complications No SCBU admissions
Current medication:	Nil

Notes

Case B1.1 Information for the patient

You are Julia Brown, 28-year old mother of Emma who is 2. She is at nursery at the moment and you just called up to request some medication for her constipation.

ICE

- You really just want some medication for Emma's constipation. You noticed she opened her bowels only a couple of times a week during last month.

Background

- You are calling to discuss medication for constipation.
- Emma never had any bowel problems before but for approximately one month it has been a nightmare. She is passing hard stools and goes to the toilet only once or twice a week.
- Your close friend Caroline works as a herbalist and she gave you some natural tea bags for constipation. You love natural remedies and believe they are healthier than 'real chemicals' but, unfortunately, Emma seems to hate the taste of the tea, so you are not pushing it too much.
- You found few tips online about constipation in children and have decided you would like to try some medication instead. Last night Emma was crying and straining on the toilet and it was impossible for you to watch her suffer.
- She was born by normal vaginal delivery and there are no other health problems. She is thriving.
- She has been complaining of recurrent tummy pain, which seems to get better after passing stool.

Information divulged freely

- You live with your husband Mark and you have three children together. Emma is the youngest. You also have 4-year old twins. They are both well.
- You are off work at the moment but you are busy enough taking care of your family. Your mum helps you at the weekends when you can finally have some time with your husband.
- You recently moved to a new place so Emma had to change nurseries.
- You love your husband. He is very busy at work though – he has his own business. He is also concerned about Emma's health, but you disagree on using natural medicine – he is very against everything your friend suggested. This attitude had prompted you to find more information on the internet and you think perhaps your husband is right and you need to talk to the doctor and get a 'real' medication that works.

Information only divulged if specifically asked

- Emma is not passing any blood and you haven't noticed any abdominal distension.
- She has no urinary symptoms / no history of soiling / no vomiting.
- You believe her diet is OK, but you are not the best cook. You find it easier and quicker to use ready meals.
- Your mum cooks very well and definitely prepares healthier meals for your children at the weekends.
- If specifically asked, you admit that your family members don't eat enough fruit and vegetables, but a lot of processed food.

- Emma's fluid regime seems to be OK; you never heard about any concerns from the nursery.
- If the doctor mentions how common constipation is you would be very surprised. If he / she is understanding and explains clearly the possible causes of constipation, you would feel that perhaps the recent relocation contributed to Emma's symptoms. If the doctor explains that one of the commonest causes of constipation is inadequate diet and insufficient fluid intake you would admit that perhaps that is something you need to address to help Emma's symptoms.
- If the doctor clearly explains that before prescribing laxatives it would be appropriate to see Emma for an examination and review, you'd ask for any reasons for this. You are happy to bring Emma for review tomorrow if your questions are adequately answered. If the explanation is not clear enough, you become more demanding and specifically ask for a script again.
- If the doctor offers a prescription you'll happily take it.

Case B1.1 **Marking scheme for the observer**

patient.info/doctor/constipation-in-children-pro
patient.info/doctor/telephone-consultations

Data gathering and diagnosis

☐	☐	☐	• Gathers information systematically and efficiently about reason for attending, to exclude other causes for the patient's presentation
☐	☐	☐	• Asks open questions
☐	☐	☐	• Identifies ICE
☐	☐	☐	• Social history important to obtain – moving house, starting a new nursery
☐	☐	☐	• Excludes 'red flag' symptoms – vomiting, abdominal distension, severe pain, urinary symptoms, pale stool

Clinical management and medical complexity

☐	☐	☐	• Uses changes in diet, lifestyle, and behavioural modifications alongside the early use of laxatives. It would be important to review and examine the child prior to prescribing
☐	☐	☐	• Recommends a balanced diet with sufficient fibre, adequate fluid intake and daily physical activity
☐	☐	☐	• Offers written, evidence-based information about constipation and its management
☐	☐	☐	• Arranges follow-up and discusses regular reviews. Bonus if suggests involvement of health visitors who can give ongoing support and have some tips on regular toilet habit

Relating to others

☐	☐	☐	• Recognises the patient's agenda and preferences and elicits a social history to be able to put problem into context
☐	☐	☐	• Communicates effectively to the patient
☐	☐	☐	• Shows empathy and understanding
☐	☐	☐	• Has a positive attitude when dealing with the problems
☐	☐	☐	• Checks for mum's understanding throughout

Case B1.2 Information for the doctor

You are a locum doctor and have been asked to telephone Beena Chattopadhyay about her daughter Geeta's results. Her usual doctor, Dr Green, is on holiday for three days.

In this case you are a doctor in surgery.	
Name:	Geeta Chattopadhyay
Age:	6
Past medical history:	none
Current medication:	Nil
Previous consultation:	**Seen by Dr Green** Presented with urinary frequency for 3 days Fever last night Came back from Spain 2 weeks ago Not eating well. Mum pushing fluids O/E looks well T 37.4 Well perfused Abdomen – soft, no masses No rash Urine – cloudy. Nitrites +, leucocytes +++ on dipstick. Imp – UTI Plan – start trimethoprim for 3/7, fluids Will be back if not better in 2–3 days MSU sent **2 days later – entry by Nurse Fiona Walker** Culture: *E. coli*: >10^8 CFU/L Sensitive to: trimethoprim / nitrofurantoin / co-amoxiclav Resistant to: amoxicillin

Case B1.2 Information for the patient

You are Beena Chattopadhyay, a 36-year old designer. You tried to phone Dr Green twice this morning. You didn't realise he was on holiday but you were hoping someone would return your call a little bit sooner.

ICE

- You are worried about Geeta, your 6-year old daughter. The nurse told you yesterday that the urine sample confirmed an infection and you are worried that this is pretty serious.
- You recently returned from holiday in Spain, so you wonder if Geeta perhaps picked up some parasites there.
- You are concerned that the antibiotics you were given are not strong enough and you believe it is impossible to treat infection in 3 days. You remember taking antibiotics for 7 days when you had a chest infection last year.
- You would like more antibiotics to make sure the infection is gone.

Background

- Geeta is your only child and she is never ill.
- When you came to see a doctor a few days ago she was 'drained' and very tired. She felt hot; you think she's been feverish on and off but you never actually checked her temperature.
- Her appetite wasn't great a few days ago but it's almost back to normal now. She was also complaining of aches in her lower tummy and her urinary frequency was unbelievable!

Information divulged freely

- You are a single mum. Very independent and confident. Dad is not involved.
- Geeta definitely picked up since she was started on antibiotics. She is back to school today and has one more day of trimethoprim left.
- Her symptoms have improved and she is eating and drinking very well since yesterday.
- As a preventative measure you'd like to give her antibiotics for at least one week, because bacteria in her bladder sounds worrying.

Information only divulged if specifically asked

- There is no family history of urinary or kidney problems.
- Geeta was born by normal delivery and there were no complications.
- She is developing and growing well.
- Her bowels are regular and there is no history of constipation.
- When the doctor explains that *E. coli* is one of the commonest causes of UTI you'd become calmer and sound more relaxed.
- When the doctor explains that this particular bacteria is sensitive to the antibiotic Geeta is already on, you'd be delighted and less stressed.
- If the doctor doesn't check your understanding you become very impatient and would have a lot of questions.
- You would accept the doctor's evidence-based explanation on current treatment for lower UTI / cystitis and reasons for 3 days course as per current NICE guidelines. If the difference between UTI and chest infection treatment is described, you'd be completely reassured.

- If you don't feel you've been reassured you'd explain that it is nothing personal but you will have to end this telephone consultation and book an appointment with Geeta's usual GP, Dr Green.
- If the doctor offers you an appointment for review and more detailed explanation you'd agree to come in.

Case B1.2 Marking scheme for the observer

patient.info/doctor/urinary-tract-infection-in-children
patient.info/doctor/telephone-consultations
https://pathways.nice.org.uk/pathways/urinary-tract-infections/management-of-urinary-
    tract-infection-in-under-16s#content=view-node:nodes-recurrent-uti

Data gathering and diagnosis

☐ ☐ ☐	• Identifies ICE and addresses mum's concerns
☐ ☐ ☐	• Is able to take a brief history over the phone
☐ ☐ ☐	• Asks questions about child's symptoms to exclude acute pyelonephritis and enquires about general health
☐ ☐ ☐	• Checks compliance with antibiotics

Clinical management and medical complexity

☐ ☐ ☐	• Clearly explains MSU results
☐ ☐ ☐	• Provides sufficient and evidence-based information on *E. coli* UTI and appropriate treatment
☐ ☐ ☐	• Offers follow-up appointment
☐ ☐ ☐	• Is able to explain difference in treatment for LRTI and UTI

Relating to others

☐ ☐ ☐	• Recognises the patient's concerns and confirms understanding
☐ ☐ ☐	• Communicates effectively
☐ ☐ ☐	• Shows empathy
☐ ☐ ☐	• Establishes rapport

Case B1.3 Information for the doctor

In this case the practice nurse has asked if you can squeeze Lucas onto the end of your call list because mum had some worries when she brought him for his immunisations. His 8-week check-up has been postponed until next week because another GP called in sick, and mum really needs to talk to someone before then.

In this case you are a doctor in surgery.	
Name:	Lucas Kowalski
Age:	8 weeks
Past medical history:	Born by NVD. Undescended right testicle documented in neonatal check.
Current medication:	Nil

Notes

Case B1.3 Information for the patient

You are Agata Kowalski, a 30-year old mum. You brought Lucas to see the nurse for his immunisations, but you booked a follow-up telephone call because you want to arrange for a doctor to examine his testicles.

ICE

- You were told after delivery that Lucas is 'missing' his right testicle but you were advised not to worry and see a GP for a usual 8-week check-up. You are quite upset and worried about this.
- After chatting to your friends you've decided you would like an ultrasound scan to see if the testicle is hidden. You also did some online reading and you are now concerned that Lucas might be at risk of developing cancer and infertility.
- You expect to be referred for an ultrasound scan.

Background

- You are an employee in a local Polish shop. Currently you are on maternity leave.
- You moved to the UK from Poland 8 years ago. You are now a British citizen.
- You live with your fiancé Josh who is a professional pianist. You have two children together: 3-year-old Tomas and 8-week-old Lucas.
- You are well and have no medical problems.
- You have two older sisters and they are both healthy. They also live in the UK.
- Your parents are in Poland and you see them 2–3 times a year. You have many close friends locally for support.

Information divulged freely

- You are concerned about your son's condition. You feel that the doctor at hospital simply left after mentioning that Lucas's right testicle is 'missing' and asked you to see a GP. You understand that doctors in hospitals are very busy but you feel disappointed that nobody took the time to explain what the condition means or simply give you some written information instead.
- Lucas is a term baby, born by NVD without any complications. You were discharged home the next day.
- You breastfeed and there are no other developmental concerns so far.

Information only divulged if specifically asked

- Recently you had a small cyst on your breast that was confirmed with an ultrasound scan. You believe a similar scan could help to visualise your son's testicle.
- Your fiancé Josh is healthy. There is no significant family history.
- If the doctor refuses to request an ultrasound scan at the beginning of the consultation, feel free to become angry and difficult.
- If the doctor is kind and understanding and provides you with some verbal and written information on maldescended testicles you'd happily listen.
- You are happy to attend a face-to-face appointment if offered but ask why the scan cannot be requested in the meantime as you don't want to be waiting long.

- If the doctor seems concerned and prefers to speak to the hospital doctor for advice you become even more worried and tearful and blame yourself for not coming earlier.
- If the doctor is not quite sure what the next step should be and suggests checking current guidelines and recommendations you appreciate the doctor's honesty and would want to see the recommendations yourself.
- If the doctor suggests to give it some time and see how things are in a couple of months, you become suspicious that the doctor just wants to finish the call. If the doctor further elaborates that in the majority of cases, the testes descend on their own with time then you'd remain calm.
- If the doctor is clear, calm and confident about the condition and explains that imaging is not routinely indicated you would want to know more. If the management plan is clearly summarised you'd be reassured and cooperate without any problems.

http://geekymedics.com/testicular-examination-osce-guide/

Case B1.3 Marking scheme for the observer

https://patient.info/doctor/undescended-and-maldescended-testes

Data gathering and diagnosis

☐	☐	☐	• Elicits ICE and desire for USS
☐	☐	☐	• Identifies mum's negative experience in hospital and offers support
☐	☐	☐	• Explores relevant family history
☐	☐	☐	• Identifies patient's understanding of her son's condition

Clinical management and medical complexity

☐	☐	☐	• Is able to explain diagnosis in a reassuring, jargon-free way
☐	☐	☐	• Discusses appropriate treatment; shows awareness that ultrasound does not change the management. If unsure, deals with uncertainty and makes plan to find out
☐	☐	☐	• Offers appropriate face-to-face appointment and explains potential for referral to Paediatric Surgeon / Urologist if the testicle was to remain undescended
☐	☐	☐	• Is aware of current recommendations regarding surgery (would usually occur around 12 months of age if indicated)
☐	☐	☐	• Offers written information

Relating to others

☐	☐	☐	• Is empathetic to patient's concerns
☐	☐	☐	• Communicates effectively to the patient
☐	☐	☐	• Avoids medical jargon
☐	☐	☐	• Explores patient's feelings and expectations
☐	☐	☐	• Maintains rapport

Case B1.4 Information for the doctor

In this case Mrs Rodrigues has booked a video consultation regarding her daughter.

In this case you are a doctor in your afternoon surgery.	
Name:	Amalia Rodrigues
Age:	5
Past medical history:	Eczema Weight 20 kg; height 110 cm (tracking normally on the 75th centile)
Current medication:	Oilatum bath oil. Diprobase emollient cream

Notes

Case B1.4 Information for the patient

You are Mariza Rodrigues, mum to 5-year old Amalia. You would like to talk to the doctor about Amalia's food allergies.

ICE

- You have been discussing food allergies with the mums at Amalia's swimming group and you think your daughter's eczema might be due to some sort of food allergy – possibly egg or nuts.
- You would like her to be tested to find out what she is allergic to.

Background

- Amalia is your only child and you live with your husband in central London. He works in the city and you are a full-time mum.
- Amalia is otherwise fit and well. You had an uncomplicated vaginal delivery and she has never had any hospital admissions or regular medications apart from her emollients.

Information divulged freely

- Amalia has suffered with eczema since she was a baby. She gets dry skin behind her knees and elbows if you don't use the diprobase.
- You never considered food allergy before until you spoke with the other mums, and they told you that sometimes milk or wheat allergies can cause skin problems.
- Amalia can sometimes be picky with her food, but you have never noticed any flare-up in her skin after eating certain foods. You have not tried eliminating foods yet, and you have called today to ask for an allergy test to see if she does have any specific food allergies.
- Amalia is growing well. She has never suffered with symptoms of colic, reflux or constipation and she doesn't complain of being tired all the time. She is not asthmatic, although her dad used an inhaler when he was a child.

Information only divulged if specifically asked

- Amalia's skin is well controlled with the diprobase and she has never had any problems with cracked / fissured skin or any concurrent infections. She does occasionally itch if it is dry and you have forgotten to apply the cream. When she was about 2 you were given a steroid cream to use because her skin was very red and itchy, but the doctor advised changing your washing powder and it settled down within a few weeks. Since then she has never had a similar flare-up.
- She has never experienced any symptoms of anaphylaxis. She has had no airway swelling or angioedema and no wheeze.
- You suffer with irritable bowel syndrome yourself, and you often find that certain foods make your symptoms worse. Your symptoms are controlled but you remember struggling for years with wind and bloating and you felt dismissed by doctors. You do not want the same thing to happen to Amalia. You think if she gets tested now when she is young she can avoid a lifetime of problems.
- If the doctor is immediately dismissive of your request for allergy testing and doesn't appear to listen to your story then you will be quite demanding and ask to be referred to a 'specialist'. If the doctor does show an interest and can reassure you that Amalia does not

have any concerning symptoms suggesting allergy, and can explain what these are, then you will feel more reassured. You would like to know what allergy testing involves and the reasons for not having it done.

- If management of the dry skin is discussed you will admit that her skin does settle down when the emollient is used regularly, and you will happily continue to use this more often.
- If explained, you would be happy to try eliminating certain foods from her diet to see if this has an effect and report back to the doctor with the results.

Case B1.4 **Marking scheme for the observer**

https://cks.nice.org.uk/cows-milk-protein-allergy-in-children
https://patient.info/doctor/cows-milk-protein-allergy-pro
http://patient.info/doctor/atopic-dermatitis-and-eczema
Food Allergy Quality Standard: www.nice.org.uk/guidance/qs118

Data gathering and diagnosis

☐	☐	☐	• Takes a detailed history to include: presence of atopy (personal and family history), symptoms of concern to mum – speed / duration / severity / frequency
☐	☐	☐	• Enquires about triggers for symptoms, and establishes how reproducible these symptoms are • Asks about feeding history and development • Asks about treatments tried and response
☐	☐	☐	• Screens for any features indicating anaphylaxis/IgE-mediated allergy (rapid onset; angioedema; wheeze/SOB; urticarial; pruritis; diarrhoea / vomiting)

Clinical management and medical complexity

☐	☐	☐	• Reassures mum that, from the history and findings, food allergy is unlikely; can discuss the typical reasons for referral to secondary care for further testing; discusses private referral options
☐	☐	☐	• Discusses the management of eczema and emollient use
☐	☐	☐	• Can discuss elimination of the suspected allergen as an option for 6 weeks and how to reintroduce foods (including safety and limitations)
☐	☐	☐	• Safety-nets by arranging follow-up and discussing the more serious symptoms of anaphylaxis or allergy-related co-morbidity to look out for

Relating to others

☐	☐	☐	• Explores mum's ICE and establishes the effect of the problem for both mum and Amalia
☐	☐	☐	• Acknowledges mum's own previous health concerns and experience with doctors and attempts to address this
☐	☐	☐	• Avoids being dismissive of mum's concerns; listens and understands and builds rapport and comes to a shared plan with the family

For children with non-IgE cow's milk allergy, the milk ladder can be used to reintroduce cow's milk protein to the diet: https://gpifn.org.uk/imap

Case B1.5 Information for the doctor

In this case you are a doctor in your morning surgery taking telephone calls.	
Name:	Kinga Fekete
Age:	15
Past medical history:	None
Current medication:	None

Notes

Case B1.5 Information for the patient

You are Kinga Fekete, a 15-year old girl, who has called to talk about contraception.

ICE

- You want a prescription for the pill.
- You are worried the doctor will make you tell your parents.

Background

- You live with your parents and younger brother.
- You attend the local comprehensive school and are currently studying for your mock exams.
- You don't smoke.

Information divulged freely

- Your periods started when you were 12 and your LMP was about a week ago (it came just after you had had sex, at the normal time for you 5/28). You have not had sex before or since then. You used a condom last week.
- You have been in a relationship for 3 months and last weekend you started having sex. He has suggested you go on the pill as he doesn't like using condoms. You agree it would be easier so have called to discuss this.
- Your parents are certainly not aware of the relationship – your mum would not be happy if she knew, as your cousin got pregnant very young and had to drop out of school. You feel she would worry about the same thing happening to you. You cannot be persuaded to tell her.
- You will continue to have sex even if not given the pill today.
- You understand all the info about the pill and seem quite knowledgeable about how to take it and the possible side-effects. You know it does not protect against STDs. You certainly don't want to consider any other methods of contraception and if asked, the reason is you don't like needles. There are no contraindications to you taking the combined pill.

Information only divulged if specifically asked

- Your boyfriend is 25 years old and he is actually a teaching assistant at the school. You know the doctor will not approve of this so at first you only state he is 'someone at school' and only reveal his job and age upon direct questioning.
- Last weekend he gave you lots of alcohol and took you back to his house. You had not really been ready to start having sex but now worry he will leave you if it does not continue. There were no other drugs involved and it was consensual. Generally your interactions outside school involve you going to his flat to drink. You have not met any of his friends or family. He is not violent or aggressive towards you.
- If the GP gives you the pill you will go away happy.
- If they express concerns about the relationship you will be very worried. Does this mean they will tell your parents? If social services are mentioned you will become very upset – this will be very embarrassing at school and surely means your boyfriend will lose his job.
- If the reasons behind the referral to social services are discussed you will accept it has to be done but remain upset at the outcome of the consultation.
- If a pill prescription is offered you understand you will need to attend either the surgery or pharmacy for a blood pressure, height and weight assessment, and you are happy to do this.

Case B1.5 Marking scheme for the observer

patient.info/doctor/contraception-and-young-people
https://patient.info/doctor/combined-oral-contraceptive-pill-first-prescription

Data gathering and diagnosis

☐	☐	☐	• Takes a detailed history including information on the sexual relationship, being mindful of the patient's age
☐	☐	☐	• Identifies the child protection issues (children and the law: learning.nspcc.org.uk/child-protection-system/children-the-law)
☐	☐	☐	• Asks relevant questions regarding oral contraception to determine if patient has any risk factors for its use, using UKMEC criteria (Quick UKMEC calculator here: www.ukmec.co.uk)

Clinical management and medical complexity

☐	☐	☐	• Discusses and refers appropriately to social services even without patient consent
☐	☐	☐	• Encourages the patient to speak to her parents
☐	☐	☐	• If the pill is prescribed – considers Fraser competence of the patient and excludes any contraindications to its use
☐	☐	☐	• Explains how to use the method, side-effects and safety nets when to stop (severe headache or painful swollen leg). Considers quick starting – see above.
☐	☐	☐	• Takes the opportunity to discuss health promotion and STD prevention

Relating to others

☐	☐	☐	• Discusses the need for social services referral in a sensitive manner
☐	☐	☐	• Tries to help the patient understand the concerns about the relationship
☐	☐	☐	• Is clear about the nature of confidentiality and when it can be breached
☐	☐	☐	• Communicates risk to the patient but maintains an awareness of her preferences

Fraser Guidelines

Contraceptive advice and treatment can be provided to a young person under the age of 16 without parental consent, using the Fraser Guidelines. To meet these criteria, health professionals need to be satisfied that prescribing is in the patient's best interests and the patient:

- refuses to tell her parents despite encouragement
- will continue to have sex, with or without contraception
- understands the advice given
- may be at risk of physical or mental health problems if contraception is not prescribed.

A duty of confidentiality is the same for children as it is for adults and may only be breached to protect the child or others from serious harm (i.e. child abuse/child protection or where required by law).

In this particular case, a referral to social services would be appropriate, but it may also be appropriate to prescribe contraception, as she is Fraser competent.

Case B1.6 Information for the doctor

In this case you are a doctor in the on-call surgery responding by telephone to an online consult submitted by Nina's father.	
Name:	Nina Stein
Age:	30 months
Online consult:	"My daughter has a cold and has had watery eyes for the last few days. I would like antibiotic drops please"
Past medical history:	Bronchiolitis; eczema
Current medication:	Nil
Allergies:	Nil

Notes

Case B1.6 Information for the patient

You are Nick Stein, a 35-year old man who is taking a call from the GP today about his daughter Nina who has had a runny nose and watery eyes for 3 days.

ICE

- Your wife Sonia asked you to get some antibiotic drops from the doctor to get rid of Nina's conjunctivitis.

Background

- Your daughter hasn't been sleeping well for three days due to congestion.
- Her eyes are watery and look inflamed. She had puffy eyelids this morning.
- She hasn't had her usual breakfast this morning but she is enjoying her banana right now.
- Nina's nursery told you about a recent outbreak of conjunctivitis and at least five children were sent home with similar symptoms.

Information divulged freely

- You are a joiner and run your own business.
- Your wife works 4 days a week as a sales assistant for John Lewis.
- Both you and your wife are healthy.
- Nina was born by ventouse delivery without any complications.
- She is up to date with vaccinations and has had no major medical problems since birth.

Information only divulged if specifically asked

- Your close friend's newborn daughter had bad conjunctivitis last month and she had swabs and two lots of antibiotic drops. You don't want to leave it until it gets worse.
- Nina's eyes are watery. Her eyelids seemed puffier this morning but they are back to normal now. She hasn't been rubbing them particularly often, as far as you have noticed.
- There is no history of sticky eyelids or purulent discharge.
- She is not complaining of any pain or discomfort and her eyes are not red.
- You have no pets at home and she has not been exposed to any potential allergens as far as you know.
- If the doctor is thorough and empathetic and explains that Nina's conjunctivitis doesn't require antibiotics, and their reasoning why not, you'd listen to the doctor's recommendations.
- If the doctor says that the condition is self-limiting you'd require more explanation.
- If the doctor prescribes antibiotic drops/ointment you'd happily accept the script and ask about how long she needs to be excluded from nursery for.
- If the doctor remains understanding and explains that the condition is typically self-limiting, you'd be relieved but still prefer to get a delayed script for antibiotics just in case. If the doctor continues to remain reassuring, confident and arranges follow-up, you'd remain calm and reassured.

Case B1.6 Marking scheme for the observer

patient.info/doctor/infective-conjunctivitis-pro
https://cks.nice.org.uk/topics/conjunctivitis-infective/diagnosis/clinical-features/

Data gathering and diagnosis

☐	☐	☐	• Takes appropriate history, establishes timing of symptoms, absence of pain, trauma, discomfort and discharge; establishes that this is an otherwise well child
☐	☐	☐	• Makes a judgement regarding examination in person; there is enough information from the photo and history to make a management plan, but arranging an in-person review may provide more reassurance for Dad (green for avoids, orange if arranges despite trying to reassure, red if arranges with no attempts to reassure and manage remotely first)
☐	☐	☐	• Enquires about recent medication, eye drops, pets; thinks about potential allergic causes

Clinical management and medical complexity

☐	☐	☐	• Diagnoses conjunctivitis (watery discharge, recent upper respiratory tract infection) and discusses viral / bacterial / allergic aetiology
☐	☐	☐	• Advises parent that the condition is usually self-limiting and expected to resolve within 1–2 weeks and that antibacterial agents have not been shown to significantly reduce duration of illness (if asked about why friend's child treated differently, is aware that conjunctivitis in neonates is treated differently and why)
☐	☐	☐	• Explains that the condition can be contagious for close contacts / family (warns not to share towels, etc.) but that school exclusion is not advised by Public Health England
☐	☐	☐	• Offers follow-up / safety-netting in place, to return if worsening symptoms / concerns

Relating to others

☐	☐	☐	• Establishes underlying reason for attendance
☐	☐	☐	• Appears alert to cues and responds to feelings and expectations
☐	☐	☐	• Elicits psychosocial context, patient centred, shows empathy
☐	☐	☐	• Provides reassurance and involves patient in management plan

Further reading

Acute conjunctivitis is more often bacterial than viral, but is self-limiting (5-7 days) and antibiotics have been shown to offer little benefit and no adverse events have been reported from not treating. Chloramphenicol is now available over the counter which suggests public health messages are not getting through (*BJGP* (2005) **55:** 924; *Lancet* (2005) **366:** 37; *BMJ* (2006) **333:** 321).

The UK Health Security Agency (UKHSA) advises that children with conjunctivitis do not need to be excluded from school (although nurseries may have their own policies on this, which GP practices should feel free to challenge; template letter example here: www.eastkentformulary. nhs.uk/media/1276/letter-to-schools-nurseries-re-conjunctivitis-jan-2019.pdf). Advice is available at: www.gov.uk/government/publications/health-protection-in-schools-and-other-childcare-facilities

Case B2.1 Information for the doctor

In this case you are a GP Registrar in your morning surgery.	
Name:	Stella Starr
Age:	41
Past medical history:	Twin pregnancy (C-section delivery 9 years ago); allergic rhinitis
Current medication:	Cetirizine 10 mg od

Notes

Case B2.1   Information for the patient

You are Stella Starr, a 41-year old lady, who is going on holiday next week and you are very worried about catching zika, so you have booked a telephone consultation with the GP.

ICE

- You and your family are off to Florida next week and you didn't realise until yesterday how close it is to South America. Remembering the news about zika from when you last went on holiday, you want to ask the doctor if it is safe to travel.
- You are also due to start your period during the holiday and you would like something from the doctor to delay this.

Background

- You work in human resources and live with your husband and twin boys.
- You are fit and well and take antihistamines for your allergies.
- You don't smoke and drink about 15 units of alcohol per week.

Information divulged freely

- You go to Florida most years during the kids' half term school holidays, but since reading so much in the media about the zika virus, you are wondering if it is safe for you to travel and if there are any precautions you should take.
- You are worried about whether it is still safe for your family to travel and if you perhaps need a vaccination against the disease. You don't know much about the disease but the coverage on TV has scared you and you want to be reassured Florida is safe.
- If the doctor is happy for you to travel, then you would also like something to delay your period.

Information only divulged if specifically asked

- Your periods are regular and you are due to start your next period on the second day of your holiday. Your husband had a vasectomy after the twins were born so you aren't interested in any other contraception if the doctor asks. You have no other sexual partners. You have never had a blood clot in your legs or lungs.
- You have been given medication to delay your period before but would appreciate a reminder from the doctor on how to use it.
- You know your children are up to date with their vaccinations and you think you and your husband are too. You never had any travel shots to go to Florida in the past but you would be happy to have any if needed.
- You are staying in a self-catered apartment so will be doing most of the cooking yourself, and you have never had any problems with diarrhoea on holiday before; however, you appreciate any travel advice the doctor may want to give you.
- You do like to sunbathe and generally use a low factor sunscreen, but make sure the kids are covered up. You will accept any advice given by the doctor regarding staying healthy while travelling.

Case B2.1 Marking scheme for the observer

www.gov.uk/government/collections/zika-virus-zikv-clinical-and-travel-guidance
https://patient.info/womens-health/periods-and-period-problems/delaying-a-period
http://nathnac.net/

Data gathering and diagnosis

☐	☐	☐	• Takes the opportunity to gather a detailed travel history
☐	☐	☐	• Enquires about the patient's menstrual cycle, gynae history, contraception use and pregnancy risk and excludes any risk factors for VTE
☐	☐	☐	• Makes reference to travellers' health resources which are available to give up-to-date health information and vaccination requirements specific to the country of travel (see *Further reading* and resources on p. 33)

Clinical management and medical complexity

☐	☐	☐	• Shows an awareness of the latest guidelines regarding zika and can discuss questions the patient may have about transmission, symptoms, vaccination and the risks to pregnant women
☐	☐	☐	• Reassures the patient that her trip is low risk for zika (or makes reference to the resources that could be checked if unsure) and takes the opportunity to encourage healthy travel. Considers vaccination / malaria prophylaxis, travellers' diarrhoea, sun exposure, sexual health, personal safety during travel
☐	☐	☐	• Is aware of methods available to delay menstruation (suggest norethisterone 5 mg tds or medroxyprogesterone 10 mg tds starting 3–4 days before period due; can be taken for up to 2 weeks and menstruation occurs on stopping), counsels patient that it has no contraceptive effects and delayed menses is not always guaranteed; also mentions small increased risk of VTE
☐	☐	☐	• Makes practical suggestions for travel: carrying regular medications in hand luggage, obtaining travel insurance, etc.

Relating to others

☐	☐	☐	• Avoids being dismissive of the patient's zika concerns. Takes time to explain any questions the patient may have
☐	☐	☐	• Discusses healthy travel without being patronising towards the patient
☐	☐	☐	• Is open and engaging and addresses ICE

Further reading

Delaying menstruation: https://patient.info/womens-health/periods-and-period-problems/delaying-a-period

Zika virus guidance:
www.rcog.org.uk/guidance/browse-all-guidance/other-guidelines-and-reports/zika-virus-infection-and-pregnancy

Discussion point

Travel health is not part of the core GP contract. For the sake of this case and learning this has not been factored into any discussion within the case, but it is worth considering how this would work in your own practices in life beyond the exam. Where do you refer patients locally for travel health queries? Do you have any practice policy on prescribing medication to delay periods? What are your thoughts on this?

Case B2.2 Information for the doctor

In this case you are a doctor in surgery.	
Name:	Hannah Stainburn
Age:	40
Past medical history:	Last consult – LMP 5 weeks ago, positive home pregnancy test, patient not sure if wants to continue with pregnancy as already has 3 children at home and may be financially difficult. She will discuss with her partner and let us know.
Current medication:	nil

Notes

Case B2.2 Information for the patient

You are Hannah Stainburn, a 40-year old social worker and mother of three, who has booked a telephone consultation with the doctor to discuss a positive pregnancy test.

ICE

- You are concerned about the risk of Down's syndrome and want to find out more about being tested.

Background

- You recently found out you were pregnant and have decided to continue with the pregnancy.
- You are very concerned about the risks of Down's syndrome in older mothers and you feel you would struggle financially to support a child with extra needs.

Information divulged freely

You want to know:
- What are the chances my baby has Down's?
- Can the baby be tested before birth? What does this involve?
- Would I be able to have a termination without my partner knowing?

Information only divulged if specifically asked

- You did try to discuss testing with your partner but he got very upset at the thought of you having an abortion. If asked, you have not told him you are calling today as you are worried he will get more upset. You would like the testing to be kept a secret from him and have decided that if needed you would get an abortion and tell him you had had a miscarriage.
- If encouraged in a sensitive way, you would be willing to have a further discussion with your partner before going for testing. You would be willing to wait until your chat with your partner before being referred and accept a follow-up appointment in one week.
- You have no prior knowledge of genes or how they are inherited. You know very little about Down's syndrome.

Case B2.2 Marking scheme for the observer

https://patient.info/doctor/prenatal-screening-for-downs-syndrome
http://patient.info/doctor/downs-syndrome-trisomy-21
www.downs-syndrome.org.uk/for-new-parents

Data gathering and diagnosis

☐ ☐ ☐	• Determines patient's prior knowledge of Down's syndrome
☐ ☐ ☐	• Elicits the social background, and any discussion regarding screening with partner
☐ ☐ ☐	• Elicits patient's ideas and concerns about Down's syndrome and her expectations of testing
☐ ☐ ☐	• Determines LMP and gains an understanding of how many weeks pregnant she is, and any other health concerns

Clinical management and medical complexity

☐ ☐ ☐	• Discusses what screening for Down's involves, i.e. she will undergo blood tests and an ultrasound as part of the screening programme, which can give her more information about the risk of Down's in her pregnancy (1 in 100 at age 40)
☐ ☐ ☐	• Covers the options and timing of amniocentesis and chorionic villus sampling and the associated risks of miscarriage of both (amniocentesis 1%; CVS 2%)
☐ ☐ ☐	• Is able to discuss Down's syndrome honestly with the patient and acknowledge health risks of the condition, but also the better prognosis of the condition now; encourages patient autonomy

Relating to others

☐ ☐ ☐	• Remains non-judgmental and sensitive to the effect of the decision on the patient's life
☐ ☐ ☐	• Provides clear explanations, giving time for the patient to ask questions
☐ ☐ ☐	• Adopts a sensitive approach to the patient's dilemma and uses time as a tool, encouraging further discussion with her partner to enable her to make the best decision for her
☐ ☐ ☐	• Communicates risk of prenatal testing effectively

Case B2.3 Information for the doctor

In this case you are a GP registrar in a routine morning surgery.	
Name:	Lara Stuart
Age:	25
Past medical history:	nil
Current medication:	Microgynon tablets

Notes

Case B2.3   Information for the patient

You are Lara Stuart, a 25-year old lady, who has called to discuss a genetics referral. You have just found out your sister carries the BRCA *gene and you want to be referred for testing.*

ICE

- You know you want a referral to be tested for the *BRCA* gene. You expect the GP to be happy to refer you to the local service.
- You are obviously upset at the news about your family history and anxious about the possible implications of the test.

Background

- You live with your fiancé and have your wedding booked for June next year.
- You work as a legal secretary in a firm in town and really enjoy your job.
- You don't smoke. You drink a couple of glasses of wine a night with a few gin and tonics at the weekend. You know you are a bit overweight – you do a weekly yoga class and plan to do more exercise prior to your wedding.

Information divulged freely

- Your sister rang you last week to tell you she had tested positive for the *BRCA* gene. You knew she had decided to have the test as she told you when she was referred. Your mum died last year of breast cancer at 50 after being diagnosed at 42 and your maternal aunt was diagnosed at 38 but is in remission. Your mum had refused *BRCA* testing at the time because she wanted to leave the decision to you and your sister if you each wanted to know. After she died your younger sister decided to go ahead and get tested and you agreed you wanted to know the results.
- You have already done your research and know there is a 50% chance you will also have the gene. You have read about the testing and options for monitoring, surgery and medication and you are certain you want a referral.

Information only divulged if specifically asked:

- You are extremely upset at your sister's news, she is only 22 and has decided to go ahead and have the surgery to remove her breasts and ovaries as she is so worried about her cancer risk.
- You know you will not go ahead with any surgery or prophylactic medication now; you are planning to wait until after you are married and hopefully had children, so plan to ask for regular mammograms and scans until you are ready to decide what to do.
- You understand the implications for any children you might have. You would let your children decide if they wanted to be tested when they were older.
- You haven't discussed this referral with your partner yet. You are not sure he will understand why you want to be tested and you think he will encourage you to not be tested. He will really struggle with a positive test result because you know he will worry every time you have a slight sniffle that this indicates that you have cancer. If the doctor strongly encourages you to discuss it with your partner you are reluctant but will eventually agree. If the doctor offers a joint appointment to discuss this with you and your partner, you agree as you feel he might be more understanding if the information comes from a doctor.

- If the GP is understanding and sympathetic to your situation you would like to ask what else you can be doing to reduce your breast cancer risk. You are taking the pill and know hormones can increase your breast cancer risk but don't want to come off it and risk being pregnant at your wedding. If the pill is a big risk would an alternative contraceptive be better? If the doctor advises any hormonal contraception would be associated with a higher risk of breast cancer but suggests the copper coil, you would be interested and take away some further information. If the doctor is not sure, you are happy for them to get back to you once they have asked their local family planning clinic.

Case B2.3 Marking scheme for the observer

The NICE CKS on Breast cancer – managing family history can be read in conjunction with this case https://cks.nice.org.uk/breast-cancer-managing-fh

Data gathering and diagnosis

☐	☐	☐	• Identifies the reason for attendance and discovers the patient has already made her decision regarding referral and testing
☐	☐	☐	• Takes a full family history of both first degree and second degree relatives, asking about all cancer diagnoses and age at onset; those in which a specific gene has been identified; presence of bilateral disease; any male breast cancer; any Jewish ancestry
☐	☐	☐	• Asks about any breast lumps / symptoms and other risk factors for breast cancer – alcohol, smoking, weight, use of the oral contraceptive pill
☐	☐	☐	• Identifies that the patient has not discussed the referral with her partner and elicits her reasons for this

Clinical management and medical complexity

☐	☐	☐	• Is able to briefly discuss the implications of testing positive for the *BRCA1* gene, including the need for monitoring for breast and ovarian cancer, and the option of prophylactic surgery or medication. Is also able to advise that the risk of any children (male or female) carrying the gene is 50%
☐	☐	☐	• Is able to advise that use of the COCP leads to a small increase in the risk of breast cancer but it has a protective effect against ovarian cancer. In carriers of the *BRCA* gene, avoidance of combined hormonal contraception is advised (UKMEC3). Can discuss alternatives and offers verbal and written advice on this and signposts to local family planning clinic or offers follow-up to discuss further
☐	☐	☐	• Is able to advise lifestyle changes to reduce breast cancer risk, such as increasing her exercise levels and reducing her alcohol consumption. Encourages breast self-examination and offers a leaflet if the patient wishes
☐	☐	☐	• Refers to a genetics service

Relating to others

☐	☐	☐	• Creates rapport with patient by empathising with her recent bad news and difficult decision
☐	☐	☐	• Sensitively encourages the patient to discuss the situation with her partner and offers to see her again with him if she wishes

Case B2.4 Information for the doctor

In this case you are a doctor in surgery taking video calls.	
Name:	Hualing Zhao
Age:	49
Past medical history:	One month ago • BP 120/89 • BMI 23
Current medication:	Nil

Notes

Case B2.4   Information for the patient

You are Hualing Zhao, a 49-year old woman, who has called the doctors to discuss your menopausal symptoms.

ICE

- You want to discuss HRT but are very fearful of the side-effects as your mother died of breast cancer.
- You are really interested in alternative methods and hope the doctor will discuss this. You worry that there is no non-hormonal alternative or that the doctor will not give this option.

Background

- You work as a shop assistant.
- You live with your husband and have 3 grown-up children.
- You don't smoke.
- You drink 3–4 glasses of wine a week.

Information divulged freely

- The flushes and sweats have been happening for about 6 months. For the past year your periods have been irregular and your last period was 4 months ago.
- You are pretty sure this is the menopause as your friends have similar symptoms. It is actually them that encouraged you to call. Your friend Mary started HRT 2 months ago and feels amazing. She has even got herself a new boyfriend!
- You are finding the flushes embarrassing; you work as a shop assistant and the uniform is quite thick so you are finding it difficult to manage.
- At home your sleep is disturbed by the sweats and your husband has been complaining about you tossing and turning. This has led to a few arguments.
- The poor sleep has made you more irritable but you deny low mood or other symptoms of depression.
- You and your husband are still having sex and you don't have any symptoms of vaginal dryness. He has had a vasectomy so you are not in need of contraception.
- Your mother had breast cancer but you have no family history of stroke/MI or endometrial cancers.
- If the doctor offers an SSRI you are dubious and wonder if the doctor feels you are depressed but if explained, you are very happy to try this and will accept either a prescription or a further appointment with written info in the meantime.
- If the doctor discusses herbal medicines you will listen but will have lots of questions about side-effects.
- If the doctor discusses HRT you will be sceptical and your gut feeling is to decline, but you will listen to the pros and cons and be happy to read more about it.

Case B2.4 Marking scheme for the observer

https://thebms.org.uk/nice-guideline/tools-for-clinicians/
https://pathways.nice.org.uk/pathways/menopause/menopause-overview#content=view-
   index&path=view%3A/pathways/menopause/menopause-overview.xml

Data gathering and diagnosis

☐	☐	☐	• Takes a history of menopausal symptoms and their impact on the patient's life
☐	☐	☐	• Identifies any contraindications to taking HRT
☐	☐	☐	• Recognises the concerns the patient has around breast cancer (BMS factsheet can help discuss risks: thebms.org.uk/wp-content/uploads/2022/12/12-BMS-TfC-Fast-Facts-HRT-and-Breast-Cancer-Risk-NOV2022-A.pdf)

Clinical management and medical complexity

☐	☐	☐	• Recognises perimenopause and discusses the risks/benefits of HRT in the context of family history of breast cancer. Aware transdermal preparations can be safely used with good effect
☐	☐	☐	• Discusses alternatives to HRT. If any information is not known, the doctor should advise when they will find out and how they will tell the patient (see smartphone link for up-to-date HRT guidance from the British Menopause Society)
☐	☐	☐	• Makes appropriate prescribing decisions and can explain these to the patient. For low mood due to menopause, NICE guidance favours HRT rather than antidepressants – see useful links above
☐	☐	☐	• Takes the opportunity to discuss health promotion and the role of lifestyle measures (exercise / alcohol, etc.) in improving menopausal symptoms and considers the role of CBT

Relating to others

☐	☐	☐	• Is able to discuss menopausal symptoms in a sensitive manner
☐	☐	☐	• Is able to respond to the patient's concerns about HRT and offer advice on both HRT and alternative options. Treats the patient as an individual and allows her to make her own informed decision regarding treatment options
☐	☐	☐	• Recognises the impact of the symptoms on the patient's life

Systemic HRT treatment

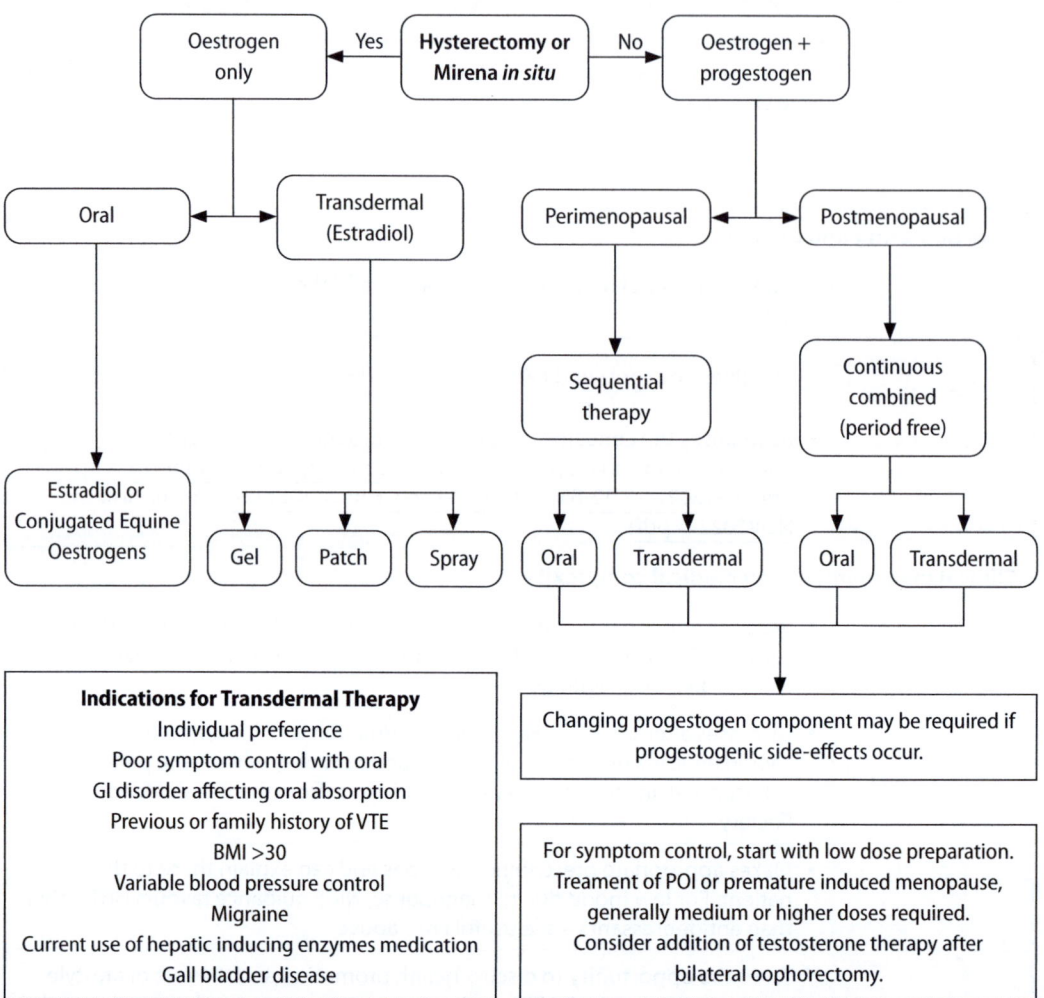

Indications for Transdermal Therapy
Individual preference
Poor symptom control with oral
GI disorder affecting oral absorption
Previous or family history of VTE
BMI >30
Variable blood pressure control
Migraine
Current use of hepatic inducing enzymes medication
Gall bladder disease

Changing progestogen component may be required if progestogenic side-effects occur.

For symptom control, start with low dose preparation. Treament of POI or premature induced menopause, generally medium or higher doses required. Consider addition of testosterone therapy after bilateral oophorectomy.

Reproduced with permission from the British Menopause Society.

Case B2.5 Information for the doctor

You are a newly qualified GP in surgery taking video calls.	
Name:	Anita Singh
Age:	31
Past medical history:	Marsupialisation for Bartholin's cyst (2011); eczema
Current medication:	Naproxen 250 mg prn, Zeroderm ointment
Telephone consultation (4 months ago):	GP Dr S: phone call from patient (not known to me), enquiring about swab and USS results – all reported as normal, reassured. Previous consult noted. Manages well with naproxen during periods. No new issues. Review as needed.
Previous consultation (6 months ago):	GP Dr K: complaining of dyspareunia in certain positions, occasional abdo ache, worse when on her period (previously seen with abdo pain in OOHs, ongoing issue), took tramadol from a friend for a few days 3 months ago as the pain was unbearable. Discouraged to do so in the future, reasons discussed in detail. Usually manages well with naproxen during periods. Admits stress at work / lack of sleep. Anxious, unable to conceive, only been trying for 6 months so reassured at this stage. Minimal PV discharge, clear – ?physiological. No urinary symptoms. Married, no problems at home. No postcoital / intermenstrual bleeding. Smear – normal last year. Examination: normal vital signs; abdo soft, normal pelvic exam, self vaginal swabs sent for reassurance, urine NAD. Imp - ?cause for abdo pain / ?stress related / ?anxiety around conceiving. Plan – arrange USS, swabs and review with results. Counselling discussed – declined at this stage.
Consultation in Out Of Hours Centre (9 months ago):	Presented with her husband with severe abdo pain for 2 days. On her period at present. Haemodynamically stable, vitals all normal. Naproxen not working. Had some loose stools. No fever. Examination – min discomfort in lower abdomen. BS normal. Urine – NAD, pregnancy test negative. Imp – menstrual cramps Plan – add short-term co-codamol, continue naproxen. See GP if not better.

Case B2.5   Information for the patient

You are Anita Singh, a 31-year old woman. You are worried there might be something wrong as you are unable to get pregnant. You have been trying for less than a year, but you are concerned and would like to get a referral to a fertility clinic. You wish to start a family as soon as possible and the fact that everyone around you seems to be getting pregnant is making you more stressed.

ICE

- You start by saying: "Sorry to bother you again but I think I need to be referred to fertility clinic".
- You've done your research and are aware that you might not qualify under the NHS criteria so are happy with a private referral.

Background

- You work as a designer and do a lot of travelling around the country.
- You love your job but recently decided to drop your hours because you are desperately trying to get pregnant.
- Your husband is a rental agent and works full time.
- You have 2 older sisters who both got pregnant in their early 20s.
- Your parents live in London, you see them every couple of months. They keep asking you if you have decided not to have children. It really affects you because you are trying to get pregnant. You and your husband haven't told them you've been trying for a while because you don't want them to worry (your mum has had 2 heart attacks in her 60s).

Information divulged freely

- You are usually well, only suffering from mild eczema in winter.
- Your mum has had 3 daughters. Your two older sisters (they are both in their 40s) were born when your mum was in her early 20s. You are not aware of any fertility problems in your family but it did take 10 years for your mum to get pregnant with you after your two sisters were born.
- One of your sisters has 2 children who are now teenagers and your second sister has a child in their early 20s.
- You don't smoke. You have the occasional Martini every few weeks.
- Your husband has asthma, otherwise he is pretty healthy. He smokes the occasional shisha when you are on holiday, otherwise he doesn't smoke. He enjoys a couple of beers at the weekend.
- Your periods are regular, your cycle is 26 days. They've always been painful for as long as you can remember. In the past ibuprofen would sort your pain but over the past year or so, you've noticed that it's simply not enough. You were given naproxen which was initially effective during your painful periods but it didn't help a few months ago, so you took some tramadol from a friend. You know it was silly but you were in agony and needed to prepare a presentation for work.
- Your periods usually last 7 days and are quite heavy.
- If the GP offers an appointment for internal examination you decline as the GP you saw last time carried this out and you are currently menstruating and don't feel comfortable doing this while you are.

- If the GP suggests that you and your husband should have some more investigations first, you'd insist on a private referral to a local fertility centre. If the GP clearly explains what tests could be done first and why, you'd be happy to have these tests first.
- If the doctor is unsure if you could be referred to a fertility clinic on the NHS but is willing to find out about current criteria, you'd be grateful if a follow-up telephone call could be arranged.
- If the GP suspects you might have endometriosis, you'd get really worried and will need more answers about what it is and how it's diagnosed. If the GP remains confident and empathetic and offers a gynaecology referral for a second opinion you'd be very happy that the doctor takes your concerns seriously.
- If the GP has some general fertility advice for you and tells you that all your tests so far (swabs and USS) are normal and you should just keep trying and give it a bit longer, you'd start crying and will keep asking about private referral to fertility clinic until the doctor agrees to arrange one.

Information only divulged if specifically asked:

- You'd admit certain sexual positions are uncomfortable. You are embarrassed to talk about it.
- If specifically asked about your bowel symptoms, you'd admit your bowel movements are usually more painful and looser during your periods but it's always been this way, so you are not sure if it's getting any worse.
- You have no urinary symptoms.
- You've never had any sexually transmitted infections.
- If specifically asked about intercourse you'd confirm you have vaginal intercourse regularly, usually three times a week unless you are on your period.
- You've been married for 5 years and have never been on any contraception; you were using the 'withdrawal method'.
- You've never been pregnant and never had any miscarriages or abortions.
- You are already taking folic acid supplements.

Case B2.5   **Marking scheme for the observer**

The NICE guidelines on Endometriosis: diagnosis and management and Fertility problems: assessment and treatment can be read in conjunction with this case:
www.nice.org.uk/guidance/ng73
www.nice.org.uk/guidance/cg156

Data gathering and diagnosis

☐	☐	☐	• Identifies reason for attendance and desire for referral
☐	☐	☐	• Takes a fertility history including: length of time trying to conceive; regularity of intercourse and any difficulties experienced; gynae history (pattern of menstrual cycle / pain / prior pregnancies or procedures / smear history); previous STIs; partners and family history
☐	☐	☐	• Checks for red flag symptoms such as postcoital bleeding, rectal bleeding, abdominal masses and enquires about general health / presence of any systemic disease
☐	☐	☐	• Considers following up with an examination and to check BMI, BP

Clinical management and medical complexity

☐	☐	☐	• Suspects possible endometriosis (cyclical pelvic pain, dyspareunia, heavy menstrual bleeding, painful bowel movements during periods) and takes appropriate steps to diagnose or exclude it. Referral to gynae clinic would be appropriate in this case. The candidate should be aware that a normal USS and examination does not rule out endometriosis and should be able to explain that diagnostic laparoscopy is the gold standard in the diagnosis of endometriosis
☐	☐	☐	• Is able to give general fertility advice (lifestyle – smoking cessation, avoidance of alcohol / illicit drugs, folic acid supplementation, having unprotected intercourse 2–3x weekly)
☐	☐	☐	• Can discuss investigations available (NICE advises against a 'blind screen' for everything and different localities will vary on what GPs can offer in primary care). The following pathway may be useful: www.ouh.nhs.uk/services/referrals/womens/fertility-clinic.aspx
☐	☐	☐	• Arranges follow-up with results / offers to see husband and explains need for semen analysis and consulting with him too
☐	☐	☐	• Explains options with regards to fertility / checks criteria for NHS referral if unsure (may differ between areas)
☐	☐	☐	• Discusses pain symptoms and analgesic options. Discusses NSAIDs being contraindicated in pregnancy. Shares with the patient that hormonal methods (such as the combined oral contraceptive pill) can be used to reduce pain, but acknowledges at present when trying to get pregnant this may not be an option

Relating to others		
☐ ☐ ☐		• Addresses ICE, empathetic towards patient concerns about fertility
☐ ☐ ☐		• Builds rapport and is able to question patient openly but sensitively about intercourse and any problems she is experiencing
☐ ☐ ☐		• Appropriately refers / arranges follow-up and safety-netting
☐ ☐ ☐		• Offers written information on both endometriosis (patient.info/health/pelvic-pain-in-women/endometriosis) and fertility (patient.info/health/infertility-leaflet).

Case B2.6 Information for the doctor

You are a GP in surgery carrying out telephone consultations.	
Name:	Joycelin Minnelli
Age:	55
Past medical history:	None
Current medication:	Nil

Notes

Case B2.6   Information for the patient

You are 55-year old Joycelin Minnelli. You have called up the GP today to discuss a problem you find very embarrassing – a "problem down below".

ICE

- You wondered if you had thrush and so tried that cream from the chemist, but it didn't work.
- You are not concerned about any sinister causes.
- You expect a thrush treatment but realise the doctor may want to do an examination as well.

Background

- You live with your husband and have 3 children in their 20s.
- You are retired but used to run your own business making jams.
- You don't smoke but drink a bottle of red wine a week.

Information divulged freely

- For the past 3–4 months you have noticed an uncomfortable dryness down below. At first you thought it was your new washing powder but changing that has not helped. Then one of your friends told you she had similar symptoms and it was thrush. You tried using Canesten cream from the chemist for one week but this did not help.
- You have no discharge.
- Your periods stopped 7 years ago and you have had no bleeding since.
- You have found over the past few years you need to go to the toilet more to pass urine. You also find you get up once during the night to go as well.
- You had all your 3 children naturally and had lots of stitches after your last son. Ever since then you have occasionally leaked a bit of urine when you cough or sneeze but it doesn't really bother you enough to raise it as an issue.
- You do have to rush a bit when you need the toilet, but don't think you have ever not made it in time.
- You would be happy to come in for an examination and swabs, but wonder if there is anything you can try in the meantime.
- If the doctor advises a hormone replacement cream you will be concerned by the use of hormones – the news says they cause breast cancer. However, you will agree to try them if their risks and side-effects are explained.
- If the doctor offers a vaginal moisturiser you will also agree to try this.
- If the doctor wishes to await swab results and contact you with these you will be happy with this plan.

Information only divulged if specifically asked

- You have been having difficulty having sex with your husband. You are very dry vaginally and you find penetration painful. Your husband is very understanding but you worry he will start to get annoyed if the problems continue. You are embarrassed to tell the doctor this and worry they will think you silly for feeling an active sex life is important. If this information is not dealt with sympathetically you will be quite upset and although you will stay on the call you will not say much and end it as quickly as you can.

Case B2.6 Marking scheme for the observer

patient.info/doctor/atrophic-vaginitis
www.bashhguidelines.org/current-guidelines/skin-conditions/vulval-conditions-2014/

Data gathering and diagnosis

☐	☐	☐	• Takes a full history of the urogenital symptoms the patient is suffering
☐	☐	☐	• Sensitively asks about the impact of the symptoms on her sex life
☐	☐	☐	• Offers an appointment to carry out a pelvic exam and swabs
☐	☐	☐	• Enquires about the presence of any other menopausal symptoms

Clinical management and medical complexity

☐	☐	☐	• Recognises and is able to explain the likely diagnosis of atrophic vaginitis to the patient
☐	☐	☐	• Offers appropriate treatment of topical oestrogens or vaginal moisturisers
☐	☐	☐	• Is aware systemic absorption is minimal using vaginal oestrogen and progestogen is not required

Relating to others

☐	☐	☐	• Puts the patient at ease when they are discussing a topic they find embarrassing
☐	☐	☐	• Sensitively discusses the impact of atrophic vaginitis on the patient's sex life
☐	☐	☐	• Appears comfortable and confident discussing sexual problems with the patient

Case B2.7 Information for the doctor

In this case you are a doctor in surgery taking video consultations.	
Name:	Ethan Black
Age:	41
Past medical history:	Tonsillectomy 17 years ago; Asthma 35 years ago
Current medication:	Seretide; Ventolin

Notes

Case B2.7 Information for the patient

You are Ethan Black, a 41-year old father of two children (7 and 4) who has called up today to discuss referral for a vasectomy.

ICE

- You expect to be referred for a vasectomy today. You are aware there might be a long waiting list if you are referred via the NHS, so you are open to discuss other options including private referral.

Background

- You and your wife Alice have both decided that you have completed your family and vasectomy sounds like a good option. Your wife can't wait to finally come off her pill.
- You are both teachers.
- You are aware that a vasectomy is a straightforward procedure (more or less) and your friend mentioned that it is easily reversible if you both change your mind.

Information divulged freely

- You have had asthma for many years but it's very well controlled on your inhalers.
- You don't smoke and your alcohol intake is approximately 20 units / week.
- You have two wonderful boys (7 and 4) and you are *almost* 100% sure that you don't want any more children. Your wife always wanted to have a girl but it just wasn't meant to be.
- You believe if you change your mind after the procedure you'd probably request reversal of vasectomy and you know it will have to be done privately.
- Alice is on the combined pill and is fed up taking it every day. She has never tried other contraceptive methods.

Information only divulged if specifically asked

- You are not aware that vasectomy is primarily considered as a permanent method of contraception.
- If the doctor informs you that you are not immediately infertile post-procedure and will have to use other contraception methods for at least a couple of months, you would require more information about this.
- You would be very interested in what the doctor has to say about vasectomy as a procedure, risks, advantages, possible side-effects and success rates.
- If the doctor mentions that unfortunately vasectomy cannot be easily reversed and should be considered as an irreversible procedure, you would be very disappointed and remain silent for a minute.
- If the doctor remains sensitive and empathetic and explains there are other methods to explore in the meantime, then you and your wife will be happy to find out more about other long-acting reversible methods of contraception (LARCs).
- Your wife Alice might be quite interested in the contraceptive implant or an IUD.
- If you are happy with the doctor's explanation you will need some time to think about your next step and will come back in a few weeks' time.
- If the doctor doesn't offer other contraceptive methods and refers you for a vasectomy you would prefer to be referred privately.

Case B2.7 Marking scheme for the observer

https://patient.info/doctor/sterilisation-vasectomy-and-female-sterilisation

Data gathering and diagnosis

☐	☐	☐	• Identifies desire for vasectomy
☐	☐	☐	• Clarifies patient's understanding about the procedure and ensures both partners agree on vasectomy request
☐	☐	☐	• Picks up on some doubts about the procedure especially after explanation about its irreversibility
☐	☐	☐	• Explores if other LARC methods have been tried
☐	☐	☐	• Clarifies that family has been completed

Clinical management and medical complexity

☐	☐	☐	• Confidently describes vasectomy, possible failure rates and when it is effective
☐	☐	☐	• Covers possible post-operative complications (chronic pain, cysts, haematoma, sperm granuloma, psychological problems…)
☐	☐	☐	• Clarifies it is a permanent method of contraception and makes sure the patient is aware that reversal success rate is low and not available under NHS
☐	☐	☐	• Makes patient aware of referral system (hospital, GPs with a special interest, private referral)
☐	☐	☐	• Offers alternatives to vasectomy and provides written information on options available
☐	☐	☐	• Offers appropriate follow-up

Relating to others

☐	☐	☐	• Remains sensitive and empathetic
☐	☐	☐	• Explores patient's health beliefs and agenda
☐	☐	☐	• Picks up on cues that patient's wife may consider alternatives
☐	☐	☐	• Develops good rapport

Case B2.8 Information for the doctor

In this case you are a doctor in surgery undertaking video consultations.	
Name:	Max Martin
Age:	65
Past medical history:	Hypertension; angina
Current medication:	Aspirin, ramipril, simvastatin, GTN spray
Social history:	Smoker 20/day, cessation advice given last year 3 weeks ago – history of blood in urine for 2/7, nocturia. No haematuria today. Lower abdo ache. Feeling well. Likely had fever last night. O/E looks well, afebrile. BP 145/80 Abdomen – soft, no masses. Urine dipstick – blood++, nitrates+, leucocytes++. No frank haematuria. Not enough urine to send MSU. Imp – UTI Plan – trimethoprim and review if symptoms persist

Notes

Case B2.8 Information for the patient

You are Max Martin, a 65-year old patient who has contacted his GP today to request more antibiotics for a UTI.

ICE

- Your wife Mary suggested contacting the doctor because you have had blood in your urine again.
- You wonder whether you needed some stronger antibiotics.

Background

- 3 weeks ago you were diagnosed with a urine infection by Dr Jones after having blood in your urine. You were treated with trimethoprim for 5 days, which magically helped.
- Last night you noticed blood in your urine again. It's clear again today but you are experiencing lower tummy ache which feels exactly like last time.
- You work in a local post office, which you have owned with your wife Mary for over 20 years.
- You are a very busy man and you are very active for your age.
- You have smoked 20 cigarettes a day for at least 35 years.
- You have two children. Your older daughter lives in France and your 30-year old son works with you.

Information divulged freely

- You believe you have another bladder infection today. You are surprised you developed it again because Dr Jones mentioned trimethoprim usually kills all bladder bugs.
- You admit you are feeling more tired lately.
- You had blood in urine 3 weeks ago for 2 days and felt very unwell then.
- Yesterday you noticed bright red blood in your urine again. It happened twice. You are much better today but your tummy is slightly 'achy' and you have no energy.

Information only divulged if specifically asked

- Your weight is stable and your appetite is good.
- You have no bowel problems.
- You've been having awful night sweats for 2 months or so.
- You have no symptoms of dysuria.
- There is no history of any recent trauma or injury.
- You have no loin pain.
- You were adopted so you don't know your family history.
- If the doctor expresses concerns about your symptoms and suggests that urgent referral to secondary care is required to rule out anything potentially serious, you would ask if the doctor means you might have cancer.
- If the doctor is honest, supportive and clear then you would agree to be referred for further investigations (cystoscopy).
- If an in-person appointment is offered you are happy with this and are also happy to hand in urine samples to the surgery.
- If the doctor seems unsure, you would become more anxious and stressed about the possibility of cancer.

- If the doctor remains supportive and confident and has clear ideas on what should happen next, you'll trust their judgment.
- If the doctor offers to see you and your wife again if any questions come up while you are waiting for a specialist review, you'd be very grateful and might come back with your family members next week.

Case B2.8 Marking scheme for the observer

patient.info/doctor/haematuria-pro
cks.nice.org.uk/topics/urological-cancers-recognition-referral

Data gathering and diagnosis

☐	☐	☐	• Identifies patient's concerns and expectations and allows patient time to talk
☐	☐	☐	• Recognises risk factors (smoker, recurrent frank haematuria in a 65-year old man, night sweats, non-specific lower abdo ache)
☐	☐	☐	• Considers need for in-person examination (without delaying further referral)

Clinical management and medical complexity

☐	☐	☐	• Considers possible diagnosis of bladder cancer until proven otherwise
☐	☐	☐	• Refers under a suspected cancer referral pathway to urology team for cystoscopy
☐	☐	☐	• Arranges relevant investigations in the meantime (bloods, urine for culture and cytology)
☐	☐	☐	• Uses safety-netting

Relating to others

☐	☐	☐	• Shows empathy and develops rapport
☐	☐	☐	• Reaches management plan through shared agreement with the patient
☐	☐	☐	• Remains positive and clearly explains reasons for urgency of referral in a way the patient can understand

Case B2.9 Information for the doctor

In this case you are a GP registrar in a routine morning surgery taking video calls.	
Name:	Alan Tyson
Age:	63
Past medical history:	Hypertension
Current medication:	Amlodipine 10 mg od

Notes

Case B2.9 Information for the patient

You are Alan Tyson, a 63-year old man with troublesome urinary problems.

ICE

- As you have grown older, you have to get up more to use the toilet at night and you wonder if this means you have prostate problems.
- You worry about prostate cancer. Your friend at work was diagnosed with prostate cancer at age 49 and you know he had similar problems to you.
- You expect "one of those blood tests" for prostate cancer.

Background

- You live with your wife May and your older son Keith (aged 42).
- You retired last year from working in a butcher's shop. You and your wife are planning a trip to Australia next year to visit your daughter who lives there.
- You have a dog who you take for long walks and you enjoy cycling. You drink a few glasses of wine a week and are an ex-smoker. You stopped smoking 5 years ago; you used to smoke 10 a day.

Information divulged freely

- For the past 3 months you have noticed you are having to go to the toilet more often to pass urine. You get up 2–3 times during the night.
- You have no pain when you go and haven't noticed any blood.

Information only divulged if specifically asked:

- You have noticed your stream is poor and you often dribble at the end of passing urine.
- You have had no burning when you pass urine and no fever or signs of infection.
- You enjoy a cup of coffee and have 5–6 cups a day including just before bed.
- You have not had any episodes of incontinence.
- You have no back pain, bony pain or weight loss.
- You have no lower abdominal pain.
- You have no erectile dysfunction.
- You are happy to come for an in-person appointment if requested and ask what will happen at this appointment.
- If the doctor mentions benign prostatic hypertrophy you are interested to know more and ask specifically if this means you will eventually get prostate cancer.
- If the doctor suggests you fill in a questionnaire about your symptoms and return for follow-up, you are happy to do this.
- If the doctor suggests blood tests you are happy to have them done – you ask specifically when you should book these tests.
- If the doctor discusses medication you are interested to hear about the options. You would be happy to take medication if the doctor felt it would help.
- If the doctor discusses your fluid intake you would be happy to try cutting down on the caffeine.

Case B2.9 **Marking scheme for the observer**

https://cks.nice.org.uk/luts-in-men

Data gathering and diagnosis

☐	☐	☐	• Takes a full history of lower urinary symptoms
☐	☐	☐	• Asks about red flag symptoms for urological cancer (unexplained haematuria, lower back pain, bone pain, weight loss): https://cks.nice.org.uk/urological-cancers-recognition-and-referral
☐	☐	☐	• Arranges appointment to perform examinations to include: digital rectal examination, abdominal examination and urinalysis (considers neurological examination and inspection of external genitalia)
☐	☐	☐	• Suggests the patient carries out an IPSS questionnaire to assess his symptoms (www.baus.org.uk/_userfiles/pages/files/Patients/Leaflets/IPSS.pdf)
☐	☐	☐	• Arranges to check U&Es and a PSA blood test given the patient's concerns, only after discussing the indications for the test, the interpretation and factors affecting it, and the implications of the results (https://prostatecanceruk.org/prostate-information-and-support/prostate-tests/psa-blood-test)

Clinical management and medical complexity

☐	☐	☐	• Correctly suspects benign prostatic hypertrophy (BPH) among the differentials and arranges in-person examination
☐	☐	☐	• Is able to explain BPH to the patient and discuss treatment options. An alpha-blocker such as tamsulosin can be offered for voiding symptoms with advice on side-effects
☐	☐	☐	• Discusses lifestyle measures such as caffeine reduction
☐	☐	☐	• Arranges appropriate follow-up and discusses urological symptoms to be aware of which require medical attention (urinary retention, haematuria, UTI)

Relating to others

☐	☐	☐	• Creates rapport with patient
☐	☐	☐	• Identifies the patient's concerns about prostate cancer
☐	☐	☐	• Explains in a clear jargon-free way the diagnosis of BPH and offers a leaflet (patient.info/health/prostate-and-urethra-problems/prostate-gland-enlargement)
☐	☐	☐	• Is understanding regarding the concern about prostate cancer and offers PSA screening with advice to the patient on the possibility of a false positive result and what would happen if the result is raised

Case B2.10 Information for the doctor

In this case you are a doctor in surgery taking video calls.	
Name:	Gina Khan
Age:	20
Past medical history:	None
Current medication:	Microgynon

Notes

Case B2.10 Information for the patient

You are Gina Khan, a 20-year old woman. You want to discuss some 'funny bleeding' you have been having for the past few months.

ICE

- You are worried about cervical cancer. You are too young to have had a smear but you read a magazine article recently about a 23-year old girl who had cervical cancer.
- You hope the GP will organise a smear to rule out cancer.
- You want to know about getting the HPV vaccine as you were not in school when it was given.

Background

- You are a 20-year old woman who is currently at university studying business management. You smoke 5 cigarettes a day and drink 3–4 vodka and Cokes on Friday and Saturday nights.

Information divulged freely

- The bleeding you are worried about has been happening for 2 months; you are finding spots of blood in your underwear 3–4 times a week and occasionally some on wiping yourself after going to the toilet. You have had a withdrawal bleed in each COCP break and need to wear 3–4 pads a day for this with no clots or flooding.
- You have remembered your pill every day so are certain you are not pregnant. You last had unprotected sex a few days ago.
- You have no lower abdominal pain or abnormal discharge.

Information only divulged if specifically asked

- You started a new relationship with a fellow business student 6 months ago. You started the Microgynon 2 months ago. Prior to this you had regular periods every month for 4–5 days.
- Before this relationship you have had two previous sexual relationships. You had an STD check about 18 months ago when you had some abnormal discharge, which was all clear.
- If the doctor will not arrange a smear you will be upset and want to know why and if you can pay for a private one. You will also ask about a referral to the gynaecologist instead. However, you will accept that bleeding is common in the first 3 months of starting the COCP if explained. If explained clearly, you will be happy to wait for it to settle down, on the understanding that if it continues you would return to be referred.
- You are happy to attend an appointment for a pelvic exam and swabs. You would accept being directed to a sexual health clinic for these as well.
- With regards to the HPV vaccine you will accept if the doctor tells you about potentially having it privately or if they say they do not know but will find out.

Case B2.10 Marking scheme for the observer

https://patient.info/doctor/breakthrough-bleeding-with-combined-hormonal-contraception

Data gathering and diagnosis

☐	☐	☐	• Takes an appropriate history of the abnormal bleeding including an appropriate sexual history
☐	☐	☐	• Offers an in-person appointment to carry out a speculum exam and pregnancy test. Triple swabs should be offered
☐	☐	☐	• Enquires about COCP use – missed pills, pill-free period and length of use

Clinical management and medical complexity

☐	☐	☐	• Discusses possible causes of bleeding, including: common occurrence in first 3 months COCP and possibility of STD. Discusses options of changing to a different pill / alternative form of contraception
☐	☐	☐	• Explains why a smear would be inappropriate – the patient is too young for the NHS cervical screening programme and the sample would not be analysed by some labs because of this. Private smear testing is available (Marie Stopes offers this for under 25s) and this can be discussed. Explaining the reasons for not testing in this age group on the NHS may be helpful in her decision (see Further reading overleaf)
☐	☐	☐	• Gives advice on the HPV vaccine and also discusses smoking cessation as this will reduce her risk of cervical cancer
☐	☐	☐	• Ensures safety-netting is in place, with clear plans on when the patient should return for review and what to do if bleeding gets worse / when colposcopy is advised

Relating to others

☐	☐	☐	• Empathises with the patient's concern about cancer and comes to a shared management plan
☐	☐	☐	• Develops good rapport
☐	☐	☐	• Gives clear explanation of management plan, including how results of the swabs will be communicated

Learning points

Cervical cancer is rare under the age of 25 and screening is not offered to younger women in the UK (in Australia it is at 18, and in the USA at 21). This is because changes to the cells of the cervix are common at this age, and these changes typically resolve without leading to cancer. Screening can sometimes lead to unnecessary further tests and worry [1].

A cervical smear is not a diagnostic test but done as part of the NHS screening programme – so should not be done routinely in patients presenting with abnormal bleeding [2,3]. These patients should be managed appropriately outside of the screening programme [4].

References

[1] https://www.gov.uk/government/publications/abnormal-vaginal-bleeding-in-women-under-25-clinical-assessment

[2] McCartney, M. Doctors and patients confuse cervical screening with diagnostic tests. *BMJ, 2014; 348: 3334 Available at* www.bmj.com/content/348/bmj.g3334.full.pdf+html

[3] McCartney, M. A tragic death but nothing to do with 'denying young women smear tests'. *Pulse, 2013* Available at: www.pulsetoday.co.uk/views/blogs/dr-margaret-mccartney/a-tragic-death-but-nothing-to-do-with-denying-young-women-smear-tests/20003266.blog

[4] www.gov.uk/government/publications/cervical-screening-programme-and-colposcopy-management/2-providing-a-quality-colposcopy-clinic

Further reading for patients:
Cervical cancer incidence statistics from Cancer Research UK:
www.cancerresearchuk.org/cancer-info/cancerstats/types/cervix/incidence/#age

Lab Tests Online provide a useful summary:
https://labtestsonline.org.uk/tests/cervical-cytology

A resource for patients that explains more about smears and HPV: www.jostrust.org.uk

The Eve Appeal: eveappeal.org.uk/gynaecological-cancers/cervical-cancer

Case B2.11 Information for the doctor

In this case you are a doctor in surgery taking video calls.	
Name:	Madeleen-Jane Lynn
Age:	32
Past medical history:	Miscarriage at 10 weeks (2 years ago) Miscarriage at 8 weeks (1 year ago) A&E attendance 2 weeks ago – PV bleeding in pregnancy, USS confirmed miscarriage at 6 weeks
Current medication:	Nil

Notes

Case B2.11 Information for the patient

You are 32-year old Madeleen-Jane Lynn. You have just had your third miscarriage. You have contacted the doctor about further testing.

ICE

- You have contacted the doctor to discuss further testing and would like a referral to the fertility clinic to discuss this.
- You are very worried there is something wrong because you don't know anyone else who has had three miscarriages. You have heard people can have clotting problems that cause miscarriages and know your grandmother and aunt both had clots in their legs – could this be the cause and how do you test for this?
- You expect your GP to refer you to the clinic.

Background

- You have been married for 5 years and started trying to get pregnant about 2 years after this.
- You work as a shop assistant and your husband works as an electrician. You have a good relationship.
- You are a non-smoker and don't drink alcohol.
- You have no past medical history.

Information divulged freely

- You have had three miscarriages. You have never been pregnant apart from on these occasions and your husband has no other children.
- You are keen to discuss any lifestyle advice the GP has to offer regarding miscarriage because there is so much online it's hard to know what is true. Specifically you want to ask:
  - Is there anything you should or shouldn't eat to help your fertility?
  - How much exercise is the "right amount"?
  - Your husband drinks about 6–7 pints of beer at the weekend – surely he should stop drinking altogether?
- You would also like to know about possible causes of recurrent miscarriage. You don't have any genetic problems which run in the family and neither does your husband, as far as you know.
- You will quickly accept any referral offered but do want to know how long the process takes.

Information only divulged if specifically asked

- You have been feeling very low since the last miscarriage. You don't sleep due to anxiety and your appetite is poor. You feel you are "obsessed" with fertility. You have even stopped seeing one of your friends who smokes, just in case. You are not suicidal. When you feel low you talk to your husband but your friends and family don't know about your troubles.
- You will accept a referral for counselling if offered. You will also be open to the idea of telling a friend or family member so you can have someone else to discuss your worries with. You will not accept medication as it may harm any future pregnancies.

Case B2.11 Marking scheme for the observer

patient.info/doctor/recurrent-miscarriage
Green Top Guideline No.17: Recurrent miscarriage, investigation and treatment of couples:
www.rcog.org.uk/en/guidelines-research-services/guidelines/gtg17

			Data gathering and diagnosis
☐	☐	☐	• Takes a history of the presenting problem including a past medical history and family history
☐	☐	☐	• Identifies the additional problem of low mood
☐	☐	☐	• Sensitively asks about the number of miscarriages and gestation, being aware that 3 or more miscarriages are defined as recurrent miscarriage

			Clinical management and medical complexity
☐	☐	☐	• Offers a referral to a miscarriage clinic and is able to either explain the possible tests which will be carried out or signposts how they will find out more information for the patient
☐	☐	☐	• Is able to discuss lifestyle and dietary advice related to fertility
☐	☐	☐	• Is able to give an overview of possible causes of recurrent miscarriage to the patient or signpost how they will get this information to the patient

			Relating to others
☐	☐	☐	• Creates a rapport with the patient
☐	☐	☐	• Discusses recurrent miscarriage and possible causes in a jargon-free way
☐	☐	☐	• Sensitively discusses the patient's low mood and possible options for managing this

Case B2.12 Information for the doctor

In this case you are a locum GP in the on-call surgery taking telephone calls.	
Name:	Jane Ramsden
Age:	32
Past medical history:	None
Current medication:	None

Notes

Case B2.12   Information for the patient

You are Jane Ramsden, a 32-year old lady, who would like emergency contraception. You open with the question "This is confidential right, you won't be able to tell anyone what I say?"

ICE

- You know about the pill being used for emergency contraception and want to be prescribed this.
- You are very worried about someone seeing the prescription or seeing you at the chemist which is why you didn't go there for advice.
- You expect a prescription to be given today.

Background

- You live with your partner of 10 years and your two children who are 5 and 2.
- You are a full-time mum at present; prior to having children you worked behind the counter at a local garage.
- You don't smoke and rarely drink alcohol.
- You are very active running around after the kids and try to go for a run twice a week.

Information divulged freely

- You want a prescription for the morning-after pill. You had sex 2 days ago and the condom broke and you certainly do not want to find yourself pregnant.
- You really don't want to go into any more details than that, surely that is all the doctor needs to know.

Information only divulged if specifically asked

- If asked in a sensitive way you confess you have been having an affair with a married man. He was a friend of yours from school and you bumped into each other again 6 months ago. It started as chatting and meeting for coffee, but now you have been meeting at his house every few weeks to have sex.
- The sex is consensual.
- Your husband had a vasectomy a year ago as you were certain your family was complete. You don't want to take any hormonal contraception as he might find the packets. You and your partner have been using condoms but realised 2 days ago the one you used had split.
- Your periods are regular and your last period was around 2 weeks ago. Your cycle is 28 days and you have a 6 day period. You have had no other episodes of unprotected sex prior to this one.
- You have not been happy with your husband for the past 2 years since your youngest child was born. He works long hours as an electrician so you feel left to do all the housework and childcare yourself. The only time you get to yourself is if you say you are going for a run as he wants you to keep active and slim.
- You would like to be tested for STIs if possible but are adamant you are not going to the family planning clinic as someone may see you. You will agree to urine and blood tests at the surgery.

- If a prescription is offered, you want to know what the side-effects may be and how effective it is. You decline any offer of a coil as you don't have time to attend for yet another appointment.
- You have no other medical problems. You have never suffered with migraines or blood clots and take no other medications.
- If the doctor discusses alternative contraception for longer term use you are interested in the implant as you feel you could hide this from your husband.
- If at any time the doctor makes a comment you feel is judgmental you will simply hang up. If they suggest you speak to your husband about your feelings or provide information about relationship counselling you are interested. You do want your marriage to work and this episode has been very stressful.

Results for the doctor

Examination provided from patient's home readings:
- BP 118/75, HR 60, BMI 22

Case B2.12 Marking scheme for the observer

The Faculty of Sexual and Reproductive Healthcare has published guidance on emergency contraception which can be read in conjunction with this case:
www.fsrh.org/Public/Public/Standards-and-Guidance/Emergency-Contraception.aspx?hkey=
8d4257db-3196-4175-8014-faa6638c42d6

Data gathering and diagnosis

☐	☐	☐	• Identifies the reason for the call as request for emergency contraception
☐	☐	☐	• Takes a history including the timing of the UPSI and the patient's usual menstrual cycle
☐	☐	☐	• Enquires about current contraception, methods used and patient's wishes moving forward
☐	☐	☐	• Asks about general health, other medical problems / medications to ensure contraception can be prescribed safely

Clinical management and medical complexity

☐	☐	☐	• Discusses methods of emergency contraception available and levels of effectiveness (copper IUD (most effective) or oral emergency contraception – levonorgestrel or ulipristal acetate (may not be effective if taken after ovulation))
☐	☐	☐	• Recognises patient's wish to have a pill rather than an IUD and can discuss both methods available. Advises the patient to call again if she vomits within 3 hours of taking the pill (2 hours if Levonelle is prescribed) to have a further dose or to reconsider having an IUD fitted
☐	☐	☐	• Advises her next period may be different: it may be earlier, later or more painful. If her period is over a week late advise she perform a pregnancy test. Advise the patient that rates of ectopic pregnancy may be higher after emergency contraception is used, so if she has any symptoms of bleeding or abdominal pain to present immediately
☐	☐	☐	• Advises the patient regarding options for longer term contraception and offers verbal and written information on subdermal implants
☐	☐	☐	• Offers testing at the surgery for STIs

Relating to others

☐	☐	☐	• Recognises the patient's reluctance to divulge details but is able to gently encourage her to open up about her situation
☐	☐	☐	• Discusses her request in a non-judgmental manner
☐	☐	☐	• Describes methods of contraception in an easy to understand way
☐	☐	☐	• Considers offering advice on improving her relationship with her husband and discusses support available locally

Case B3.1 Information for the doctor

In this case you are a doctor in surgery doing telephone consultations.	
Name:	Joseph Mattison
Age:	42
Past medical history:	nil
Current medication:	nil
Last consultation:	
Health check:	BP 126/88; BMI 27
Blood results:	Total cholesterol 8.1 mmol/L HDL cholesterol 2.8 mmol/L LDL cholesterol 5.3 mmol/L Triglycerides 2.0 mmol/L

Notes

Case B3.1 Information for the patient

You are Joseph Mattison, a 42-year old man, calling to discuss your cholesterol results as requested.

ICE

- You are expecting the doctor to tell you that your cholesterol was high and that you need to lose weight.
- You are concerned about your cholesterol results because your mum died of a heart attack at 45; you have been planning for a while to get your cholesterol and blood pressure checked because you remember she had problems with both of these.

Background

- You live with your wife and two children (aged 12 and 9).
- You stopped smoking 5 years ago after being a 20 a day smoker for 10 years.
- You drink around 2 bottles of wine a week.
- Playing golf at the weekends is your only form of exercise. Your diet is fairly good although you have takeaway meals a couple of times a week and indulge in puddings at the weekend.

Information divulged freely

- You decided to get your cholesterol checked because you are getting older and one of your friends recently had a heart attack. You know you're a bit overweight and you don't exercise enough so you expect the result to be high.
- Your mum died of a heart attack at 45 after being on tablets for her blood pressure and cholesterol for a few years.

Information only divulged if specifically asked

- You are very concerned to hear your cholesterol is so high. Even more so if the doctor mentions "genetics" as you have two children – should they be tested and how likely are they to have this?
- Your mum had a brother who you think maybe suffers from angina but you don't have much contact with him. You have no other family history of cardiac disease.
- You are otherwise well with no symptoms at all.
- You will agree to have a fasting test if the doctor suggests this. You also agree to any further blood testing the doctor suggests but would appreciate knowing why the tests are being done.
- You are keen to hear about any suggestions the doctor has for reducing your cholesterol. You agree to reduce your alcohol intake, aim to exercise more and eat better. You ask if you do all these things, can you avoid medication?
- You are interested to hear more about the medication you may be prescribed. You know from a colleague that statins give you lots of muscle aches and he had to stop taking his. You also saw on the news about them causing diabetes. If the doctor explains the need for medication and explains adequately about the side-effects, you accept a prescription. You are also happy to be referred to the lipid clinic for a prescription instead of being given one today.
- You have no signs of tendon xanthomas, corneal arcus or xanthelasma.

Case B3.1 Marking scheme for the observer

The NICE guidelines can be read in conjunction with this case:
https://cks.nice.org.uk/hypercholesterolaemia-familial

Data gathering and diagnosis

☐	☐	☐	• Takes a history, enquiring about any cardiovascular symptoms / risk factors and about the patient's diet and lifestyle
☐	☐	☐	• Enquires about family history of heart disease / sudden death and specifically asks about MI in a 1st degree relative (parents / siblings) <60 or a 2nd degree relative (grandparents / aunts / nieces) <50
☐	☐	☐	• Identifies that the blood results are abnormal and require action
☐	☐	☐	• Identifies that the patient has a raised BMI
☐	☐	☐	• Identifies the patient's concerns about his children due to the genetic nature of this condition
☐	☐	☐	• Asks about symptoms of thyroid disease and diabetes to rule out secondary causes of hypercholesterolaemia

Clinical management and medical complexity

☐	☐	☐	• Advises the patient to have a fasting blood test and suggests that TSH, U&Es, HbA1c and LFTs are also carried out to rule out secondary causes of high cholesterol and check liver function before starting a statin. A baseline ECG can also be requested
☐	☐	☐	• Suspects familial hypercholesterolaemia and uses a clinical tool advised by NICE such as the Simon Broome or the Dutch Lipid Clinic Network Criteria to assist in making this diagnosis (https://thefhfoundation.org/diagnostic-criteria-for-familia-hypercholesterolemia); avoids using a CV risk calculator such as QRISK2 which underestimates CV risk
☐	☐	☐	• Suggests a referral to a lipid clinic for genetic testing and management and says that the clinic can discuss and advise on testing of his children
☐	☐	☐	• Discusses treatment and informs the patient that this is lifelong. Offers a prescription for atorvastatin 20 mg daily or advises this is the likely outcome of the clinic. Discusses common side-effects such as muscle aches
☐	☐	☐	• Addresses his concerns about diabetes and describes how the use of statin can increase the risk of developing high sugar levels and type 2 diabetes; advises annual HbA1c test will be part of his annual review and if this is raised, this will be discussed with him
☐	☐	☐	• Discusses reducing his modifiable risk factors and addresses alcohol intake and weight loss to improve his cholesterol and reduce his risk of heart disease and diabetes

Relating to others			
☐	☐	☐	• Creates good rapport with patient
☐	☐	☐	• Can offer a jargon-free explanation about the genetics of familial hypercholesterolaemia (an autosomal dominant condition, therefore his children have a 50% chance of inheriting the condition)
☐	☐	☐	• Treats this case as breaking bad news with a warning shot and "chunks and checks" information given
☐	☐	☐	• Offers an appointment to discuss the condition further with himself and his family if he wishes to do so

Case B3.2 Information for the doctor

In this case you are a doctor in surgery calling a patient with the results of recent investigations.

Name:	Walter White
Age:	66
Past medical history:	Hypertension Current medication: Ramipril 10 mg od Bisoprolol 1.25 mg od
Last consultation:	2 weeks ago: Presented with SOB for past 2/12, mainly on walking up one flight of stairs, no cough, no chest pain or palpitations, ex smoker (stopped 10 years ago) OE: HS normal, chest few bibasal creps, pitting ankle oedema to midshin, SpO$_2$ 97%, bloods inc BNP, CXR then review with results. FBC: Normal U&Es, LFTs, CRP: normal NT-pro-BNP: **2100** ng/L (normal <400 ng/L) CXR: signs consistent with pulmonary oedema

Notes

Case B3.2 Information for the patient

You are Walter White, a 66-year old man. You have called today to discuss your results.

ICE

- You are very worried about lung cancer as you used to smoke. One of your good friends died of lung cancer last year.
- You are hoping the doctor gives you good news about your X-ray. You are not really sure why the blood tests were done but hope these do not show anything too serious.

Background

- You live with your wife and you are a retired teacher. You stopped smoking 10 years ago after smoking 10 a day for 30 years. You drink about 1–2 bottles of wine a week. You are reasonably active – you walk in the local area a lot and play golf once a week.

Information divulged freely

- You came to the doctors a few weeks ago to discuss your feeling of being out of breath. You first noticed it climbing the flights of stairs in your house a few months ago but now it is starting to be a problem on the golf course and you are struggling to keep up with your friends.
- You have not noticed a cough and have not had any chest pain. You had noticed your legs were a bit swollen but had not thought much of it until the other doctor asked last week.
- You sleep with 3 pillows at night and admit you have woken up feeling short of breath in the past month.

Results for the doctor

Your nephew is a physician associate and examined you this morning – he wrote down his findings for you to share with the GP.

- SpO_2 97%, PR 80, regular, RR 20
- HS normal
- BP 130/80
- Chest – coarse creps both lung bases
- Pitting oedema both legs to midshin

Case B3.2 Marking scheme for the observer

https://patient.info/doctor/heart-failure-diagnosis-and-investigation
https://patient.info/doctor/heart-failure-management
https://cks.nice.org.uk/topics/heart-failure-chronic/management/

Data gathering and diagnosis

☐	☐	☐	• Takes an appropriate history of the patient's shortness of breath and identifies symptoms of heart failure (exertional dyspnoea, orthopnoea, paroxysmal nocturnal dyspnoea plus peripheral oedema)
☐	☐	☐	• Identifies the patient's concerns about lung cancer and addresses these while making a diagnosis of heart failure
☐	☐	☐	• Listens to the examination findings reported by the patient's nephew and recognises their relevance to the diagnosis

Clinical management and medical complexity

☐	☐	☐	• Considers the need for additional investigations (ECG / other bloods / urinalysis / spirometry)
☐	☐	☐	• Talks through the investigations and explains the diagnosis of heart failure to the patient and how it is managed
☐	☐	☐	• Urgent cardiology referral (ideally within 2 weeks) due to BNP level
☐	☐	☐	• Provides safety-netting by informing the patient which symptoms warrant seeking more urgent medical review
☐	☐	☐	• Reviews Walter's current medication – starts a loop diuretic for symptom control; considers statins/antiplatelet therapy and a cardiovascular risk assessment

Relating to others

☐	☐	☐	• Establishes good rapport with the patient
☐	☐	☐	• Gives clear explanation of diagnosis and further management
☐	☐	☐	• Avoids use of jargon
☐	☐	☐	• Allows time for the patient to ask questions

Case B3.3   Information for the doctor

In this case you are a doctor in surgery carrying out telephone consultations.	
Name:	Gareth Johnson
Age:	48
Past medical history:	Gout Hypercholesterolaemia
Social history:	Smoker 15/day
Current medication:	Atorvastatin 10 mg on

Notes

Case B3.3 Information for the patient

You are Gareth Johnson, a 48-year old man with ongoing symptoms of indigestion. Last night you couldn't sleep because of horrible retching and your wife asked you to finally speak to a doctor.

ICE

- Your wife Jane asked you to call because you are complaining of daily indigestion and constant retching. She feels 'you need sorting'. You are not worried, but would like to try some medication because Gaviscon is not working any more. Your friend Andrew recommended omeprazole – he's been on it for years and you would like to try it.

Background

- You have worked as a lorry driver for over 20 years and love your job.
- You live with your wife and two children. Your wife is an excellent cook.
- Last year your cholesterol was high so you are taking some medication for it at night.

Information divulged freely

- You have had indigestion for many years and use Gaviscon for it. Usually it works but lately you've noticed it's not making any difference.
- Every morning you wake up with a horrible taste in your mouth. It makes you feel sick at times.
- You have a large appetite and you enjoy spicy meals.
- You know you should eat healthier but you just can't stand tasteless salads.

Information only divulged if specifically asked

- You smoke 15 cigarettes a day and have a few cans of beer every night.
- You have gained 6 kg over the past 8 months.
- You have 2–3 cups of coffee every day.
- Your bowels are regular.
- You have occasional burning pain in your upper tummy, which usually lasts a few minutes and gets better if you eat something.
- You have no dysphagia.
- If the doctor offers medication to try (omeprazole or lansoprazole) you'd be delighted because that's what you were you hoping for anyway.
- If the doctor suggests your long-standing symptoms might be caused by bacteria (*Helicobacter pylori*) you'd want to know more about it.
- If the doctor comments on your lifestyle and smoking you'd ignore them, because you know best what's good for you. If the doctor remains understanding and calm and clearly explains in a non-judgmental manner why your current lifestyle might be responsible for the worsening of your symptoms, you'd listen and be more open to suggestions.
- If the doctor remains positive and supportive and offers further resources to improve your diet you'd be interested, but will have a chat about it with your wife first.

Case B3.3 Marking scheme for the observer

patient.info/doctor/gastro-oesophageal-reflux-disease
patient.info/doctor/helicobacter-pylori-pro
www.nice.org.uk/guidance/cg184

Data gathering and diagnosis

☐	☐	☐	• Explores ICE
☐	☐	☐	• Covers red flags (dysphagia, haematemesis / melaena, vomiting, weight loss)
☐	☐	☐	• Takes appropriate history

Clinical management and medical complexity

☐	☐	☐	• Is able to identify triggers for dyspepsia (weight gain, alcohol intake, smoking, coffee, spicy food)
☐	☐	☐	• Considers possible diagnosis of duodenal / peptic ulcer and considers testing for *Helicobacter pylori*
☐	☐	☐	• Follows current guidelines and considers 1 month trial of PPIs
☐	☐	☐	• Is able to address lifestyle and diet – offers smoking cessation advice, reducing alcohol, weight reduction and avoiding fatty foods – considers involving dietitian or weight management service, depending on local availability
☐	☐	☐	• Safety-netting and offers follow-up

Relating to others

☐	☐	☐	• Establishes good rapport and remains supportive and non-judgmental
☐	☐	☐	• Encourages patient's contribution in decision making and management plan
☐	☐	☐	• Ensures patient's understanding

Case B3.4 Information for the doctor

In this case you are a doctor in surgery carrying out video consultations.	
Name:	Jonathan Butler
Age:	42
Social and family history:	married, 2 children
Past medical history:	13 years ago ACL reconstruction 2 months ago BP: 134/80 BMI: 30 Smokes: 10 cigarettes / day Alcohol: 20 units / week
Current medication:	nil

Notes

Case B3.4 Information for the patient

You are Jonathan Butler, a 42-year old bank manager who is talking to the GP today to request surgery to cure your snoring.

ICE

- You don't really want to have surgery – it is your wife who is keen. You do want the problem to improve and hope the doctor can offer some alternative treatment options.

Background

- Your wife, Vicky, has complained about your snoring for many years but she usually manages to get some sleep by wearing earplugs.
- Over the last fortnight you have had to attend a few social events at work which involved consuming more alcohol than usual, and Vicky complained your snoring was much worse. Despite wearing earplugs, she was unable to get to sleep, which caused some arguments this week.
- Vicky has a friend at work who underwent surgery for snoring and it was Vicky that actually made the appointment for you to discuss this.

Information divulged freely

- Your snoring never wakes you up nor disturbs your sleep.
- Your wife has never noticed you choking or heard you stop breathing during the night.
- You wake up feeling refreshed and have no problems concentrating at work and don't ever fall asleep during the day.
- You have never had any nasal injuries or problems with nasal congestion.
- You often entertain clients at work and regularly have a couple of pints of beer with colleagues after work, then share wine with your wife at the weekends.
- You smoke 10 cigarettes a day and have done so since your 20s.
- You stopped playing football after injuring your knee 13 years ago and have put on weight since then.
- Your mood is good and you are generally happy at work and with family life.

Information only divulged if specifically asked

- You will admit you are not keen on the idea of surgery.
- You are willing to address any lifestyle issues (including cutting down on smoking and drinking) if the doctor suggests it will help the problem.

Results for the doctor

Remote examination attempted whilst being aware of the limitations.
- BMI 30
- Nose – no polyps, no septal deviation, tonsils shrunken, normal oropharynx / mandible / neck examination. Complete visualisation of uvula and soft palate possible

Case B3.4 Marking scheme for the observer

patient.info/doctor/snoring-pro
https://cks.nice.org.uk/topics/obstructive-sleep-apnoea-syndrome/

Data gathering and diagnosis

☐	☐	☐	• Gathers information systematically and efficiently about reason for attending, including ICE
☐	☐	☐	• Takes an appropriate snoring history, enquires about symptoms of OSA and considers using the Epworth Score (www.asthmaandlung.org.uk/conditions/obstructive-sleep-apnoea-osa/epworth-sleepiness-scale)
☐	☐	☐	• Obtains an alcohol and smoking history
☐	☐	☐	• Attempts a remote examination (pointing out its limitations) and arranges an in-person follow-up as needed: BMI; brief ENT exam to observe any nasal blockage, tongue / tonsillar size

Clinical management and medical complexity

☐	☐	☐	• Discusses lifestyle measures which will improve his symptoms: smoking cessation, reducing alcohol intake, weight reduction and exercise
☐	☐	☐	• Offers patient options to stop snoring. Practical advice would include avoiding alcohol before bed and sleeping on the side. Discusses mandibular advancement devices / OTC treatments if appropriate
☐	☐	☐	• Makes patient aware of relative risks of surgery and emphasises lifestyle advice as first-line treatment
☐	☐	☐	• Offers links to support groups (e.g. https://britishsnoring.co.uk) and arranges a follow-up appointment

Relating to others

☐	☐	☐	• Correctly establishes that the patient would rather avoid surgery
☐	☐	☐	• Explores the impact of the problem on the patient's life and relationship with his wife
☐	☐	☐	• Provides explanations that the patient can understand

Case B3.5   Information for the doctor

You are a locum GP in a busy afternoon surgery undertaking telephone consultations.	
Name:	Eileen Bulmer
Age:	78
Past medical history:	Last consultation: Head and neck examination normal Otoscopy – normal, canal clear of wax Hearing grossly normal on whisper testing. Tuning fork tests – normal Ongoing tinnitus – no red flags Hypertension
Current medication:	Amlodipine 5 mg od, simvastatin 20 mg on

Notes

Case B3.5 Information for the patient

You are Eileen Bulmer, a 78-year old retired shopkeeper.

ICE

- You have had tinnitus for years and were told 'nothing can be done' but it has been getting worse over the past few months and starting to prevent you from sleeping. You are certain there must be a serious problem. You have been having panic attacks and avoiding going out with your friends. You aren't sure what the doctor can do, but you want it to stop.

Background

- You are a 78-year old widow and have suffered with mild tinnitus for many years, but it was just a minor nuisance until now. When it first started you saw Dr Brown, the senior partner at the surgery, and you know that there's nothing that can be done for tinnitus.
- Your husband Tony died 5 years ago and you still miss him terribly. You have kept busy with the church events since he passed, but lately you have been avoiding social events and staying in.
- You have a daughter who lives in Northern Ireland and you talk on the phone every couple of weeks, but have never been particularly close. Your friends from bingo are your biggest support and they have been worried about you as you have stopped joining them. They have encouraged you to contact the surgery today.

Information divulged freely

- You don't feel like your hearing has changed at all, but you wonder if you need a hearing test, because the tinnitus can be noisy at times.
- You are sorry to be wasting the doctor's time for a problem you already know can't be helped, but your friend Betty insisted you make an appointment.

Information only divulged if specifically asked

- You have never suffered with dizziness and the buzzing is in both ears.
- You are not prone to ear infections or wax build-up.
- You don't suffer with headaches or any other symptoms.
- If asked about medications you take, you say you have been taking a baby aspirin every night for the last 2–3 months on the advice of your friend Betty who told you it would protect your heart.
- You admit you have not been yourself recently. You have been feeling more lonely at home in the evenings, but you feel very anxious going out to bingo, as it is difficult to hear the numbers being called over the buzzing sound.
- The more anxious you feel, the worse the buzzing gets. It is getting you down, but you have never had any thoughts about suicide and if medications for depression are mentioned, you are not keen.

Case B3.5 Marking scheme for the observer

patient.info/doctor/tinnitus-pro
www.nice.org.uk/guidance/ng155

Data gathering and diagnosis

☐	☐	☐	• Takes a systematic history and asks relevant questions to determine if further investigation is needed (i.e. unilateral tinnitus; acoustic neuroma; vertigo / deafness; Ménière's)
☐	☐	☐	• Considers possible underlying causes such as wax, drugs, head injury and medications
☐	☐	☐	• Discovers the effects of the problem on the patient's mood
☐	☐	☐	• Appreciates the need for an up-to-date examination in person

Clinical management and medical complexity

☐	☐	☐	• Recognises the effect of the problem on the patient's wellbeing and makes efforts to address this
☐	☐	☐	• Considers referral for CBT and / or to ENT to consider a hearing test / hearing aid and to see a hearing therapist
☐	☐	☐	• Discusses reasoning for aspirin use and recognises salicylates as a possible cause of tinnitus
☐	☐	☐	• Demonstrates a positive attitude towards the condition, emphasising that although there may not be a 'cure' there are various strategies that can be used to minimise symptoms
☐	☐	☐	• Shows awareness of resources available to help patients such as support groups, psychological therapies, masking devices

Relating to others

☐	☐	☐	• Elicits psychological and social information to put the problem in context
☐	☐	☐	• Responds to the patient's expectations and feelings
☐	☐	☐	• Includes the patient in formulating a management plan
☐	☐	☐	• Is sensitive to the effects of the problem on the patient's life

Case B3.6 Information for the doctor

In this case you are a doctor in surgery calling a patient in response to her online consult.	
Name:	Caroline Miller
Age:	31
Past medical history:	Migraine
Online consult:	"I've got a rash on my hands and I'm worried about scabies"
Current medication:	Takes OTC paracetamol and ibuprofen prn

Notes

Case B3.6 Information for the patient

You are Caroline Miller, a 31-year old healthcare assistant. You work in a care home. You noticed an itchy rash on both hands few days ago and it's getting worse.

ICE

- You are concerned you have scabies. Your best friend Amy works as a healthcare assistant on a paediatric ward and saw exactly the same rash in a patient with scabies. You expect the doctor to prescribe you a treatment for scabies.

Background

- You are a happily married 31-year old woman. You have two children – they are healthy.
- Your husband Dave works as a builder and thought it might be some kind of allergy but you have never been allergic to anything.
- It started with small pimples on both hands 2 days ago and it's driving you crazy with itch. It kept you awake all night.
- Yesterday you showed it to your friend Amy who is convinced it must be scabies. You trust Amy, she works with children and knows exactly what she is talking about.

Information divulged freely

- You are normally fit and well and only suffer from occasional migraines once a year or so.
- You are not allergic to anything.
- You used some Fucidin cream from work but it didn't make any difference.

Information only divulged if specifically asked

- Your family members have no symptoms.
- You dyed your hair two weeks ago. You've been using the same dye for many years.
- Your work ordered new gloves a few weeks ago and you had to use them 3 days ago for the first time. You used to have thick blue gloves, which were better and didn't make any white marks on your hands.
- You are not impressed with your new gloves, they are too thin. Your boss commented they are cheaper though.
- If the doctor picks up on the fact that it might be an allergy to latex in the new gloves you would be very unsure and comment that you don't have any allergies.
- If the doctor clearly explains the possibility of contact dermatitis / allergy and describes why scabies is less likely in your instance (distribution, family members are symptom-free) you would change your opinion and become more open to the doctor's suggestions.
- If the doctor suggests avoiding using the new gloves and suggests appropriate treatment and follow-up, you would appreciate their help and will agree to come back if symptoms persist.

Results for the doctor

Please show the doctor this photograph when requested.

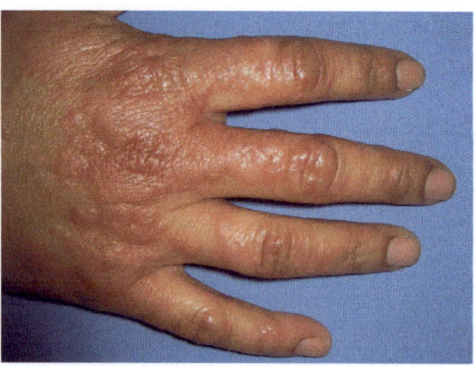

Reproduced from *Dermatology Made Easy 2e* (© Scion Publishing Ltd).

Case B3.6 Marking scheme for the observer

patient.info/doctor/contact-and-occupational-dermatitis
https://cks.nice.org.uk/dermatitis-contact

Data gathering and diagnosis

☐	☐	☐	• Identifies patient's agenda
☐	☐	☐	• Gathers adequate information on symptoms to exclude scabies (asks about symptoms in any contacts / distribution and attributes of the rash) and asks the patient to send a photo
☐	☐	☐	• Identifies possible triggers (likely latex allergy in this case)

Clinical management and medical complexity

☐	☐	☐	• Considers likely diagnosis of contact dermatitis rather than scabies
☐	☐	☐	• Discusses appropriate treatment (emollients, topical steroids, avoid triggers); if unsure – deals with uncertainty and makes a plan to review in person
☐	☐	☐	• Offers support and suggests involving occupational health department at work
☐	☐	☐	• Watch and wait approach is reasonable. Offers follow-up and if symptoms persist with suggested treatment, dermatology referral for patch testing may be appropriate

Relating to others

☐	☐	☐	• Explores the patient's concerns about scabies and is able to offer reassurance and formulate a management plan that is acceptable to both patient and doctor
☐	☐	☐	• Communicates effectively to the patient
☐	☐	☐	• Avoids jargon and has a good rapport and a positive attitude towards helping the patient

Case B3.7   Information for the doctor

In this case you are a doctor in surgery undertaking telephone consultations.	
Name:	Emily Ferguson
Age:	22
Past medical history:	Nil
Current medication:	Nil

Notes

Case B3.7   Information for the patient

You are Emily Ferguson, a 22-year old student. You are very distressed about losing your hair over the past 6 months. Two nights ago your partner noticed a clump of hair on the pillow and it was very embarrassing. You have developed a bald patch behind your right ear, which is getting bigger and you are trying to hide it as much as you can.

ICE

- You know you have alopecia. You searched about it online and know enough about your condition. You have also joined an alopecia society. You expect to be referred to a dermatologist for steroid injections because it might help with the regrowth of your hair.

Background

- You are a biochemistry student.
- You are in a new relationship with Richard. He has no idea about your problem and you are embarrassed to talk about it, even after he saw the hair on your pillow.
- You are well otherwise.
- You have 2 older brothers and they are both healthy.
- Your mum has thyroid problems.

Information divulged freely

- You noticed you started losing your hair approximately 6 months ago. Initially it was just a small amount but it's getting worse.
- You developed a round bald patch behind your ear and you are very distressed your partner might notice it.
- You have already tried topical steroid cream but you realised it has to be an injection instead, which is available in dermatology clinics and you believe it is your only hope.

Information only divulged if specifically asked

- You have been feeling really low lately. You don't feel like going out and you are losing concentration easily.
- You are worried that the alopecia will get worse and you will end up being bald for the rest of your life.
- You don't have any suicidal ideas but you do wonder sometimes what your purpose in life is.
- You are very open to the doctor's suggestions about 'chatting therapy'. You are not depressed, just sad it happened to you.
- You would refuse antidepressants if they were offered.
- You have no history of mental health problems or deliberate self-harm.
- If the doctor is not sure about your condition you would be very nice and understanding and give them a chance to deal with uncertainty.
- If the doctor is judgmental and not convinced that steroid injections will work and offers a watchful waiting approach, you would become very argumentative and decide to see another GP.
- If the doctor is sensitive, offers support and understanding and suggests you should perhaps involve your partner and family, you would strongly consider it.

- You would accept more information on alopecia, possible causes and prognosis if the doctor were keen to discuss it with you.
- At the end of this consultation you expect to be referred to dermatology. You will not accept any other alternatives.

Case B3.7 Marking scheme for the observer

patient.info/doctor/alopecia
https://cks.nice.org.uk/alopecia-areata

Data gathering and diagnosis

☐	☐	☐	• Elicits ICE – takes a history of the problem and arranges an in-person examination to ensure no other skin problems are present
☐	☐	☐	• Identifies what has she already tried for alopecia
☐	☐	☐	• Explores relevant family history
☐	☐	☐	• Identifies patient's understanding of alopecia
☐	☐	☐	• Explores patient's mental state and assesses for possible depression

Clinical management and medical complexity

☐	☐	☐	• Is able to explain diagnosis of alopecia and is aware of autoimmune pattern of this condition
☐	☐	☐	• Discusses appropriate treatment; if unsure, deals with uncertainty and makes a plan to find out more
☐	☐	☐	• Discusses referral to secondary care. Is realistic about treatment options and comes to an agreement with the patient regarding ongoing management
☐	☐	☐	• Arranges review, perhaps arranges blood tests to exclude thyroid disease
☐	☐	☐	• Offers counselling therapy

Relating to others

☐	☐	☐	• Is empathetic to patient's concerns
☐	☐	☐	• Communicates effectively to the patient
☐	☐	☐	• Avoids medical jargon
☐	☐	☐	• Explores patient's feeling and expectations
☐	☐	☐	• Maintains rapport

Case B4.1 Information for the doctor

In this case you have been asked to call back Mrs Stanton, the neighbour of your patient Maria Lopez.

In this case you are a doctor in surgery.	
Name:	Maria Lopez
Age:	88
Past medical history:	COPD, hypertension, glaucoma (severe visual impairment), depression
Current medication:	Salbutamol, tiotropium HandiHaler, Serevent Accuhaler, latanoprost eye drops on, brimonidine eye drops bd, hypromellose eye drops prn, amlodipine 10 mg od, simvastatin 40 mg on, omeprazole 20 mg od, co-codamol 30/500 prn, Movicol sachets prn, sertraline 50 mg od
Recent consultation:	Seen by Dr Joseph 2 weeks ago who documented: Discharged from hospital yesterday – reviewed as requested by A&E discharge summary. Neighbour called ambulance over the weekend as patient having increasing SOB. Mild exacerbation of COPD. Started on antibiotics / steroids and discharged home with friend; GP follow-up advised. Hospital staff note patient not using inhalers regularly. Seen at home – cough persists but breathing improved and neighbour says better since starting antibiotics. Long-standing problems with poor vision – last seen by ophthalmology 2 years ago – declines further referral. Says 'they can do nothing for me'. Examination: RR 18 SpO$_2$ 96% on air afebrile mild wheeze throughout chest, good air entry Vision: can finger count both eyes Capacity assessment: patient able to retain / understand / communicate – has capacity Plan: Spacer device issued and instructed on how to use inhalers properly. Discussed rescue antibiotics to prevent future admissions. Discussed arranging for help at home but declines, says has neighbour to help and doesn't want strangers involved. Review prn (Note: patient has given verbal consent for Mrs Stanton to collect medication and speak to the surgery on her behalf)

Case B4.1   Information for the patient

You are Frances Stanton, a concerned friend, speaking to the doctor about your neighbour Maria Lopez, an 88-year old lady who you visit every day.

ICE

- You think Maria needs some home help but you know she is not keen on the idea. You are calling the doctor for some advice.

Background

- You have lived next door to Maria since you moved to the area 3 years ago, but you have only started helping her out over the last 6 months.
- You're quite happy to help out, but you do have your own problems at the minute. Your husband's health is up and down and you are due to go for a knee replacement next month, so you really won't be able to pop in to see Maria until you have fully recovered from that.

Information divulged freely

- You became friendly with Maria over your shared love of gardening, and although she could never see all that well, you used to see her in the garden every day. You noticed she stopped going outside about a year ago, so you would go round for a cup of tea most mornings. She has no other family, she never married and all her other relatives live in Spain.
- You now go round every morning and make sure she has had some breakfast. You do her shopping for her and try to help her with her medicines, but you are not really sure you are giving her them properly because she has so many.
- You know she has a few medical problems, but it's her chest you have been worried about lately. You were there when the other doctor gave her a new device to use to make taking her inhalers easier, but with her poor vision, you think it has made things more complicated for her. You didn't like the other doctor – he told you off for calling an ambulance for Maria, and said she could have been treated by the GP at home, but you didn't know what to do for the best.
- Maria's vision has been poor for years, but she refused to see anyone. It does make it difficult for her seeing her medications properly, and she is looking a little bit more dishevelled these days.
- She mobilises around the house without any problems, but she has no confidence leaving the house any more.

Information only divulged if specifically asked

- You are struggling with the responsibility of being there for Maria, and you feel guilty calling the surgery, but you know you are not going to be around when you go in for your knee replacement. You're also looking after your husband who had a heart attack recently. You are not registered at this practice, but would agree to go and see your own doctor to talk about support available if asked.
- You know Maria is quite stubborn and has refused offers of help before; however, you think if you suggest it when the doctor is there, even as a short-term measure while you have your operation, then you think she might agree, and you would really like a home visit from the doctor to talk to Maria about this. You asked the other doctor about this but he said that Maria had refused so there was nothing he could do – you want to ask the doctor about this.

- You would love Maria to have some help with medications and if a dosette box is suggested, you have never heard of this and would love to hear more.
- You have never been in a situation like this before and are not really sure how 'getting help' works so you are interested to hear about any options available.
- If the doctor refuses to talk to you because you are not the patient, then you will get very angry and feel that no-one cares about Maria. If the doctor explains that due to confidentiality there are certain things they are unable to discuss, but makes alternative arrangements to discuss them with Maria present, you are quite happy, although it will need to be a home visit because Maria will refuse to come to the surgery.

Case B4.1 Marking scheme for the observer

patient.info/doctor/community-care
patient.info/doctor/mental-capacity-act
http://patient.info/doctor/telephone-consultations

Data gathering and diagnosis

☐	☐	☐	• Establishes the identity of the caller and her relationship to the patient. Is aware of issues of confidentiality when discussing the patient and takes care not to divulge any clinical information
☐	☐	☐	• Gathers information regarding Maria's situation and difficulties and also appreciates the problems Mrs Stanton is facing
☐	☐	☐	• Establishes the social situation of the patient and what, if anything, has been tried before to help the patient

Clinical management and medical complexity

☐	☐	☐	• Recognises multiple medical and social problems and makes a plan to visit the patient to discuss further
☐	☐	☐	• If asked, mentions possible help available such as dosette box for medication, a review / rationalisation of medications and inhalers, involvement of social services to assess for further help such as carers / pendant alarms/ keysafe
☐	☐	☐	• If asked, provides an explanation about capacity and what this means, and why the previous doctor did not organise any help
☐	☐	☐	• Appreciates an element of carer strain and attempts to address this with offers of respite care, discussion of the support available for carers

Relating to others

☐	☐	☐	• Has an awareness of patient confidentiality and thinks about what information is divulged. Can still talk generically about the sort of options and help available for the patient without breaching confidentiality over the telephone
☐	☐	☐	• Explores the impact of these problems on both Maria and Mrs Stanton
☐	☐	☐	• Has a positive attitude to Mrs Stanton's concerns and works towards a shared management plan, while being aware that there is a need to involve Maria in the plan ultimately

Case B4.2 Information for the doctor

In this case you are a doctor in an afternoon clinic taking video consultations.	
Name:	Shona Riley
Age:	73
Past medical history:	Osteoporosis
Current medication:	Alendronic acid 70 mg weekly, Accrete D3 1 tablet bd
Results:	DEXA scan (6 months ago) BMD T-score: -2.8 osteoporosis Normal renal function, bone profile, TFTs, FBC and inflammatory markers

Notes

Case B4.2 Information for the patient

You are Shona Riley, a 73-year old retired dentist who has called the doctor today to discuss a change of medication.

ICE

- You stopped taking the bisphosphonate medication a few months ago because it was upsetting your stomach and you would like to know what the alternative options are. You also think you should have another DEXA scan because you feel your osteoporosis may have got worse since stopping the medication.

Background

- You are a retired dentist and live with your husband Leonard.
- You are otherwise quite well, but have suffered with indigestion quite a lot in the past.

Information divulged freely

- You were started on alendronic acid about 6 months ago after someone in the practice organised a DEXA scan for you.
- You remember being told that your 'risk score' had been assessed as high so a scan was advised, and this picked up that you had osteoporosis.
- You took the medicine as advised, but stopped a few months ago because it was upsetting your stomach. You have not vomited blood or had black stools, but you suffered with severe indigestion after taking the medicine so decided to stop.
- You want another scan to see if your bones have got worse.
- You smoke 5 cigarettes a day and drink 1 or 2 glasses of wine most nights.
- You have always been thin, and you do try to walk every day for exercise.

Information only divulged if specifically asked

- You remember when you were working as a dentist that you saw a patient with osteonecrosis of the jaw due to bisphosphonates and you are really not keen on being on this medication. You don't want to try an alternative bisphosphonate.
- You went through the menopause in your early 50s and you didn't use any HRT.
- You have been quite well throughout your life, and don't recall ever taking oral steroids for prolonged periods.
- When you were taking the alendronate you made sure you had it first thing in the morning on an empty stomach. You knew not to eat for 30 minutes, and to stay upright, and you used to use that time to clean the kitchen.
- If the doctor is unsure about other treatments for osteoporosis you are happy for them to get back to you after a discussion with colleagues. You are equally happy to be referred to secondary care for a further opinion.

Case B4.2 **Marking scheme for the observer**

https://pathways.nice.org.uk/pathways/osteoporosis
patient.info/doctor/osteoporosis-pro
patient.info/health/bisphosphonates

Data gathering and diagnosis

☐	☐	☐	• Asks about relevant risk factors for osteoporosis. Discusses risk factors covered in FRAX scoring (low BMI, smoking, diet, exercise, excessive alcohol, medication use (e.g. steroids), co-morbidity (e.g. RA, thyroid disease, early menopause) (https://frax.shef.ac.uk/FRAX/tool.aspx?country=9)
☐	☐	☐	• Checks that the patient is taking bisphosphonate correctly (take once a week on the same day, first thing in the morning before eating; swallow whole and drink a large glass of water; stand / sit upright for 30 minutes after taking) (www.patient.info/medicine/alendronic-acid-for-osteoporosis-fosamax)
☐	☐	☐	• Elicits patient's concerns and preferences

Clinical management and medical complexity

☐	☐	☐	• Negotiates with patient to avoid a further DEXA scan, and is able to provide reasons for this (results will not influence treatment, only 6 months since last scan, NICE guidance advises not to monitor treatment with DEXA scans)
☐	☐	☐	• Considers an alternative bisphosphonate. Aware of alternative treatment options such as strontium, denosumab, raloxifene and makes appropriate prescribing decisions (if unsure, negotiates a plan acceptable to the patient such as further discussion with colleagues / secondary referral)
☐	☐	☐	• Uses opportunity for health promotion relevant to osteoporosis: smoking cessation, weight-bearing exercise, reduced alcohol intake, BMI 20–25, calcium/Vit D from diet / supplements)

Relating to others

☐	☐	☐	• Explores the patient's health beliefs and concerns and addresses them appropriately
☐	☐	☐	• Works in partnership to find a shared management plan
☐	☐	☐	• Provides explanations the patient understands
☐	☐	☐	• Backs own judgment regarding repeat DEXA scanning with appropriate evidence

Case B4.3 Information for the doctor

In this case you are a doctor in surgery taking telephone consultations.	
Name:	Jagoda Williams
Age:	78
Past medical history:	Hypertension
Current medication:	Ramipril 5 mg od
Last consultation:	Hypertension review – BP 130/85 Bloods taken for routine monitoring
Results:	Hb **10.0** (12.0–15.0 g/L) MCV **78** (80–100 fL) Plt 220 (150–400 x 10⁹/L) WCC 8.0 (4.0–11.0 x 10⁹/L) Na 136 (135–145 mmol/L) K 3.8 (3.5–5.0 mmol/L) Ur 5.6 (3.0–6.5 mmol/L) Cr 99 (60–125 µmol/L) eGFR **80** (>90 ml / min) LFTs normal Ferritin **9** (14–200 mcg/L) Previous results from 1 year ago – Hb normal

Notes

Case B4.3 Information for the patient

You are Jagoda Williams, a 78-year old widow, who has called today for blood results.

ICE

- You received a call yesterday asking you to make a telephone appointment to discuss your blood results. You have worried all night as you know having high blood pressure can damage your kidneys and you are sure this is what the doctor is going to tell you. You certainly don't want to have to go on dialysis like your friend Fred.

Background

- You live alone with your dog Barney for company and apart from the high blood pressure you think you are very well for your age. You moved to the UK from Poland with your family after the war, and your sister's family still live over there, but you don't really keep in touch. Your son lives in Dubai but you don't like to worry him as he is always so busy with work. Your husband John died 10 years ago, and you do miss him, but are independent and keep busy with activities at church and the Women's Institute.

Information divulged freely

- You came for your annual blood test with the nurse last week. You have been told before that your kidneys don't work as well as they used to, and you always worry each year that they are going to get worse.
- Your friend from church, Fred, has to have dialysis three times a week and you have seen how it has taken over his life. You are adamant that you want nothing like this and want to make this clear to the doctor.
- You usually see Dr Hannington when you come to the surgery and he knows you well – he diagnosed your husband with lung cancer and treated him until he died. You're not very happy about speaking to a new doctor who doesn't know you, but you wanted to find out about these results as soon as possible.

Information only divulged if specifically asked

- If asked, you have regular bowel motions and eat three meals a day, containing plenty of fruit and veg. You would be happy to take a supplement.
- You have no heartburn, nausea and have not had any black stools or bleeding from your back passage.
- You have been very pleased to lose some weight recently. Over the last 2 months half a stone slipped off without you even trying and you have bought a new dress for the fundraising dance at church.
- You have been feeling tired recently, but you have been helping to organise this dance, and you are 78 and expect to feel more tired at this age.
- When the doctor explains your results, you have no idea what this might mean and wonder if it is related to your kidneys. You are shocked if they suggest this may be due to a cancer.
- You are happy to come in for an in-person appointment but do want to know what will happen at this appointment. You are also happy to carry out a stool test but would like to know if this is negative does that mean you don't have cancer?

- Your initial reaction is to decline further assessment – you don't like the sound of any camera tests and would rather not have them.
- If the doctor clearly explains the risk of cancer and reasoning for further investigation then you will accept this.
- You become a little tearful when cancer is mentioned, as it brings back memories of your husband.

Case B4.3 Marking scheme for the observer

https://cks.nice.org.uk/anaemia-iron-deficiency
patient.info/doctor/iron-deficiency-anaemia-pro

Data gathering and diagnosis

☐	☐	☐	• Gathers information about upper and lower GI symptoms to explain the blood results (e.g. enquires about dietary iron intake, NSAID use, obvious blood loss, family history of cancers)
☐	☐	☐	• Interprets the blood results as showing iron deficient anaemia and shows an awareness of the likely causes of this

Clinical management and medical complexity

☐	☐	☐	• Manages risk appropriately – offers in-person appointment for exam including DRE which is often required for referral. Advises FIT test and is able to advise up to 10% of patients will have a negative test but still have colorectal cancer.
☐	☐	☐	• Shows awareness of the 2-week rule criteria for lower GI malignancy and arranges appropriate investigations and examinations for this; explains the reasoning for this to the patient
☐	☐	☐	• Discusses iron replacement (ferrous sulphate 200 mg od), its common side-effects and sources of iron from the diet

Relating to others

☐	☐	☐	• Elicits patient's agenda and reassures about renal concerns while building rapport
☐	☐	☐	• Discusses the results as a 'breaking bad news' scenario – elicits patient's understanding, avoids ambiguity and is clear about concerns but gives time for questions
☐	☐	☐	• Acknowledges patient's experience of dealing with cancer with her husband and shows responsiveness to her feelings. Discusses support available and encourages her to talk to her son / friends
☐	☐	☐	• Demonstrates respect for others and equality of care for all – avoids becoming offended or defensive when the patient clearly states preferences for another doctor
☐	☐	☐	• Communicates risk to patient clearly

Further reading

Suspected cancer: recognition and referral (NICE guidelines NG12)
www.nice.org.uk/guidance/ng12/chapter/1-recommendations-organised-by-site-of-cancer

Guidelines for the management of iron-deficiency anaemia
www.bsg.org.uk/clinical-resource/guidelines-iron-deficiency-anaemia-in-adults

Rapid Referral Guidelines by Macmillan Cancer Support (July 2015)
www.macmillan.org.uk/healthcare-professionals/cancer-pathways/prevention-and-diagnosis/
    rapid-referral-guidelines

Case B4.4 Information for the doctor

In this case, a request has been made to call this patient by her daughter who lives in Scotland. She has advised that her mother has been having problems with her memory and she is worried she may have dementia. She has told her mum you will be calling today.

In this case you are a GP Registrar taking telephone calls.	
Name:	Jane Russell
Age:	81
Past medical history:	Hypertension – last check-up 1 year ago CKD 2
Current medication:	Ramipril 10 mg od – note last prescription issued 6 months ago

Notes

Case B4.4 Information for the patient

You are 81-year old Jane Russell and you live alone in your own home. You were not aware the doctor was calling and as far as you are aware you have no health problems.

ICE

- You don't feel you have any health problems.
- You have certainly heard of "Alzheimer's" because your friend Mabel died with it last year. Mabel's family put her straight into a horrible nursing home the moment they found out and you would be worried your daughter would do the same to you if you became ill.
- You are sure you can show the doctor there is nothing to be worried about and hopefully they won't call again.

Background

- You have lived in this house for 35 years. Your husband died 6 years ago of lung cancer. Since then you have been by yourself with no carers helping.
- Your daughter lives in Scotland – she hardly ever visits. You are not close although you do get on when she does visit.
- You have many friends in the area – your neighbours are very helpful (although you can't seem to remember their names at the minute) and often get your shopping for you. You go to bingo once a week and like visiting the local café for tea and a scone.

Information divulged freely

- You are adamant you have no memory problems. You remember all about your childhood and happily chat about your work at the biscuit factory and your younger years, unless interrupted by the doctor.
- If the doctor wants to ask some memory questions you will agree to them. If not properly explained, then the questions the doctor is asking frustrate you – you might not know which month or year it is but that does not mean you have dementia. If they explain the reason for the memory tests then you will go along with them, although you might not manage many answers. If they offer to come back to carry out some testing this is also OK.

Information only divulged if specifically asked

- If the doctor asks about your medication you say you don't take any medication – you are fit and healthy.
- If they mention your blood pressure you are sure you had it checked at the surgery just last week and so say that it doesn't need to be checked again.
- There was an incident a few weeks ago where you decided to go to the café but got lost – you ended up getting in a taxi to get back home, but surely most people your age will have a few moments like this?
- You will only tell the doctor about Mabel if dementia is specifically mentioned.
- You will listen to their concerns about a possible diagnosis but remain certain you do not have it. If they explain the treatments available and also discuss homecare rather than nursing homes you will be more open to testing. You will accept blood tests first, but would be prepared to have someone come to the house to talk to you more as well. You would like some help around the house as it can get quite messy. You also like the idea of going to a day centre as you like chatting to people.

Case B4.4 Marking scheme for the observer

www.nice.org.uk/guidance/ng97
patient.info/doctor/dementia-pro

Data gathering and diagnosis

☐	☐	☐	• Takes a full social history with focus on social support
☐	☐	☐	• Attempts to carry out a mental state examination or arranges to follow up at a later date to carry out formal testing of the patient's memory.
☐	☐	☐	• Establishes patient's ideas around her daughter's contact with the surgery and if she has any specific memory concerns
☐	☐	☐	• Elicits patient's fears about going into a nursing home

Clinical management and medical complexity

☐	☐	☐	• Demonstrates awareness of blood tests which should be carried out when considering a dementia diagnosis (FBC, U&Es, Ca, LFTs, glucose, TFTs, ESR, B12 and folate; consider urinalysis, ECG, CXR)
☐	☐	☐	• Carries out a medication review, considering those medications that can contribute to symptoms
☐	☐	☐	• Offers appropriate social support including referral to social services for homecare and discusses the voluntary services available in the area
☐	☐	☐	• Can advise on a referral to the memory services including information on what to expect from the referral
☐	☐	☐	• Discusses possible treatment options for Alzheimer's in a clear way with no jargon

Relating to others

☐	☐	☐	• Creates rapport with the patient
☐	☐	☐	• Is able to keep the patient focused on the questions whilst allowing her to tell her story
☐	☐	☐	• Is able to identify and address the patient's anxiety and concerns around a dementia diagnosis

Case B4.5   Information for the doctor

In this case you are a locum GP in the on-call surgery making video calls.	
Name:	Irene Bird
Age:	79
Past medical history:	Hypertension; anxiety
Current medication:	Amlodipine 5 mg od, diazepam 5 mg nocte, Calcichew 500 mg od, simvastatin 40 mg nocte

Notes

Case B4.5 Information for the patient

You are Irene Bird, a 79-year old woman, whose daughter Mandy has set up a video call for you (she has left the room because you asked to speak to the doctor alone) because you had another fall last night and hurt your wrist.

ICE

- You think it is only a wrist sprain and think Mandy is making a bit of a fuss.
- You have had a few falls recently, but feel this is due to your age and you haven't felt it was anything serious to be worried about.
- You are really consulting to keep your daughter happy, but you would be willing to try anything the doctor suggests that may be helpful to stop you falling, because it is a nuisance.

Background

- You have lived alone since your husband died 15 years ago and have always managed well. You cook, clean and look after yourself. Your daughter who lives nearby helps you with the weekly shopping.
- You do have arthritic hips but you mobilise independently and have never needed walking aids and don't want them.
- You are a retired teacher. You don't smoke or drink any alcohol.

Information divulged freely

- You had a fall last night when you got up to pass urine during the night. It was dark and you slipped on the rug in the hallway when you were walking to the bathroom. You were able to get yourself up and walk immediately.
- You fell onto your outstretched hand and had no pain in your wrist at the time but noticed it was sore this morning when you were making tea for Mandy, who had come to take you shopping.
- You have never really felt dizzy or off-balance, and only seem to fall at night time, but your walking has become slower as you have got older – your arthritis makes you less agile.

Information only divulged if specifically asked:

- You definitely just tripped and find this is always the case when you fall. You have never had any preceding chest pain, dizziness, palpitations or shortness of breath before falling. You have never had any weakness or numbness of your limbs and no tremor. You have never lost consciousness and you have never banged your head or hurt yourself more than you did last night.
- You have fallen possibly 3 or 4 times in the last 6 months. You feel that is because it is winter and it's dark and you don't always put the light on when you get up to go to the bathroom at night.
- You have worn glasses for years and Mandy took you to get your eyes tested a few months ago – there was no change to your prescription and no problems found. You don't always put your glasses on when you go to pass urine at night.
- You have taken the diazepam at night for many years after another GP diagnosed you with anxiety when your husband died. It helps you to sleep but it does make you feel off-balance if you get up to use the toilet at night. You would be willing to take less of this if the doctor asks.

- You have never had any memory problems.
- You are managing well at home by yourself and don't feel you need any extra help. Mandy is there if you need her. You would be willing to go to a falls clinic and would be happy to try any practical suggestions the GP may have to stop you falling.
- Your daughter can take you to a minor injuries unit or A&E this afternoon if the doctor feels an X-ray is needed. You are also happy to attend for an in-person appointment for an exam and blood pressure if offered.

Case B4.5 Marking scheme for the observer

NICE has a helpful guideline on the assessment of falls which can be read in conjunction with this case: https://cks.nice.org.uk/falls-risk-assessment#!scenario

Data gathering and diagnosis

☐	☐	☐	• Takes a history to determine the nature of the falls to distinguish between a mechanical fall and a collapse (circumstances, frequency, associated / preceding symptoms, eyewitness accounts covered)
☐	☐	☐	• Excludes head injury and fracture with targeted questions
☐	☐	☐	• Identifies that Irene has fallen several times and asks about her risk factors for falling (to consider: frailty, visual / cognitive impairment, conditions that affect mobility / balance (Parkinson's disease, diabetes, stroke, arthritis, incontinence, hypotension, medication, alcohol use)

Clinical management and medical complexity

☐	☐	☐	• Considers a referral to a 'falls clinic' for a multifactorial risk assessment (to include an assessment of gait and balance and chronic conditions affecting this, vision assessment, osteoporosis risk, cognitive assessment, cardiovascular assessment, continence assessment, medication review and assessment of home hazards)
☐	☐	☐	• Discusses as part of the assessment that investigations may be carried out (either at GP surgery or falls clinic depending on local setup) such as blood tests to exclude diabetes, lying / standing blood pressures and ECG
☐	☐	☐	• Can suggest some practical measures to reduce the risk of falls, such as ensuring rooms are well lit, installing non-slip mats, installing fall / pendant alarms, removing clutter, engaging in exercise to improve strength and balance and wearing well fitted shoes / slippers
☐	☐	☐	• Reviews the patient's medications and identifies the use of antihypertensives and benzodiazapines as possible contributing factors to her falls and considers reducing the diazepam / stopping it at night
☐	☐	☐	• Discusses first aid measures to ease the wrist sprain (simple analgesia, rest, ice, considers wrist support)

Relating to others

☐	☐	☐	• Considers the personal circumstances of the patient and assesses if any extra help is required; considers walking aids / grab rails / home modifications
☐	☐	☐	• Identifies that the patient is appeasing her daughter, but is able to address the multiple falls and encourage the patient to seek help with this
☐	☐	☐	• Can answer any questions Irene may have about what will be assessed at a falls clinic
☐	☐	☐	• Can signpost patient to useful local services (fall alarms / council, etc.)

Case B4.6 Information for the doctor

In this case you are a doctor taking a telephone call from your patient's wife.	
Wife will be phoning on behalf of the patient	
Name:	William Hanssen
Age:	78
Past medical history:	Prostate cancer – invasive, under oncology for chemotherapy COPD
Current medication:	Nil
Drug history:	Paracetamol 1 g qds Zomorph 10 mg bd Oramorph 10 mg/5 ml. Takes 5 ml prn for pain, max 4 hourly Tamsulosin 0.4 mg od Current inhalers: Atrovent od, Ventolin prn, Seretide bd

Notes

Case B4.6 Information for the patient

You are Margaret Hanssen, wife of William Hanssen, and you are ringing today to ask for some antibiotics for your husband's urine infection.

ICE

- You want antibiotics as you are certain he has a water infection.
- You don't want anything further from the doctor today.
- You are not concerned – he has had many urine infections before.

Background

- You live at home with your husband.
- You have no outside care for Bill but plenty of family in the area who often come to visit.
- Neither of you smoke or drink.
- You are in good health.

Information divulged freely

- Your husband was diagnosed with prostate cancer last year and has been undergoing chemotherapy. The doctors decided he was not fit for surgery due to his COPD but he is being tried on some new inhalers and they might consider surgery later on. His last chemo was 2 weeks ago.
- You were told by the specialist it was an invasive form and you should prepare yourself for the worst.
- He hasn't really been well for the past week or so. He has mainly been resting in bed, but is still able to get up and walk to the toilet.
- Yesterday he was complaining of some lower abdominal pain.
- Today when he woke up he seemed confused – he did not know who you were at first and still seems muddled now.
- He has not had a temperature; you have checked with the thermometer the hospital gave you and it's 36.5°C. He has not had paracetamol.
- His bowels are fine. He is passing urine and not complaining of pain. He is going more often than usual.
- He has had urine infections in the past and tends to get confused with them. The doctors at the hospital warned you about the danger of infections with the chemo and said if he had one he would need urgent antibiotics from the GP.
- He has eaten some breakfast and you were pleased to see him drinking plenty of water; he had several cups.
- If the doctor offers a script, you will happily accept and are willing to bring a urine sample down if needed.
- If the doctor advises your husband should be reviewed you question why; really you have both had enough doctor's visits at the minute and would prefer to be left alone.
- If the doctor mentions concerns about possible immunosuppression you remember the specialists telling you he would have a fever with this. You also wonder, is it not too long after the chemo to get this?
- If the doctor mentions high calcium you start to get concerned. Why would this happen and what would need to be done about it?

- If you feel there is a reasonable explanation of why the doctor wants to visit you will agree but you will not accept hospital admission without being seen by the GP first.
- If you feel it is unclear why the doctor is concerned then you will again request a script for antibiotics and assure the doctor that you will call back if Bill gets worse.

Case B4.6 Marking scheme for the observer

patient.info/doctor/oncological-emergencies
patient.info/doctor/telephone-consultations

Data gathering and diagnosis

☐	☐	☐	• Takes a history of current symptoms and the background illness
☐	☐	☐	• Appreciates the need for a clinical assessment in person rather than over the telephone
☐	☐	☐	• Considers differential diagnosis including hypercalcaemia and sepsis

Clinical management and medical complexity

☐	☐	☐	• Arranges review of patient in a timely manner and communicates this effectively to patient's wife
☐	☐	☐	• If unable to convince the wife a visit is needed, considers alternative options that may be acceptable to the patient, such as getting a trusted Macmillan nurse to attend with you
☐	☐	☐	• Avoids simply prescribing the requested antibiotic. Recognises complex history and potential for serious illness

Relating to others

☐	☐	☐	• Clearly explains why the patient needs to be seen without using too much jargon
☐	☐	☐	• Creates rapport with the patient's wife
☐	☐	☐	• Appreciates the wife's concerns and her reasons for not wishing to be seen but communicates this to her sensitively
☐	☐	☐	• Enhances autonomy and comes to shared management plan

Case B4.7 Information for the doctor

In this case you are a GP registrar. You have been asked to have a telephone consultation with the daughter of Muriel Hamilton, who is a resident in the local care home.

Name:	Muriel Hamilton (daughter Maureen calling to discuss her case)
Age:	95
Past medical history:	Alzheimer's disease Congestive cardiac failure Hypertension Vertebral collapse, osteoporosis
Current medication:	Fentanyl 25 mcg / h (one patch applied every 72 hours) Lisinopril 10 mg od Furosemide 40 mg od Adcal-D$_3$ 2 a day Alendronic acid 70 mg once weekly
Last consultation:	One month ago: Dr Stevenson: asked to review by care home staff, general decline. Worsening dementia, now non-verbal. Reduced oral intake. Weight loss ++. Family aware of decline, want her to remain in care home. Review as needed. Yesterday : Dr Stevenson: decline +++. Now unresponsive. Staff giving mouth care only. For end of life care. Routine medication stopped. Family aware and daughter has requested meeting to talk about her mum. Reception to arrange.

Notes

Case B4.7   Information for the patient

You are Maureen Hamilton, a 55-year old lady, and you have called today to discuss your mum's end of life care.

ICE

- You would like to discuss what the next steps in your mum's care are so you can tell the family what to expect.
- You have no concerns about her current care but do have worries about what happens now she is no longer able to take her medication by mouth.
- You expect a full discussion about the medication your mum takes and what the doctor can give instead.

Background

- You live with your husband and have three grown-up children who live elsewhere.
- You also have a brother who lives in Australia and a sister who lives in the Highlands.
- Your mum had a sister who sadly passed away 3 years ago.
- You have always been close to your mum and have tried to visit her as often as possible in the care home since she moved there 10 years ago.

Information divulged freely

- You have been told by the staff at the care home that yesterday the GP stopped all her oral medication. You are a little concerned about this. You know when she previously had to stop her furosemide because of a diarrhoeal bug, her legs filled up with fluids and she became breathless.
- You are also concerned about her pain; she has struggled with back pain for many years and she has a pain patch on. You want to ask if this can stay in place or does she need to have something else?

Information only divulged if specifically asked:

- You have taken an active role in your mum's care. Before she went into the care home you visited her at home every day and took charge of all her medications. You made sure you knew what they were all for and knew all about her health conditions.
- You have known for months that she has been in decline since she stopped chatting to you about her day and wasn't interested in her food.
- You are very happy with her care at the home, the staff know her very well and look after her well.
- You have discussed her emergency care plan before and know you want her to stay in the home to die as she is comfortable there. She also has a DNACPR in place.
- You know your mum would be upset at her current condition and feel she has no quality of life.
- If the GP discusses the furosemide you are open to her trying without and understand any breathlessness would be treated with alternative medications such as morphine. You understand she is unable to take the medications by mouth any more.
- If the GP advises the fentanyl patch can stay, you are very relieved; would this be increased if she had more pain?

- If the GP discusses anticipatory medication you ask what the medications are and how they will be given. You know nothing about these medications but want to be as informed as possible.
- You will also ask if your mum is getting dehydrated now that she is not drinking; does the GP think she should have some IV fluids?
- You also ask if your brother should start travelling back from Australia.

Case B4.7 Marking scheme for the observer

> Most trusts have palliative care guidelines you can access. The following handbook from the North of England Cancer Network can be read in conjunction with this case:
> www.northerncanceralliance.nhs.uk/wp-content/uploads/2018/11/NECNXPALLIATIVEXCAREX2016-1.pdf

			Data gathering and diagnosis
☐	☐	☐	• Identifies the issues the patient's daughter Maureen wants to discuss during the consultation
☐	☐	☐	• Identifies that Maureen is happy with her mum's care and wishes her to remain in the care home
☐	☐	☐	• Ensures Maureen is aware and understands that her mum has had treatments stopped and palliative care has commenced

			Clinical management and medical complexity
☐	☐	☐	• Reassures about the cessation of oral medication. Can discuss alternative medication for breathlessness such as morphine / midazolam / glycopyrronium (alternatively furosemide sc could also be considered)
☐	☐	☐	• Advises that fentanyl patch can remain in place and be used as pain relief in her end of life care. Advises if the patch needs to be removed, the equivalent dose of morphine will be provided by subcutaneous injection or syringe driver
☐	☐	☐	• Discusses the use of anticipatory medication: morphine for pain relief and breathlessness, cyclizine or levomepromazine for nausea, midazolam for anxiety and glycopyrronium or hyoscine for respiratory secretions. Advises how these medications will be given, i.e. subcutaneously
☐	☐	☐	• Explains what a syringe driver is and why this may be needed
☐	☐	☐	• Discusses the use of subcutaneous fluids in palliative patients. Reduced oral intake is part of the natural dying process and it would be reasonable for the GP to suggest continuing mouth care (especially as Muriel is prone to fluid build-up), but if they feel it is justified (dehydration leading to delirium / distress) a prescription for subcutaneous fluids could be discussed. The following may be helpful: www.westmidspallcare.co.uk/wp-content/uploads/Subcutaneous-hydration-in-palliative-care-v2.4-Final-2.pdf
☐	☐	☐	• The doctor can offer to discuss Muriel's care with the palliative care team if they require advice regarding medication, or if the family wish to do so

			Relating to others
☐	☐	☐	• Creates rapport with Maureen; acknowledges how she is feeling about the situation and listens to her concerns
☐	☐	☐	• Sensitively discusses end of life care and what to expect in her mum's final days
☐	☐	☐	• Shows an awareness that end of life discussions are difficult, and is guided by the family's wishes alongside the clinical presentation; clarifies what has been discussed to ensure mutual understanding
☐	☐	☐	• Offers reassurance that should Muriel become distressed, or if the family have any concerns, then they know who to contact (GP/OOH/palliative care if involved)

Case B4.8 Information for the doctor

In this case you are a doctor in surgery carrying out video consultations.	
Name:	John George
Age:	75
Past medical history:	Hypertension High cholesterol
Current medication:	Stopped statins last year due to side-effects Stopped antihypertensives as home BP readings were normal

Notes

Case B4.8   Information for the patient

You are John George, a 75-year old man who is speaking to the doctor today via a video call to discuss a 'funny do' you had yesterday.

ICE

- You really just want a check-up. You are not really concerned about the event but don't want it to happen again. You expect the doctor to reassure you.

Background

- You had a 'funny do' yesterday. It started just after lunch; you had felt well all morning and then suddenly you found yourself unable to raise the soup spoon to your mouth. You tried to tell your wife what was happening but she didn't seem able to understand you. You decided it would be best to go have a rest and when you got up half an hour later you felt back to normal. This has never happened to you before. You experienced no chest pain, shortness of breath or palpitations. You know your blood pressure is high and cholesterol is high but you are otherwise well.

Information divulged freely

- You live with your wife – she suffers from Alzheimer's and has been getting worse over the past year. You have no outside help as you know she wouldn't want this. You help her get washed and dressed. You do the shopping and clean the house. You have no nearby family.
- You are very surprised if the doctor mentions a 'mini stroke'. Your first thoughts are about who will take care of your wife if you become unwell.

Information only divulged if specifically asked

- You are very grateful if the doctor explains that carers for your wife could be put in place straight away if you were admitted to hospital. You are willing to consider further help at home in the meantime but want to discuss it with your wife first.
- If the doctor specifically mentions driving you will be very upset as you rely on your car for shopping and appointments. However, if the doctor points out in a sensitive way the reasons not to drive and alternatives available such as patient transport and delivery of food shopping, you accept this.
- You are very happy to attend a TIA clinic as you want to keep yourself as healthy as possible for your wife.
- You are an ex-smoker of 15/day – you stopped when you retired nearly ten years ago. You rarely drink any alcohol. You used to work in retail.

Results for the doctor

The patient had measured his blood pressure just before the call and was able to give a pulse reading from his smartwatch:
- BP 138/90
- Pulse 80 – regular rhythm, no AF clinically
- A limited remote neuro exam shows no facial droop and no limb weakness or sensory loss

Case B4.8 **Marking scheme for the observer**

patient.info/doctor/transient-ischaemic-attacks
https://cks.nice.org.uk/topics/stroke-tia/

Data gathering and diagnosis

☐	☐	☐	• Gathers information systematically and efficiently about reason for the call and considers differential diagnoses for his presentation
☐	☐	☐	• Considers the likely diagnosis of a TIA and demonstrates through history taking they are ruling out a stroke (time of onset, duration and intensity of symptoms, presence of focal neurological deficits); scoring systems such as ABCD2 no longer to be used
☐	☐	☐	• Within the confines of a remote consult, performs a focused assessment (BP and pulse) to rule out any persisting neurological symptoms: the Face Arm Speech Test (FAST) is a validated assessment tool; appreciates an in-person assessment is ultimately needed in this case
☐	☐	☐	• Takes a social history and recognises John's caring responsibilities

Clinical management and medical complexity

☐	☐	☐	• Management reflects an appropriate assessment of risk – as symptoms occurred in the last 24 h, referral for specialist assessment and investigation is advised by NICE within 24 h
☐	☐	☐	• Start aspirin 300 mg as John has no contraindications
☐	☐	☐	• Ensures John (and any relatives) are aware of the symptoms of stroke and understand that they should call 999 if symptoms develop
☐	☐	☐	• Gives advice regarding driving and informing the DVLA (advises not to drive until reviewed by specialist)

Relating to others

☐	☐	☐	• Recognises the patient's agenda and preferences and elicits a social history to be able to put his problem into context
☐	☐	☐	• Explores the impact this has on the patient's life and takes a sensitive approach to the issue of driving
☐	☐	☐	• Communicates risk effectively to the patient
☐	☐	☐	• Enhances patient autonomy by discussing solutions to the patient's concerns (i.e. carers for his wife; patient transport)
☐	☐	☐	• Avoids jargon and has a good rapport and a positive attitude towards helping the patient

Case B5.1 Information for the doctor

In this case you are a doctor in surgery taking video calls.	
Name:	Craig Childs
Age:	27
Past medical history:	Hodgkin's lymphoma (completed chemotherapy and radiation therapy 5 years ago and remains disease-free)
Current medication:	

Notes

Case B5.1 Information for the patient

You are Craig Childs, 27 years old and unemployed. Your mum made this appointment for you to speak to the GP because she is worried about your mood.

ICE

- "Life is crap". You're nearly 30 and feel you haven't achieved the things you wanted to in your life. You are tired of your misery bringing everyone else down and feel everyone would be better off if you weren't around any more.
- You don't think the doctor will be able to do anything for you, and are only there to placate your mum.

Background

- You are a 27-year old ex-army recruit. You were diagnosed with Hodgkin's disease when you were 21 and had to leave the army to undergo treatment. You were given the all clear about 4 years ago and were discharged from follow-up.
- You live at home with your mum (your dad died when you were a teenager and your elder sister works as an interpreter in Japan).
- You have felt low since leaving the army, but you split up with your long-term girlfriend 3 months ago and started to feel worse after this. You quit your bar job soon after this and have been spending the days playing on the Xbox and not leaving the house.
- You got drunk at home a few nights ago. Your mum came home early and found you with several boxes of paracetamol about to attempt an overdose. She has asked you to speak to the doctor about your problems today.

Information divulged freely

- You feel your life is hopeless. You joined the army after leaving school and had started training for the Royal Artillery. You were progressing well when you were diagnosed with Hodgkin's and had to leave.
- You loved the army and have not had any consistent work since leaving, as you feel you don't have any transferable skills. You have worked as a waiter and a barman in various places but hate the idea of doing a job like that for the rest of your life.
- You have never had any mental health problems in the past and have no regular medication.

Information only divulged if specifically asked

- You do feel depressed and have felt this way for a long time. It probably started when you were diagnosed with Hodgkin's lymphoma, but you stayed very positive throughout your treatment and were keen to stay strong and not show any signs of weakness. As time went on, you lost interest in the things you used to love, which is why you felt your girlfriend left you, and since your relationship ended 3 months ago, things have been getting worse.
- You left your job because you didn't see the point of going into work doing something you hate. You have been feeling lethargic and felt you could never concentrate when you were there anyway.
- You feel like you have let your family down. Your sister is successful and your family all supported you when you were ill, and now you feel you have failed them all by not having a high-flying career. You know your girlfriend left you because you were constantly negative and had no interest in doing anything fun any more.

- You have no problems sleeping; you probably sleep too much. You stay up late playing on the Xbox and sleep during the day, but lately even playing on the Xbox is starting to bore you.
- You haven't noticed a change in your appetite, but you have put on weight since leaving the army and you miss being as fit as you used to be.
- You generally avoid alcohol, but 2 nights ago you drank almost a whole bottle of bourbon by yourself. It was the anniversary of when your dad died, and you had collected 5 boxes of paracetamol with the intention of taking an overdose. You thought your mum was going to be out, but when she came home early and found you drunk with the pill boxes, you felt incredibly guilty that you almost tried to kill yourself.
- You have never tried to hurt yourself before, and although you promised your mum that 'you wouldn't do anything stupid' you still feel life is pretty hopeless and don't really see another way out.
- If specifically asked about future suicidal intent you will go quiet and look at your feet. You have done some research online and thought about hanging yourself, but you really don't want to mess it up, you want it to 'be quick'. If you were still in the army you would just use a gun, but you don't have access to one any more. An overdose seems like the best option to you as you think you will just fall asleep and not wake up. If probed by the doctor, then you will admit you have been thinking about it, but haven't made any fixed plans.
- You have not experienced any hallucinations and you don't smoke or use any other recreational drugs.
- You are not particularly keen on medication after going through chemotherapy, but you would be willing to try antidepressant medication. Talking therapies are not really 'you' but you are open to suggestions if the doctor thinks they are going to help.
- If the doctor discusses a psychiatric assessment, you are initially dismissive and decline this. However, if the doctor explains their concerns about your suicidal ideation and risk of hurting yourself, or mentions 'being sectioned' then you will agree to speak to the mental health team and have questions about what this will involve.

Case B5.1 Marking scheme for the observer

https://patient.info/doctor/suicide-risk-assessment-and-threats-of-suicide

Data gathering and diagnosis

☐	☐	☐	• Establishes history, social situation/support available, alcohol/drug use
☐	☐	☐	• Assesses severity of depression and identifies that patient has multiple risk factors for suicide
☐	☐	☐	• Asks about intent, protective factors and makes an assessment of mental state
☐	☐	☐	• Asks about physical symptoms of depression

Clinical management and medical complexity

☐	☐	☐	• Discusses a diagnosis of depression, offers an explanation and checks understanding
☐	☐	☐	• Recognises the patient is at high risk of further suicide attempts. Discusses involvement of local mental health services and considers compulsory assessment under the Mental Health Act if this is refused. Aims to encourage the patient to agree to a voluntary assessment
☐	☐	☐	• Discusses treatment options for depression – medications, talking therapies, exercise, sleep hygiene, self-help resources available – and ensures adequate follow-up is in place

Relating to others

☐	☐	☐	• Establishes rapport, asks questions sensitively without rushing patient
☐	☐	☐	• Finds out the patient's ICE and reasons for presenting
☐	☐	☐	• Elicits information regarding the patient's situation to put problems into context, and explores impact on his life
☐	☐	☐	• Acts in an open, non-judgmental manner
☐	☐	☐	• Communicates risk effectively and makes attempt to reach a shared management plan
☐	☐	☐	• Ensures patient safety and mentions 24-hour support through the crisis service/local mental health team

Case B5.2 Information for the doctor

In this case you are a newly qualified GP in a morning surgery taking video consultations.	
Name:	Tess Cowper
Age:	27
Past medical history:	Spontaneous vaginal delivery 10 days ago, 2nd degree tear sustained (first pregnancy)
Current medication:	Nil

Notes

Case B5.2   Information for the patient

You are Tess Cowper, a 27-year old woman, who gave birth to baby Larissa 10 days ago. Your husband has become concerned about your behaviour and made this appointment on your behalf. You present as extremely energetic and talkative, speaking rapidly and changing topic frequently.

ICE

- Your husband has taken Larissa out in her pram while you are on the video call. He has been concerned about your behaviour and asked you to speak to the doctor.
- You become quite agitated after waiting for the video call to start, and you change the subject frequently.

Background

- You live with your partner Russ, a musician, and this is your first child.
- You are a stylist for a magazine but are on maternity leave at present.
- This was an unplanned pregnancy and it has interrupted your career plans, but now Larissa is here you realise that she is special and this was all meant to be.

Information divulged freely

- You had a long labour, but it was beautiful. You had a second degree perineal tear which was stitched with dissolving stitches. The midwife checked this last week and advised that you would need further review of this. You have minimal pain and no discharge or sign of infection.
- You had a lot going on leading up to the birth of Larissa. You worked until the week before delivery preparing a huge magazine shoot. You moved house a few weeks prior to that and have been sorting everything out to do with that. You also lost your grandmother who you were close to and travelled to the other side of the country for the funeral while heavily pregnant.
- You are breastfeeding and are up every few hours overnight doing this and you love it, it is going very well.
- You have lots of plans at the moment to make your fortune and aim to use all the time you have being on maternity leave to start writing your novel.

Information only divulged if specifically asked:

- You are not feeling at all depressed – the opposite in fact, you have never felt better.
- You have not been sleeping. The insomnia started prior to the birth, but since delivering you are only managing the odd hour of rest here and there.
- If specifically asked you do admit to feeling tearful and overwhelmed when you first brought Larissa home to your new house. You could not sleep due to anxieties about her stopping breathing, but you now realise that you were overreacting and you feel pretty invincible. You are still not sleeping but you are making the most of being awake overnight to chat to all your friends in different parts of the world who are awake too.
- If asked about visual hallucinations you deny this. If asked about auditory hallucinations you laugh. You do keep hearing a voice in your head when you are breastfeeding at night telling

you that you are the 'Chosen One' and Larissa is special. You feel this is your internal wisdom as a mother telling you this and it makes you feel elated.

- You have never had any mental health problems in the past. You have never taken any psychiatric medication or had inpatient mental health treatment.
- You are not aware of any family history of perinatal mental health problems.
- You have not had any alcohol since you became pregnant and you do not use drugs.
- If the doctor thinks you need to see a psychiatrist you are not willing to do this unless your baby and husband can come with you. If the doctor explains their reasoning sensitively and kindly and reassures you, then you will agree.

Case B5.2 **Marking scheme for the observer**

The NICE Pathway on antenatal and postnatal mental health (Updated April 2018)
https://pathways.nice.org.uk/pathways/antenatal-and-postnatal-mental-health
The RCGP have perinatal mental health resources here:
www.rcgp.org.uk/representing-you/policy-areas/perinatal-mental-health

Data gathering and diagnosis

- Identifies the reason for the call and focuses on the mental health presentation
- Clarifies the patient's psychiatric history to cover: any personal history of mental illness including any inpatient care or any severe perinatal mental illness in a first degree relative
- Asks about mood, hallucinations, thoughts of harming herself or others
- Asks about sleep, how she is managing feeding her baby
- Asks about social support and the quality of interpersonal relationships (mother; baby; partner). Enquires about where the baby is today

Clinical management and medical complexity

- Recognises the patient is presenting with psychotic features (delusions about the baby, grandiose thoughts, pressured speech, tangential thinking, auditory hallucinations) which is a psychiatric emergency
- Advises referral for immediate psychiatric assessment (within 4 hours), ideally in a specialist mother and baby unit
- Is able to provide Tess with an honest explanation of your concerns, what postnatal psychosis is and why you would like to offer her help
- Safety nets at the end of the consult by arranging for a nurse to sit with Tess until her husband returns and the referral has been arranged

Relating to others

- Creates a good rapport with patient and demonstrates empathy
- Is aware of the fear of stigma around mental health problems in the postnatal period and the fear that their baby may be taken into care, and that this may cause a reluctance to disclose
- Uses a reassuring manner to allay Tess's fears. Explains that a mother and baby unit should be available, meaning mum can stay with baby
- Asks to involve Tess's husband and offers to call him so he can accompany her to hospital. Considers providing leaflets for Tess and her family to learn more about the condition www.rcpsych.ac.uk/mental-health/problems-disorders/post-natal-depression?searchTerms=postnatal%20depression

Case B5.3 Information for the doctor

You are the on-call GP calling back a nurse at the local nursing home who wishes to speak with you about Gladys White.

Name:	Gladys White
Age:	88
Past medical history:	AF 13 years ago Left hip replacement 16 years ago Osteoporosis 19 years ago Hypertension 17 years ago Hysterectomy (for menorrhagia) 30 years ago
Current medication:	Lisinopril, furosemide, warfarin, alendronic acid, paracetamol, senna and lactulose (prn)
Social history:	Bethlehem nursing home for last 12 years 1 week ago – telephone encounter – Staff nurse Caroline – requested zopiclone. Gladys seems more agitated today, couldn't sleep last night. Eating and drinking well. Not complaining of any pain. No other concerns. Prn review.

Notes

Case B5.3   Information for the patient

You are Caroline Foster, a 28-year old staff nurse who is phoning today to request lorazepam for Gladys who has been more agitated lately.

ICE

- You would like to request lorazepam to help Gladys with agitation, because she was very aggressive towards another resident yesterday. You expect the doctor to prescribe it without any problems because you use this quite frequently with other residents.

Background

- You have been looking after Gladys for a couple of years now.
- You phoned the surgery last week when Gladys had a bad night and asked for zopiclone, which helped, but you need something extra to give her during the day if required.
- You look after 15 residents with one healthcare assistant and have to keep an eye on everyone.

Information divulged freely

- You are concerned about Gladys's memory. She didn't recognise you this morning, which is very unusual.
- She seems very aggressive towards the other residents. Last night she walked into Dorothy's room (another resident) and accused her of stealing her diamond ring. She was shouting and it took a while to calm her down. However, the point is that Gladys doesn't have a diamond ring and doesn't usually behave like that.
- You believe it's probably memory deterioration. You have already checked her urine and her observations. Everything is normal.
- She is eating and drinking well.
- You would like to try some lorazepam for a few days and see if it helps.

Information only divulged if specifically asked

- Gladys has no family.
- There is no history of cough. She was not complaining of any pain.
- Her mobility is good. She had a fall a few weeks ago and has been using a stick since.
- She takes her medications regularly. Her recent INR was 3.3.
- You were on annual leave when Gladys had a fall. When you checked in the nursing notes it said that Gladys tripped over in the bathroom a few weeks ago and fell forward. Nobody witnessed the fall, but she had a small bruise on her leg and forehead since, which is getting better.
- If the doctor offers lorazepam you are thankful, ask for the script to be faxed to your local pharmacy and finish the conversation.
- If the doctor is concerned and wants to visit Gladys, you mention that you have already checked her and she is not septic.
- If the doctor shares with you their concerns about Gladys being on warfarin, the recent fall and confusion / agitation and mentions the risk of possible subdural haematoma, you'd become very concerned and apologise that you never considered it and would be grateful for the doctor to come in and visit Gladys.

Case B5.3 Marking scheme for the observer

patient.info/doctor/subdural-haematoma-pro
patient.info/doctor/rapid-tranquilisation
patient.info/doctor/telephone-consultations

Data gathering and diagnosis

			• Identifies reason for phone call and explores ICE
			• Identifies the seriousness of the symptoms in the context of abnormal behavioural change
			• Makes good use of open and appropriate closed questions

Clinical management and medical complexity

			• Considers diagnosis of possible subdural haematoma (patient on warfarin, recent fall, new agitation/confusion, worsening of mobility) or other cause for the change in behaviour
			• Arranges urgent home visit to assess the patient further
			• Prescribing a sedative without a face-to-face review would in this case be marked negatively

Relating to others

			• Develops good rapport with the nurse
			• Shows clear communication skills and backs up own judgment appropriately; explains reasoning clearly to the nurse
			• Demonstrates effective communication skills in a non face-to-face setting

Case B5.4 Information for the doctor

In this case you are a doctor in surgery taking video consultations.	
Name:	Amira Aziz
Age:	16
Past medical history:	Acne Eczema
Current medication:	Locoid cream prn

Notes

Case B5.4 Information for the patient

You are Amira Aziz, a 16-year old girl who called to speak to a new GP Registrar today to discuss your mood.

ICE

- You are feeling very low.
- You have nobody to talk to about your feelings because you don't trust anybody, not even your own family. They are too busy anyway. You wonder if you should see a psychologist or psychiatrist because your thoughts are 'killing' you.

Background

- You live with your parents. You are an only child.
- You can't talk to your parents, despite being very close to your mum. You are worried they'll think that you are a failure.
- You are one of the top students in your class.
- You enjoy school but lately you have not been able to concentrate.
- You do have some good friends but you don't trust them. You were friends with Peter for over 3 years, but recently your relationship has broken down somewhat.
- You are pretty sure Peter is gay even though he is not quite sure himself yet.
- You are not in a relationship.
- Your appetite is not great. Perhaps you lost some weight.

Information divulged freely

- You've been feeling depressed for 3–4 months. You had an argument with your best friend Peter about something silly. You haven't spoken to him since.
- You see him at school every day and are waiting for him to make the first step. You are too proud to do it yourself.
- You wanted to see a school counsellor, but she is on long-term sick leave.
- Your mum is a midwife and your dad is a chef in a local restaurant.
- You are not seeing your own doctor today, because he is friends with your father.
- You don't have any suicidal plans or ideas and you never self-harmed.
- You love your family and you would never take your own life. You just want to find the 'light at the end of the tunnel'.

Information only divulged if specifically asked

- You don't want your family to know that you are not feeling very well, because your mum just had a miscarriage and has enough to worry about.
- You can't sleep very well and are waking up in the middle of the night.
- You haven't been able to relax for weeks. It's like you are always stressed about everything: your family, Peter, making sure you are the best at school so your parents are proud of you, attending piano lessons twice a week.
- If the doctor specifically asks if you take any illicit drugs, you'd admit that you smoke marijuana occasionally with your friends. Lately you've been smoking it a couple of times a week, because it helps you to feel relaxed and not worry about things too much. You call it a short-term escape from daily problems.

- You believe you are not addicted, because you don't smoke every day and you can stop any time you want.
- You don't drink alcohol.
- You don't do any exercise. You don't see the point – you are fit enough.
- If the doctor is empathetic and clearly explains potential harmful side-effects of cannabis including depression, you'd be surprised and listen to the doctor's suggestions.
- If the doctor discusses Child and Adolescent Mental Health Services (CAMHS) assessment, you are initially dismissive and decline this. However, if the doctor explains their concerns and gives you more information on what CAMHS can offer including counselling, you will agree to be referred to see them.
- If the doctor suggests talking to your family you'd get very upset.
- If the doctor remains supportive, emphasises confidentiality and offers you follow-up, you'd calm down and agree.

Case B5.4 **Marking scheme for the observer**

patient.info/doctor/cannabis-use-and-abuse
patient.info/doctor/depression-pro

Data gathering and diagnosis			
☐	☐	☐	• Explores ICE
☐	☐	☐	• Establishes history, social situation / support available, alcohol / drug use
☐	☐	☐	• Screens for depression and identifies triggers (argument with best friend, cannabis use) and protective factors (family)
Clinical management and medical complexity			
☐	☐	☐	• Discusses a diagnosis of depression, offers an explanation and checks understanding
☐	☐	☐	• Considers referral to CAMHS, offers support and arrangement of regular follow-up
☐	☐	☐	• Addresses cannabis use and offers involvement of the Drug and Alcohol Team (if required)
☐	☐	☐	• Suggests and encourages involvement of family members
☐	☐	☐	• Discusses management options – CAMHS assessment / counselling, lifestyle, exercise, sleep hygiene, relaxation techniques
Relating to others			
☐	☐	☐	• Is open and non-judgmental
☐	☐	☐	• Involves the patient in management plan
☐	☐	☐	• Is empathetic and able to communicate effectively so the patient understands

A note on cannabis

Following the UK Government's announcement in 2018 to reschedule certain cannabis-based products for medicinal use, you may have patients making appointments to discuss this further with their GP. NHS England and the RCGP have prepared guidance for clinicians regarding what this actually means in practice:

www.gmc-uk.org/ethical-guidance/learning-materials/information-for-doctors-on-cannabis-
    based-products-for-medicinal-use

www.england.nhs.uk/long-read/cannabis-based-products-for-medicinal-use-cbpms/

Case B5.5   Information for the doctor

In this case you are a GP registrar in a routine surgery taking video consultations.	
Name:	Martin Neptune
Age:	22
Past medical history:	Right shoulder dislocation (6 years ago)
Current medication:	Nil

Notes

Case B5.5 Information for the patient

You are Martin Neptune, a 22-year old man, who has been advised to speak to the GP by your dentist, who noticed you had erosions on your teeth, prompting you to admit that you have been making yourself vomit for several years. You have never discussed this with a professional before and think it is time you did so.

ICE

- You want to make sure you haven't harmed your body in any other way by making yourself sick and would like to be checked out.
- You feel more in control of your behaviour right now, but would be willing to engage in any therapy the GP may offer you.

Background

- You went to the dentist a few weeks ago complaining of very sensitive teeth. The dentist told you that many of your teeth were eroded and you admitted that you often make yourself vomit. The dentist was great and encouraged you to make this appointment today with the GP.
- You live with your parents and younger sister after recently returning home from university.
- You work for NHS 111 as a call handler, mainly doing night shifts.

Information divulged freely

- You have been making yourself vomit since you were 16. You used to do it almost every day but now only do it once or twice per week, typically after having a food binge.
- You generally lead a healthy lifestyle. You go to the gym once a week and know about and stick to a healthy eating plan, but you are prone to having food binges – mainly after a long night shift at work.
- During the binges you will load up on unhealthy snacks from the vending machine at work and gorge on them during your break at night.

Information only divulged if specifically asked

- You wouldn't describe yourself as depressed. You feel you were when you were younger, which is why you think this started, but you feel OK at the moment, you just don't want to become overweight. You do not feel suicidal and never have.
- You do have some regrets about your career. You played basketball for the county when you were younger and had dreams about becoming a professional. However, you dislocated your shoulder and stopped playing altogether. Since your injury, you felt that you started to get chubby and, to control this, you started to make yourself vomit. This has been ongoing since then.
- You did a marketing degree at university and have dreams about starting your own business eventually, but right now you are living at home and doing the 111 night shifts to save some money while you search for the perfect job.
- Your typical diet is porridge or bircher muesli for breakfast, a sandwich, fruit and crisps for lunch or as your overnight work meal, and typically meat / veg for your main meal of the day. If you do have snacks you ordinarily stick to fruit. When you binge you will get about 6 chocolate bars and 3 packets of crisps and a fizzy drink and eat them all in one go.

- After your binges you feel ashamed and almost immediately go to the toilet and put your fingers down your throat to make yourself vomit.
- You have never used laxatives or any other drugs to help you to vomit.
- Your family don't know about your problem and you feel embarrassed to discuss it with them. You feel your family would be supportive. They never said anything, but you feel they were disappointed that you never 'made it big' with your basketball.
- You have never been abused. Your mum suffers with anxiety and takes pills every day and your sister is always on a diet, but you know of no other mental health problems in your family.
- Apart from the problem with your teeth you haven't had any other problems from vomiting. You have never noticed any blood in your vomit. You occasionally have abdominal pain and a sore throat after purging but this is never long-lasting.
- You don't smoke and you rarely drink alcohol and have never used any recreational drugs.
- If the doctor suggests an in-person appointment for an examination, blood tests or other investigations you are keen to have these, but question what they are looking for.
- If the doctor offers a referral to the eating disorders team you feel apprehensive as you don't feel you have an eating disorder like anorexia, but if it is explained that this service will be able to provide specific support to help you with this problem, then you will be willing to engage with this.
- You are happy to follow-up with the GP as requested.

Case B5.5 Marking scheme for the observer

> NICE has helpful guidance on eating disorders which can be read in conjunction with this case: www.nice.org.uk/guidance/ng69
> Or see the BMJ Best Practice topics (Dec 2018): https://bestpractice.bmj.com/topics/en-us/441

Data gathering and diagnosis

☐	☐	☐	• Understands reasons for the call and ICE
☐	☐	☐	• Takes a history, asking about both physical symptoms (teeth erosions, BMI, GI bleeding, etc.) and mental health, including any risks to self or signs of abuse and family history. Asks about use of laxatives and excessive exercise
☐	☐	☐	• Enquires about previous contact with services and any prior support or counselling he has received
☐	☐	☐	• Establishes social situation, living arrangements and support networks available to him

Clinical management and medical complexity

☐	☐	☐	• Recognises that Martin is suffering from bulimia nervosa and can discuss what this is and describe the help available to him
☐	☐	☐	• Suggests arranging an appointment for blood tests (renal function / electrolytes), ECG and checking physical health for signs of malnutrition / electrolyte disturbances
☐	☐	☐	• Discusses referral to the local eating disorders team to enable Martin to engage with a specific bulimia nervosa focused guided self-help programme
☐	☐	☐	• Discusses involving his family to enable them to support him
☐	☐	☐	• Arranges GP follow-up to monitor physical health and provide ongoing support and suggests he continues to see his dentist regularly to monitor his teeth
☐	☐	☐	• Signposts to support groups such as Beat (www.beateatingdisorders.org.uk)

Relating to others

☐	☐	☐	• Creates rapport with patient
☐	☐	☐	• Consults in an open, non-judgmental manner
☐	☐	☐	• Identifies psychological background to his bulimia (sporting injury) and reflects on this with the patient
☐	☐	☐	• Communicates management options effectively and offers leaflets / written weblinks of support groups available

Case B5.6 Information for the doctor

In this case you are a doctor in surgery telephoning a patient with her recent blood results.	
Name:	Maryam Kharoushi
Age:	40
Past medical history:	None
Last consultation:	1 week ago: TATT, sleep OK, no low mood, for bloods and review with results. Blood results: U&Es – normal LFTs – ALT, alk phos & bilirubin normal Hb – 129 (115–160 g/L) MCV **105** (80–100 fL) WCC & platelets normal B12, folate & ferritin normal TSH normal

Notes

Case B5.6   Information for the patient

You are Maryam Kharoushi, a 40-year old woman, who is speaking to the doctor to discuss her blood results.

ICE

- You think you're probably hypothyroid as one of your friends had this and she was also tired a lot.
- You are not really concerned about anything more serious.

Background

- You are originally from Iran and have been unable to return there for political reasons, but you settled into the UK many years ago.
- You live alone after your husband left you about one year ago.
- You have no family in the area; both your children are grown up and live away from home.
- You don't smoke. You don't do much exercise.
- You work at a nearby law firm as a receptionist.

Information divulged freely

- You have been feeling tired for about 3 months. You sleep well, around 8 hours a night.
- You don't feel low or anxious.
- You have no specific symptoms such as weight gain, urinary or bowel symptoms. You have regular periods but they are not heavy.
- You have lots of friends in the area but they all have their own families so you don't see much of them outside of work.

Information only divulged if specifically asked

- You have been drinking more alcohol than normal since your husband left. You are alone in the evenings and find it a way to pass the time.
- You know there are guidelines for alcohol and don't want the GP to think you are an alcoholic so you will try to avoid answering the questions about your consumption, answering 'not much', 'a few glasses', etc.
- If the GP asks you direct questions about how much and what you drink you will eventually answer. You drink one bottle of red wine every day with no other spirits or beers.
- You don't drink in the mornings and have gone without alcohol for a few days in the past and did not experience any unpleasant physical symptoms.
- If the GP advises this is too much alcohol to be drinking you will point out your liver was functioning fine so surely it is not too much. You know people at work who drink the same amount.
- If the GP points out your alcohol intake may be contributing to your symptoms you will accept this and will have a think about cutting down. You will ask if the GP has any advice on how to do this but decline any input from the drug and alcohol team.

Case B5.6 Marking scheme for the observer

https://patient.info/doctor/alcoholism-and-alcohol-misuse-recognition-and-assessment
www.nice.org.uk/guidance/cg115

			Data gathering and diagnosis
☐	☐	☐	• Takes an appropriate 'Tired all the time' history including systemic enquiry (for more detail: https://geekymedics.com/tiredness-history-taking-osce-guide/)
☐	☐	☐	• Identifies alcohol excess and screens for any physical symptoms of alcohol misuse (withdrawal symptoms, signs of liver disease, AF, injuries from falling when intoxicated)
☐	☐	☐	• Asks about mood and mental health
☐	☐	☐	• Takes a social history, picking up on her recent relationship breakdown
☐	☐	☐	• Assesses if the alcohol use is harmful use or dependence. Considers using an alcohol screening tool
			Clinical management and medical complexity
☐	☐	☐	• Discusses reducing alcohol intake and specific strategies to achieve this
☐	☐	☐	• Offers support in the practice or via drug and alcohol team
☐	☐	☐	• Discusses local counselling support available / CBT online. Support groups such as Alcoholics Anonymous
☐	☐	☐	• Arranges a follow-up appointment to assess progress
			Relating to others
☐	☐	☐	• Discusses alcohol intake in a sensitive, non-judgmental manner
☐	☐	☐	• Is able to gently establish specific alcohol intake from a patient who does not wish to disclose this information
☐	☐	☐	• Discovers patient's social background to put the drinking into context
☐	☐	☐	• Communicates risk of alcohol misuse effectively to patient

Case B5.7   Information for the doctor

In this case you are a locum undertaking telephone consultations.	
Name:	Borys Shevchenko
Age:	35
Past medical history:	None
Current medication:	Nil
Last consultation:	2 weeks ago: marital stress, poor sleep, not coping at work, agreed to zopiclone to help. Pt advised this is short-term only.

Notes

Case B5.7 Information for the patient

You are Borys Shevchenko, a 35-year old man, who has called today to request some more medication.

ICE

- You want some more of the medication given to you by your GP 2 weeks ago.
- You know the last doctor said it was short-term only but you still need it and don't think another few weeks will be a problem.
- You are concerned the GP might refuse to give you more – you were really struggling without it.

Background

- You work as a broker in the City.
- You have been married for 10 years.
- You used to go to the gym 3 times a week but recently have stopped. You don't smoke.
- At the moment you are drinking every night – usually half a bottle of wine.

Information divulged freely

- Your work has been very busy recently and you found yourself arguing more with your wife at home. This escalated when she accused you of having an affair. You are sleeping in separate rooms and fight every night.
- You were having problems with sleep for about 6 weeks before you came to the GP. You struggled to get to sleep and you were having 2–3 hours a night.
- During the day you were very tired. Your concentration was poor and your work was suffering as a result. Your boss had taken you aside to ask if anything was wrong and this was what prompted you to call the surgery.
- You don't feel low, just fed up and stressed at all the arguing.
- The GP gave you some medication to take each night to get to sleep and it really helped. You were able to sleep and this meant you performed better at work.
- If the GP gives you another script then you will be very pleased.
- If the GP does not give you a script you will become upset; you want to know exactly why you can't have more. You understand about addiction but surely another few weeks won't hurt?
- If the GP still will not prescribe the medication, you want to know what else you can do. You accept you could cut down on your alcohol and could get to the gym more. You will also accept you and your wife do need to sit down and discuss the future of your marriage; maybe some marriage counselling would be a good idea.

Case B5.7   Marking scheme for the observer

patient.info/doctor/insomnia
https://cks.nice.org.uk/insomnia
https://cks.nice.org.uk/benzodiazepine-and-z-drug-withdrawal

Data gathering and diagnosis			
☐	☐	☐	• Explores the history, including screening for any signs of depression or physical causes of patient's insomnia
☐	☐	☐	• Identifies the social and occupational impact of insomnia
☐	☐	☐	• Elicits the patient's ideas and expectations regarding his problem
☐	☐	☐	• Finds out if the patient has tried any other strategies to address his problem

Clinical management and medical complexity			
☐	☐	☐	• Gives advice regarding addictive nature of sleeping tablets and advises against long-term use
☐	☐	☐	• Is able to advise on sleep hygiene measures and lifestyle advice which may help with sleep
☐	☐	☐	• Offers appropriate referral to counselling services such as 'CBT-I' (CBT for insomnia: www.cntw.nhs.uk/services/nctalkingtherapies/what-do-nc-talking-therapies-offer/cbt-i-cbt-for-insomnia)
☐	☐	☐	• Considers offering the patient blood tests to screen for anaemia and hypothyroidism

Relating to others			
☐	☐	☐	• Creates a rapport with the patient
☐	☐	☐	• Discusses insomnia in a non-judgmental, sensitive manner
☐	☐	☐	• Sensitively approaches the topic of marriage counselling (www.relate.org.uk)
☐	☐	☐	• Remains positive about alternative treatment options for his problems and offers a follow-up appointment to check in

Case B5.8   Information for the doctor

In this case you are a GP Registrar in an afternoon clinic taking telephone calls.	
Name:	Michelle Douglas
Age:	30
Past medical history:	Chronic back pain
Current medication:	Tramadol 50 mg Take 1–2 up to 4 times a day 100 tablets Last script: 9 days ago Gabapentin 300 mg Take one 3 times a day 90 tablets Last script: 9 days ago

Notes

Case B5.8 Information for the patient

You are Michelle Douglas, a 30-year old woman, who has called to request some more medication. You are annoyed at having to call in because your medication is on your repeat prescriptions. You tried to ask for it at the chemist but they said you had to speak to the doctor first.

ICE

- You want your medication and you don't see any reason why the doctor cannot give it to you.

Background

- You live with your husband and 2 children. You don't work as your back pain stops you.
- You smoke 10 cigarettes a day.
- You drink one bottle of wine per week.

Information divulged freely

- You have had chronic lower back pain for 10 years. A previous GP in the practice started you on tramadol and then on the gabapentin. This combination seems to work. It allows you to sleep and look after your children.
- You have no interest in changing your medication at present.
- If the GP points out it's only been 9 days since your prescription you will be surprised and start to make excuses, such as you must have lost some or maybe the chemist didn't give you all the tablets last time.
- You are absolutely certain you are taking the correct amount and you are down to the last few tablets in each pack. However, you will also ask why it would be a problem if you took a few extra every now and then.
- You need a prescription today – you will not accept if the GP wants to review your script orders or speak to the chemist. Without your medications you know the pain will come back and you will not be able to pick your children up from school or make their dinner.
- You deny selling any of your medication and are sure no-one else has access to it.
- If the GP gives you your normal script you will be happy.
- If they give you a reduced script to allow time to review your notes and make a review appointment you will grudgingly accept. You do want assurances they are not going to suddenly stop your medication as you really need it.
- You will accept a minimum order date on your prescriptions or removal from repeats whilst the GP reviews your notes.
- If offered you will decline a pain clinic referral. You will also be completely against attending a review with the drug and alcohol team or other support services as you are not a drug addict.

Case B5.8 Marking scheme for the observer

patient.info/doctor/opioid-abuse-and-dependence
patient.info/doctor/assessment-of-drug-dependence
https://cks.nice.org.uk/opioid-dependence

Data gathering and diagnosis

☐	☐	☐	• Takes an appropriate history of pain and reviews medications
☐	☐	☐	• Identifies the potential overuse of medications and elicits reasons for this
☐	☐	☐	• Discovers patient's social setup
☐	☐	☐	• Explores the patient's mood / mental health

Clinical management and medical complexity

☐	☐	☐	• Explains potential problems of medication overuse
☐	☐	☐	• Agrees a plan with the patient to monitor medication use to reduce the chance of overuse, including involving the medicines management team and any local reduction programmes
☐	☐	☐	• Encourages rehabilitation and considers alternative approaches to managing her pain such as re-exploring physiotherapy / review by specialist pain teams

Relating to others

☐	☐	☐	• Discusses medication overuse in a sensitive, non-judgmental manner
☐	☐	☐	• Comes to an appropriate plan which doctor and patient can both agree on, avoiding conflict where possible
☐	☐	☐	• Acknowledges the impact of the problem on the patient's life and is able to communicate the risks of medication overuse effectively, and suggest alternative solutions

Case B5.9   Information for the doctor

In this case you are a GP registrar in a routine afternoon surgery undertaking telephone consultations.	
Name:	Mario Plaza
Age:	57
Past medical history:	None
Current medication:	None
Last consultation:	• Temp 37.1°C, HR 98, RR 18, SpO$_2$ 97%, BP 140/90, GCS 15 – alert, orientated, nil confusion • Nil tremor, nil jaundice or clubbing, no pallor or bruising, nil stigmata of liver disease • Abdomen soft, non-tender, no masses palpable, no ascites New patient check carried out on joining the surgery in 2009: BP 140/91, BMI 25, ex-smoker, alcohol 14 units per week

Notes

Case B5.9   Information for the patient

You are Mario Plaza, a 57-year old man, who has called about a prescription for your heartburn.

ICE

- You have suffered with heartburn for months but have been too busy to come to the doctors.
- You typically take Gaviscon but this just doesn't work. A colleague suggested a medication called lansoprazole and you are calling to request a trial of this.

Background

- You work as a human resource manager for a large airline. You worked as cabin crew for years but moved to a land-based role 5 years ago.
- You live alone and have no partner or children, which suits your busy lifestyle.

Information divulged freely

- You have been experiencing heartburn for about 6 months, mostly in the evenings after eating and drinking. You have been using Gaviscon daily for the last month but this is not working for you any more.
- You describe the pain as a discomfort and burning sensation in the epigastric area with no radiation elsewhere. You do occasionally feel bloated and suffer with a lot of wind.
- You are generally a very well person and have no other medical problems and take no medication apart from the Gaviscon. You occasionally take paracetamol if you have a hangover, but you don't take ibuprofen or any other NSAIDs.
- You are very busy both at work and socially. Your role involves a lot of travelling and there are frequent social events you have to attend.

Information only divulged if specifically asked

- You occasionally feel nauseous and you have vomited sometimes; the most recent episode of this was last night. You only vomit after having a little too much alcohol to drink. You have never noticed blood or coffee ground in your vomit and you have not had any black tarry stools or fresh rectal bleeding.
- You have not had any problems swallowing and have not noticed food sticking in your throat.
- You have not lost any weight recently.
- You have had no chest pain, palpitations or shortness of breath.
- If asked about alcohol, you admit to drinking a bit more than you should. You drink a bottle of wine most nights, and often more than this if you are at a social event (typically 5–6 gin and tonics as well as the wine). You feel in control of your drinking and could easily stop if you wanted to, but you enjoy it, and it is expected at these social events.
- You have never had an 'eye opener' drink first thing in the morning and you have never missed work because of alcohol. Your sister has raised concerns about your drinking before, but she has a very different lifestyle to you, and your colleagues and friends have a similar drinking pattern to you, so you are not worried.

- You have fallen over on particularly heavy nights out before, but you have never sustained more than a few cuts and bruises. You do feel guilty about your drinking on these occasions and you have had nights out where you have no memory of the end of the evening.
- You have never had any tremors or symptoms of withdrawal if you do not drink, and you have never had a seizure or any hallucinations.
- Your mood is good. You occasionally suffer from insomnia and sometimes feel anxious, but you are happy in your job and with your social life.

Case B5.9 **Marking scheme for the observer**

https://cks.nice.org.uk/cirrhosis#!scenario and https://cks.nice.org.uk/alcohol-problem-drinking
https://cks.nice.org.uk/topics/alcohol-problem-drinking

Data gathering and diagnosis

☐	☐	☐	• Takes a history to ask about red flags for dyspepsia (GI bleeding, dysphagia, recurrent vomiting, unintentional weight loss) and identifies alcohol as the likely cause for his symptoms
☐	☐	☐	• Recognises a harmful level of alcohol consumption and uses a recognised alcohol screening test to assess (https://www.gov.uk/government/publications/alcohol-use-screening-tests)
☐	☐	☐	• Considers other causes for his dyspepsia and enquires about diet, smoking and use of medications such as NSAIDs, steroids, bisphosphonates, calcium antagonists and nitrates
☐	☐	☐	• Enquires about mood and mental health
☐	☐	☐	• Recognises that an examination is required, checking for any abdominal masses, signs of confusion or alcohol withdrawal and any stigmata of alcoholic liver disease, and arranges a face-to-face appointment

Clinical management and medical complexity

☐	☐	☐	• Considers further investigations for both the dyspepsia and to exclude any liver disease: FBC, U&Es, LFTs, proteins, clotting factors, *H. pylori* testing
☐	☐	☐	• Discusses Mario's drinking habits and the link to dyspepsia as well as other medical problems; offers structured brief advice (see CKS weblinks)
☐	☐	☐	• Offers a prescription for a PPI for 1 month for empirical acid suppression while awaiting test results and arranges a face-to-face follow-up review
☐	☐	☐	• Discusses psychological therapies available locally, such as cognitive behavioural therapy, and suggests referral to this and the local alcohol service for support
☐	☐	☐	• Offers dyspepsia lifestyle advice (smoking / alcohol cessation, dietary advice)

Relating to others

☐	☐	☐	• Creates rapport with the patient by being frank but non-judgmental about his drinking
☐	☐	☐	• Elicits social background and understands the reasons for the drinking patterns
☐	☐	☐	• Communicates risk of alcohol misuse effectively to the patient
☐	☐	☐	• Encourages patient to engage with alcohol services or to continue to be supported by the GP. Arranges appropriate follow-up to monitor progress

Case B6.1 Information for the doctor

In this case you are a doctor in surgery doing a video consult.	
Name:	Lucy Oliver
Age:	28
Past medical history:	Consultation 2/52 ago – positive home pregnancy test, LMP 8/52 ago, planned pregnancy, refer midwife
Current medication:	nil

Notes

Case B6.1 Information for the patient

You are Lucy Oliver, a 28-year old gym instructor who has a video consultation with the doctor today regarding abdominal pains.

ICE

- You are very concerned about this being a miscarriage as your sister suffered a miscarriage around this stage of pregnancy. You would like to be referred to the hospital to have a scan today; however, you promised you would pick your sister's children up from school so need to go and do this before going to the hospital.
- Your opening statement: 'I have been getting some stomach pains for the past 2 days so thought I better call in for advice'.

Background

- You are a 28-year old gym instructor, recently married and this is your first pregnancy. You are otherwise fit and well and your last period was 8 weeks ago.

Information divulged freely

- You have a constant sharp pain in the left side of your abdomen. These pains have been intermittent for the last 2 days but have been continuous since this morning.
- You feel nauseous and very tired, because the pain stopped you from sleeping last night.
- You have no bowel or bladder symptoms and have not noticed any vaginal bleeding.
- You do not smoke or drink any alcohol.

Information only divulged if specifically asked

- You have not been pregnant before and were taking the contraceptive pill previously, but stopped this to become pregnant.
- You have had no previous abdominal surgery.
- If asked specifically about sexually transmitted infections you admit you had a hospital admission when you were 18 with pelvic inflammatory disease which was due to *Chlamydia*.
- If the doctor suggests this may be an ectopic pregnancy you are surprised as you don't know much about these. You would like to know if this will affect the pregnancy and also if you will require surgery.
- If the doctor suggests you go directly to the Emergency Department at your local hospital you are certain you can't go as you need to pick up your sister's children. If the seriousness of the situation is made clear you will go to A&E and arrange for another friend to pick up the children. If you do not feel the potential outcome of a ruptured ectopic is made clear then you will continue to remain adamant that you will attend the hospital later.
- If the doctor does not suggest ectopic pregnancy but discusses another cause such as miscarriage, your questions about the pregnancy remain the same and you will accept next day referral for scan.

Results for the doctor

If asked, you tell the doctor that you have a home blood pressure monitor and this provides the following measurements:
- HR 110; BP: 95/69

Case B6.1 **Marking scheme for the observer**

https://pathways.nice.org.uk/pathways/ectopic-pregnancy-and-miscarriage
patient.info/doctor/ectopic-pregnancy-pro

Data gathering and diagnosis
☐ ☐ ☐ • Takes an appropriate pain history and considers risk factors in the history relevant to ectopic (i.e. previous chlamydial infection)
☐ ☐ ☐ • Considers ectopic pregnancy as a likely diagnosis
☐ ☐ ☐ • Attempts basic remote examination by asking if patient can check pulse/BP

Clinical management and medical complexity
☐ ☐ ☐ • Recognises an acutely unwell patient and arranges immediate hospital admission
☐ ☐ ☐ • Involves the patient in the decision and makes her aware of the risks of the situation
☐ ☐ ☐ • Can explain what investigations the hospital is likely to carry out and how an ectopic is usually managed
☐ ☐ ☐ • Discusses appropriate follow-up

Relating to others
☐ ☐ ☐ • Communicates risk effectively to the patient, including the risk of tubal rupture, heavy bleeding and even death if left undiagnosed
☐ ☐ ☐ • Responds to the patient's agenda but remains clear about the need for immediate assessment
☐ ☐ ☐ • Addresses patient's concerns and builds rapport

Group discussion point

We wrote this case over ten years ago for the first edition of our 'CSA Workbook'. In this scenario, our management was to arrange an ambulance to take this patient to hospital due to the concerns of a potential rupture of an ectopic pregnancy.

The NHS we now work within is a very different place. One of the more difficult aspects of being a GP today, is the moral injury we face working within an imperfect system.

It is now not uncommon for GPs to ask patients to make their own way to hospital, in the knowledge it will be quicker and safer than waiting hours for ambulance transport. Reports of GPs taking patients to hospital themselves are also not new (www.gponline.com/gps-forced-drive-patients-hospital-ambulance-delays-raise-risk-practices/article/1873994).

Discuss in your group any cases you have dealt with where you would ideally have arranged ambulance transfer, but had to compromise due to system pressures.

Consider the geography of your practice and how scenarios may differ in rural Cumbria versus central London.

Further reading

Medicolegal implications for GPs facing ambulance delays: https://nwssp.nhs.wales/ourservices/legal-risk-services/legal-risk-services-documents/general-medical-practice-indemnity-gmpi-docs/application-of-the-scheme-for-gmpi-where-there-are-ambulance-delays-in-the-community-final-pdf

Case B6.2 Information for the doctor

You are a locum GP carrying out telephone consultations in your afternoon surgery.	
Name:	George Smith
Age:	76
Past medical history:	COPD – last FEV_1 30% and SpO_2 93% Hypertension – last BP 140/90 Last consultation 3 months ago: • exacerbation of COPD – cough and SOB worsening past 3 days • usual ET 50 yards • manages activities of daily living at home alone • start antibiotics & steroids • review as required.
Current medication:	Seretide, Ventolin, ramipril

Notes

Case B6.2   Information for the patient

You are 76-year old George Smith. You called the surgery to request your usual antibiotics and steroids for your bad chest and the receptionist insisted on putting you down for a call from the doctor.

ICE

- You are apologetic and feel you are wasting the doctor's time. You have had COPD for a long time and usually get infections 3–4 times a year which are treated with antibiotics and steroids. You are not really concerned because you are used to your COPD now. You expect the doctor to give you the medications as normal.

Background

- Usually your COPD is pretty bad – you can't walk up a full flight of steps and can only walk to the front door without being short of breath.
- You live alone with your dog Digger. Your son lives nearby and he does your shopping. You usually get to the surgery on the number 10 bus which leaves from outside your house.
- You take your inhalers every day. You do not smoke any more, having stopped seven years ago.

Information divulged freely

- The past two days have been much worse though – you are SOB at rest and it has made sleeping, preparing your meals and dressing yourself very difficult.
- You have not had a cough.
- Your chest is tight – it does feel very uncomfortable and you have taken some paracetamol.

Information only divulged if specifically asked

- This is not following the pattern of your usual infections. Usually you would cough up lots of phlegm and your chest does not normally feel this tight.
- If asked specifically, your left leg has also been painful when you have been walking around the house. It did look swollen before you got dressed this morning.
- If the doctor mentions a hospital admission you adamantly refuse. There is no one to look after your dog Digger and when your late wife went into the hospital she never came out.
- If the doctor explains more about a potential blood clot you ask about treatment. When medication is mentioned you ask why you can't have this at home. When a scan is mentioned you ask why your son can't take you up for this scan tomorrow when he is off work.
- You fully understand what the doctor is telling you and are polite but insistent you will not attend. You will still refuse admission even if the possibility of death is mentioned.
- You will accept an in-person review or home visit to discuss this further. You would also accept interim anticoagulation therapy and referral for a scan in the day case unit tomorrow. You will also accept bloods or a chest X-ray if these are suggested. If a clot is never mentioned and a script for antibiotics and steroids is given, you are very pleased.

Results for the doctor

If asked, you tell the doctor that you have a home blood pressure monitor and oxygen sats monitor and these provide the following measurements:

- HR 110
- BP: 120/80
- SpO_2 88%

Case B6.2 **Marking scheme for the observer**

patient.info/doctor/pulmonary-embolism-pro
cks.nice.org.uk/topics/pulmonary-embolism

Data gathering and diagnosis

☐	☐	☐	• Gathers information from the patient about reason for calling the surgery
☐	☐	☐	• Considers differential diagnosis including possible PE. Avoids collusion with the patient to accept that this is 'just my bad chest again'
☐	☐	☐	• Calculates a 2-level PE Wells score using the information available
☐	☐	☐	• Social history important to obtain in this case
☐	☐	☐	• Attempts remote 'examination' asking the patient for vital signs

Clinical management and medical complexity

☐	☐	☐	• Discusses management of likely PE, including immediate referral to hospital
☐	☐	☐	• Respects patient autonomy and provides safety-netting when it becomes clear the patient will not attend hospital
☐	☐	☐	• Discusses anticoagulant therapy (oral vs. injectable) – further investigations recommended including CTPA
☐	☐	☐	• Assesses capacity in context of refusal of admission

Relating to others

☐	☐	☐	• Recognises the patient's agenda and preferences and elicits a social history to be able to put his problem into context
☐	☐	☐	• Develops good rapport with the patient
☐	☐	☐	• Communicates risk effectively to the patient
☐	☐	☐	• Gives clear explanations of possible diagnosis / prognosis and need for urgent treatment
☐	☐	☐	• Avoids jargon and has a good rapport and a positive attitude towards helping the patient

Case B6.3   Information for the doctor

In this case the Emergency Department nurse in a large teaching hospital has triaged a patient to your list who has been complaining of intermittent dizziness for several months. He was booked for a follow-up call with you before he left the Emergency Department.

You are the GP working in an out of hours centre based in a large teaching hospital.	
Name:	Arnold Layne
Age:	75
Past medical history:	Notes from triage nurse: Intermittent dizziness, not able to wait to see GP; booked follow-up call Examination: Alert, GCS 15; BP 109/60; HR 50 regular; SpO$_2$ 100% OA; examination otherwise unremarkable 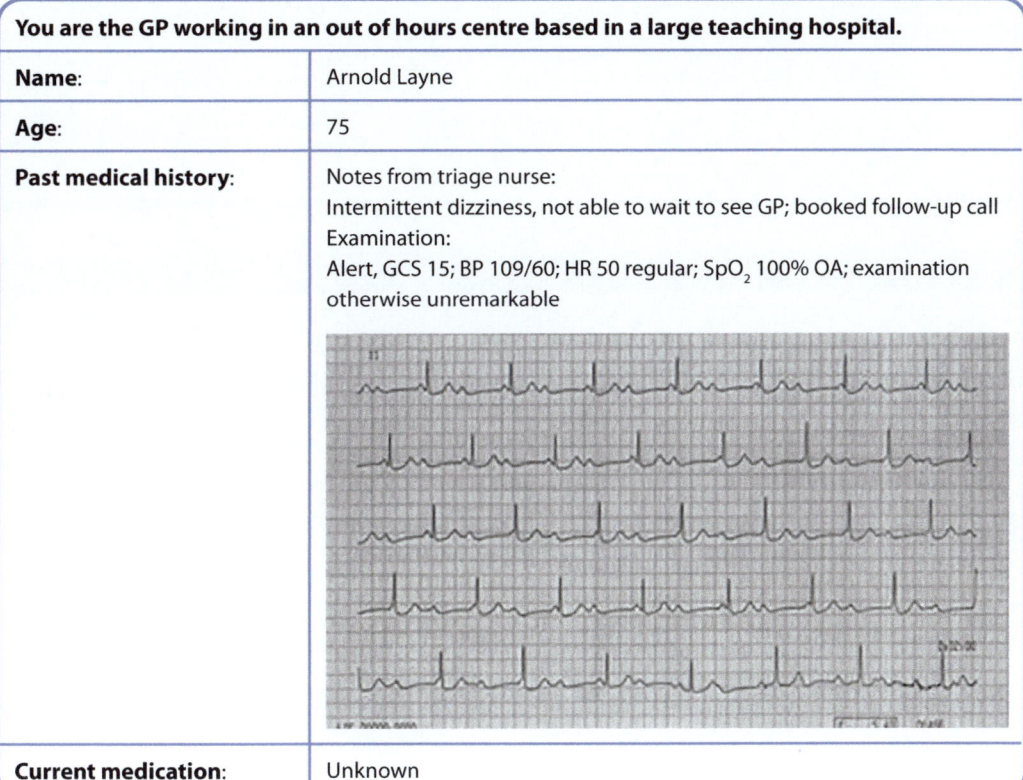
Current medication:	Unknown

Case B6.3   Information for the patient

You are Arnold Layne, a 75-year old man, who has been having intermittent dizziness for a couple of months. It was worse than usual tonight and you thought you were going to pass out which is why you decided to go to the Emergency Department.
Opening line: "The nurse said that you need to check the ECG they took"

ICE

- You don't want to waste anyone's time. You are well aware of the pressures on the NHS and, after speaking to the busy triage nurse, you are feeling guilty for going to the Emergency Department when you probably should have waited to see your own GP.
- You have been quite concerned about your symptoms and have booked a routine appointment to see your own GP, but that isn't until next week. This evening you really did feel quite bad which is why you came to hospital, but now you feel like you were making a fuss over nothing and will quite happily wait to see your own GP if the doctor thinks you are OK.

Background

- You consider yourself fit and well and have been enjoying your retirement with your wife. She was out with her book group tonight when this happened and she is with you at home now.
- You worked as a sommelier before you retired and still enjoy a glass of wine (a glass a day). You have never smoked.

Information divulged freely

- You have been feeling lightheaded on and off for nearly 2 months. You have not noticed any particular pattern to these symptoms and you have not passed out.
- You have an appointment to see your GP next week, but this evening while you were sitting watching the news, you suddenly felt very dizzy and lightheaded. You considered calling an ambulance because you felt like you were going to pass out, but this settled after a few minutes so you called a local taxi firm you are friendly with, and they brought you straight to hospital.
- You currently feel fine with no symptoms.
- You are very sorry for wasting anyone's time.

Information only divulged if specifically asked

- You have a list of your current medications with you and will describe this to the doctor if asked (aspirin 75 mg od; simvastatin 40 mg on; bisoprolol 2.5 mg od; ramipril 5 mg od).
- You had a 'mild heart attack' about a year ago and were started on these medications after this. You have had no problems since then.
- You have not experienced any chest pain or palpitations during these episodes, but you have sometimes felt short of breath and you did feel breathless earlier today when you were watching the news.
- You have been otherwise well and if the doctor asks about any other symptoms you will deny any other problems. You have had plenty to eat and drink today and have taken your medications as normal – you are due your evening medications now and if the doctor asks, you wonder if you should take them (your simvastatin and bisoprolol are due).

- You expect the doctor to ask you to see your GP next week and you would be happy with that plan. If the doctor tells you that you should go back to the Emergency Department you will be very surprised and insist that you have already been there and they ruled out anything serious. You feel sure you were wasting the time of the emergency team and are very reluctant to go back there, especially if the GP seems unsure. If the reasons behind this decision are explained then you will eventually feel reassured and you will feel better that you haven't been a time waster and you will agree to go. If the doctor is uncertain then you will remain reluctant to be admitted and opt to follow up with your own GP next week.

Case B6.3 Marking scheme for the observer

patient.info/doctor/bradycardia
Bradyarrhythmia guidance from the Resuscitation Council: www.resus.org.uk/pages/periarst.pdf

Data gathering and diagnosis

☐	☐	☐	• Takes a detailed history and elicits his previous MI and current medications
☐	☐	☐	• Identifies the presence of complete heart block on the ECG or seeks an opinion on it from a colleague
☐	☐	☐	• Asks about adverse signs (chest pain; breathlessness; dizziness) and recognises that the patient has been experiencing these
☐	☐	☐	• Makes a fresh, unbiased assessment and avoids being falsely reassured that the patient has already been seen in the Emergency Department. Remains open to the possibility of a potentially life-threatening diagnosis for the symptoms

Clinical management and medical complexity

☐	☐	☐	• Recognises that the patient has an abnormal heart rhythm which requires further inpatient assessment
☐	☐	☐	• Arranges for transfer to the Emergency Department for monitoring and cardiology review
☐	☐	☐	• Is aware that the patient is taking a beta-blocker which could be contributing to the bradycardia and ensures that the patient doesn't take his evening dose of bisoprolol
☐	☐	☐	• Displays clinical confidence and shows a willingness to pursue a management plan that may differ from that initiated by colleagues

Relating to others

☐	☐	☐	• Discusses the situation and management plan openly with the patient and tactfully addresses any questions the patient may ask regarding why he is going back to the Emergency Department when he was re-directed from there earlier
☐	☐	☐	• Avoids being disparaging towards colleagues but also shows confidence in their own diagnostic skills
☐	☐	☐	• Is able to reassure the patient that he is not a 'time waster'
☐	☐	☐	• Communicates risk to the patient while maintaining an awareness of his preferences

---

Further reading

Useful ECG articles: patient.info/doctor/ecg-identification-of-conduction-disorders

Case B6.4 Information for the doctor

In this case you are a GP registrar in an emergency surgery and the patient has a video call.	
Name:	James Wells (Dr)
Age:	68
Past medical history:	Nil
Current medication:	Nil
Last consultation:	2 days ago: cellulitis left leg after scratching leg whilst gardening. Start flucloxacillin 500 mg qds for 7 days and review if not improving or if cellulitis is spreading

Notes

Case B6.4 Information for the patient

You are James Wells, a retired obstetrician, who has called for review as the cellulitis on your leg is getting worse. Your opening line is: "Just a quick one doc, I need some different antibiotics for my cellulitis and then I'll be out of your hair".

ICE

- You know exactly what you want, which is different antibiotics. You must be resistant to these ones as your cellulitis is spreading past the line the last doctor drew.
- You are not concerned. You know what cellulitis is and just want it treated so you can get back to your garden.
- You expect the doctor to do exactly what you want since you are a trained doctor too and you are sure your plan is the best one.

Background

- You live with your wife; your three grown-up children all live away.
- You retired about 5 years ago having worked in obstetrics for 30 years.
- You don't smoke but drink around 3 bottles of wine a week.
- You are a keen traveller and are off on holiday to Greece in 1 week.

Information divulged freely

- You are clear from the start of the consultation that you simply want new antibiotics. If the doctor asks more specific questions you try to distract them with comments like "Look I know how busy you guys are these days, so just sort the script and I'll be gone". You are not angry at the doctor but more dismissive of any concerns there is anything more serious wrong.
- You are otherwise fit and well with no regular medications or medical conditions and you rarely come to see the GP.

Information only divulged if specifically asked:

- If specifically asked and after a large sigh, you will admit you haven't been feeling all that well but you do have cellulitis so you expected that.
- Only if asked specifically will you admit to the following symptoms: nausea, reduced appetite (if pushed, you admit you've only had 2 cups of water yesterday and nothing yet today, you have noticed your urine is darker and you have gone less often – you last passed urine this morning), dizziness on standing, lethargy, fever and rigors last night.
- The rash has extended past the line the last GP drew and is now extending up into your groin.
- You have had no coryzal symptoms or shortness of breath, no headache or new rash elsewhere, you have no abdominal pain, no diarrhoea or vomiting and no symptoms suggestive of a urinary infection.
- If the GP mentions sepsis you laugh and say: "Just because it's all over the news doesn't mean every patient has it".
- If further attempts to explain are seen as patronising you will simply thank the doctor and end the call, saying you will call your friend at a nearby surgery to get him to write a script.

- If the GP advises you on the latest guidelines for cellulitis and sepsis and explains that your symptoms warrant further treatment then you will reluctantly agree that you may need IV antibiotics.
- If the GP discusses hospital referral you are very against this as it is a 40 minute drive away and you know how long waiting times are in your local emergency department. You have heard about ambulatory care and the possibility of having IV treatments at home or elsewhere in the community and you would be willing to do this. If the GP can offer you the option of blood tests and IV treatment more locally then you are pleased and will agree to this plan. You will also accept an in-person review but would still like to know what the options will be at this review.
- If the GP insists on hospital referral you are very reluctant but if you feel the doctor explains the reasons why without sounding patronising and gives what you feel to be "professional courtesy" then you will agree.

Results for the doctor

If asked, you have your own blood pressure monitor, pulse oximeter and thermometer at home, with the following results:

- Temp 38.9°C
- HR 110 regular
- BP 100/60
- SpO_2 98%

Case B6.4 Marking scheme for the observer

The NICE Clinical Knowledge Summary on Acute cellulitis (https://cks.nice.org.uk/cellulitis-acute) and the NICE Quality Standard for Sepsis (cks.nice.org.uk/topics/sepsis) can be read in conjunction with this case.

The smartphone app 'microguide' is available to download and provides antibiotic guidelines for all NHS localities: www.microguide.eu

			Data gathering and diagnosis
☐	☐	☐	• Manages to take a good history in a reluctant patient (previous diagnosis of cellulitis but worsening despite 2 days of antibiotics; elicits spreading erythema, fever with rigors and poor urine output) and briefly considers alternative sources of infection
☐	☐	☐	• Asks the patient if they can help by providing measurement of temperature, heart rate, blood pressure and oxygen saturations
☐	☐	☐	• Uses a risk stratification tool to aid recognition of sepsis. Recognises the presence of several 'amber flags' in this patient and notes deterioration despite already taking oral antibiotics (could also use https://sepsistrust.org/wp-content/uploads/2018/06/GP-adult-NICE-Final-2.pdf)
			Clinical management and medical complexity
☐	☐	☐	• Is able to advise on management of early sepsis, i.e. hospital referral / ambulatory care, referral for blood tests and IV antibiotics today
☐	☐	☐	• Is able to advise on the reasons IV rather than oral antibiotics are recommended. In this case symptoms have worsened and he has developed systemic symptoms
☐	☐	☐	• Highlights that sepsis is a severe condition which can develop quickly and may be life-threatening. The Eron Classification system is suggested by NICE to guide admission and treatment decisions for cellulitis: app.pulsenotes.com/medicine/infectious-diseases/notes/cellulitis#
☐	☐	☐	• Is able to discuss alternative options with the patient and advise on local services such as IV antibiotics in the community or ambulatory care, but in view of the presence of 'amber flags' and the fact he has already deteriorated, continues to advise a hospital assessment where access to immediate blood testing and treatment will be available

Relating to others

☐	☐	☐	• Creates rapport with patient by discussing the case in a professional manner
☐	☐	☐	• Identifies the patient's agenda early on and refers back to this agenda often (wants alternative oral antibiotics and nothing more)
☐	☐	☐	• Is able to explain sepsis in a clear way without appearing patronising to another healthcare professional
☐	☐	☐	• Considers showing the patient the latest guidance on both cellulitis and sepsis to demonstrate the thinking behind the management decision
☐	☐	☐	• Acknowledges the patient's medical background but avoids colluding with the patient by prescribing alternative antibiotics without adequately exploring the history; comes to a shared management plan

Case B6.5 Information for the doctor

In this case you are a doctor in the on-call surgery undertaking a video consultation.	
Name:	Derek Ruffalo
Age:	61
Past medical history:	nil
Current medication:	nil

Notes

Case B6.5 Information for the patient

You are Derek Ruffalo, a 61-year old taxi driver who has booked an emergency video call with the doctor today to see about your painful foot.

ICE

- You never contact the doctor and you want them to sort this pain out pronto!

Background

- You have worked for a local taxi firm for the past 5 years, mainly on the night shift. Your wife is a healthcare assistant in a nursing home and also tends to work night shifts. You have no children but do have 2 dogs. You never go to the doctors so consider yourself quite healthy.

Information divulged freely

- You have had pain in your left foot since yesterday. You took the dogs for a walk the day before, which is usually your wife Jean's job. You don't remember injuring the foot, but it's possible you might have strained it during the walk.
- The pain is definitely getting worse rather than better and paracetamol hasn't worked. You'd like something stronger because you couldn't sleep last night. You are on your days off and need to get some sleep before your night shift tomorrow.
- You work night shifts on the taxis so you only drink on your days off, and even then you have one or two shots of whisky.
- You do tend to drink a lot of Coke when you are at work. You quit smoking a few years ago after Jean's sister died from lung cancer, and since then you have put some weight on. You tend to eat crisps and chocolate in the cab when you are waiting for a job.
- You don't do much exercise but you do take the dogs out for a walk on your days off – Jean takes them the rest of the week.
- You don't like taking medicines and you are proud of the fact you never come to the doctors.

Information only divulged if specifically asked

- You have never had anything like this before, and there is no pain in any of your other joints.
- You have had no fever and feel well in yourself.
- If the doctor mentions gout then you remember that your dad used to suffer with gout, but you do have some questions about what it actually is.
- You are happy to take anything the doctor can recommend if it is going to get rid of this pain. You have never had any problems taking ibuprofen before and don't suffer with any stomach problems.
- If the doctor mentions taking medicines to prevent future attacks you are not keen. You think this is a one-off and shouldn't happen again.
- If the doctor mentions changes to your lifestyle you will initially get a little defensive. You work night shifts and have no time to eat as well as you should and you definitely have no time for exercise. You stopped smoking – what more does the doctor want?!
- If the doctor discusses the risk of cardiovascular problems in the future and the link with gout and sensitively mentions your blood pressure, you will start to listen.

- If the doctor asks you what you think you could improve in your lifestyle rather than dictating to you, you will concede that you do eat a lot of 'rubbish' when you are at work and you could cut down on the amount of Coke you drink. You always feel tired doing night shifts, but you do feel better when you take the dogs out, so you could do that a bit more often. Jean keeps telling you to lose some weight and you know you should really.
- You will reluctantly agree to an appointment to have blood tests if the doctor mentions it, and you will agree to come back for the results and to have your blood pressure checked at the surgery.

Results for the doctor

The patient has a blood pressure monitor and knows his height and weight, so reports the following results if asked:

- BP 148/95
- BMI 27
- Pulse 65
- The patient is also happy to show the doctor the affected foot and lower leg: left 1st MTPJ – erythematous and mild swelling noted. Nil sign of cellulitis / ascending infection

Case B6.5 Marking scheme for the observer

patient.info/doctor/gout-pro
https://cks.nice.org.uk/gout

Data gathering and diagnosis

☐	☐	☐	• Elicits history suggestive of gout, considers differential diagnosis of septic arthritis
☐	☐	☐	• Asks about lifestyle – alcohol, fizzy drinks, weight / exercise
☐	☐	☐	• Asks about any contraindications to NSAID use
☐	☐	☐	• Asks about BP, BMI and also asks the patient to video the affected foot and lower leg

Clinical management and medical complexity

☐	☐	☐	• Discusses clinical diagnosis of gout, safety-nets to exclude septic arthritis, suggests arranging a separate appointment for blood tests including FBC, U&E, glucose/HbA1c/lipids. (Urate can be done but note this has no value in the diagnosis of gout, only when decision made to treat with urate-lowering drugs)
☐	☐	☐	• Discusses treatments of acute gout (NSAIDs, colchicine, prednisolone) including rest, elevation, ice
☐	☐	☐	• Addresses non-drug management – weight loss, restricting purine-rich foods / alcohol / fizzy drinks
☐	☐	☐	• Discusses role of urate-lowering drugs
☐	☐	☐	• Recognises the link between gout and metabolic syndrome and considers a cardiovascular / diabetes risk assessment. Recognises high BP and organises follow-up appointment to review

Relating to others

☐	☐	☐	• Discusses gout and its treatment in a jargon-free way
☐	☐	☐	• Explores the patient's health beliefs and gently communicates risk of cardiovascular complications with current lifestyle
☐	☐	☐	• Enhances patient autonomy by discussing options and coming to shared management plan
☐	☐	☐	• Elicits social information to place problem in context and help the patient more effectively

357

B7.1

Health disadvantages and vulnerabilities, including veterans, mental capacity, safeguarding, and communication difficulties

Case B7.1 Information for the doctor

In this case you are a GP Registrar in surgery taking video consultations.	
Name:	Kemi Ademola
Age:	4 months old
Past medical history:	Born by vaginal delivery. No complications.
Current medication:	Paracetamol prn
	3 recent discharge summaries from A&E:
	Last month – brief discharge summary from A&E – attended with mum, cut on left cheek following an accidental fall from bed. Steristrips applied. Reassured.
	2 weeks ago – seen with ?father, who appears drunk and distressed. Says he was attacked by his friend on the street and had to hold Kemi tight in his arms just to protect her from the attacker. Police involved. O/E child well, alert. Obs stable. Small bruise noted on right forearm. Reviewed by Paeds – spoken to family. Sent home with paracetamol.
	2 days ago – attended with mother with ?bruise on back – couldn't wait. Self-discharged.

Notes

359

B7.1

Health disadvantages and vulnerabilities, including veterans, mental capacity, safeguarding, and communication difficulties

Case B7.1   Information for the patient

You are Shola Ademola, a 20-year old mother of 4-month old Kemi. You called up to get some paracetamol for Kemi's bruise on her back. Your daughter is with your partner at the moment and they are out of the house.

ICE

- You called to get some painkillers for your daughter. Your daughter is well but you noticed some bruising on her back a few days ago and she seems more miserable and tearful. You thought paracetamol might work.
- Deep down you are terrified that your partner might do something awful. He is back on heroin and is verbally abusive to you. He smashed the window in the kitchen this morning.

Background

- You live with your current partner Emmanuel and your daughter in his home. You met him 3 months ago and he suggested you should move in to his beautiful house. You didn't hesitate and everything was great until 1 month ago.
- You love him and he is a good guy, but you weren't aware of his previous drug problems.
- You are not in touch with Kemi's real dad.
- You are close to your mum but she lives in Nigeria. You try to speak every week on the phone; however, she is getting married soon and is very busy with organising the wedding.

Information divulged freely

- You ran out of paracetamol and went to A&E 2 days ago. You couldn't wait too long because Emmanuel was getting impatient and wanted you to come back home.
- You believe Emmanuel cares about you but, unfortunately, his behaviour significantly changed since he started taking drugs. You want him to change and get better because you love him.
- He seems to love Kemi too, but he is not very attached to her.

Information only divulged if specifically asked

- Emmanuel seems to be OK with your daughter but a few weeks ago you noticed that his friends made some funny comments about Kemi when she was asleep. They also took her to the pub once without your permission and she was very unsettled when they came home, which made you very angry.
- You are getting more worried about your partner's impulsive behaviour. He never physically attacked you but you are absolutely terrified something might happen to you and your child if you won't bring home money for his drugs. He asked you to get some cash sent over from your mother otherwise 'he'll be very disappointed'. You are not sure what he meant, but you realised that you and your daughter might be in danger and you don't know what to do and are terrified to go back home.
- If the doctor is empathetic and asks in a sensitive way about your concerns and Kemi's safety you'd start crying and admit that you suspect Emmanuel might have injured your baby. You can't prove it though, because you didn't see it happen, and you don't want to lose Emmanuel. You feel like you are constantly failing.

B7.1

Health disadvantages and vulnerabilities, including veterans, mental capacity, safeguarding, and communication difficulties

- If the doctor is non-judgmental and caring, and suggests it would be reasonable to involve the police due to safety concerns, you'd agree.
- If the doctor is judgmental and makes assumptions you'd absolutely disagree with the police involvement, start shouting and end the call.
- If the doctor remains understanding and explains in a sensitive manner that there are concerns about the safety of your child and that perhaps Kemi's bruises might be related to possible physical abuse, you'd agree and realise you should have called sooner.
- If the doctor also clearly explains that it is very important to make sure that your child is transferred to a place of safety and he/she is obliged to breach confidentiality and contact social care workers and healthcare professionals immediately until more facts and history could be obtained, you'd cry but will cooperate, because you understand this is the right thing to do.
- You are willing to accept a call back later on after the GP has discussed this with the safeguarding lead, if this is offered.
- If the doctor doesn't clearly explain reasons for contacting social workers and healthcare professionals you will start shouting, and if the doctor becomes confrontational you will end the call. However, if the doctor remains calm and addresses your concerns, you will also calm down and cooperate.
- Your partner will be back around lunchtime and then he will go to work, so you would be able to bring Kemi to the surgery later this afternoon or take her to the paediatric ward if this is offered. If not, you understand you need to go to a friend's house and wait for the social worker to call.

361

B7.1

Health disadvantages and vulnerabilities, including veterans, mental capacity, safeguarding, and communication difficulties

Case B7.1 **Marking scheme for the observer**

https://patient.info/doctor/safeguarding-children-how-to-recognise-abuse-or-a-child-at-risk
https://patient.info/doctor/safeguarding-children-referral-and-management-of-an-abused-
or-at-risk-child

Data gathering and diagnosis

☐	☐	☐	• Identifies patient's agenda
☐	☐	☐	• Elicits mum's concerns and asks specific questions about safety of both mum and Kemi
☐	☐	☐	• Identifies risks to a child and suspects child maltreatment (recurrent A&E attendance, recent cut, bruising in a child who is not independently mobile)
☐	☐	☐	• Identifies and thinks about concerns in the previous medical records

Clinical management and medical complexity

☐	☐	☐	• Discusses plan of action with senior colleague, practice lead for safeguarding or named professional
☐	☐	☐	• Clearly identifies reasons for both breaching confidentiality and contacting social care workers and healthcare professionals
☐	☐	☐	• Offers police involvement in order to maintain mum's and child's safety
☐	☐	☐	• Arranges home visit and explains to mum reasons for possible admission and review on paediatric ward until safeguarding procedures are in place
☐	☐	☐	• Offers supportive services (e.g. domestic violence support; signposts to drug and alcohol input for partner)

Relating to others

☐	☐	☐	• Picks up on cues to recognise mum's concerns and understands the complexity of the situation
☐	☐	☐	• Has a non-judgmental approach
☐	☐	☐	• Avoids confrontational approach and remains supportive and caring despite patient's questioning and possible anger
☐	☐	☐	• Checks for understanding and involves the patient in the decision making

363

B7.2

Health disadvantages and vulnerabilities, including veterans, mental capacity, safeguarding, and communication difficulties

Case B7.2 Information for the doctor

In this case you are a doctor in surgery. Abby has a video call booked to speak to you with her older sister Hayley. The computer system is down today so you don't have access to her previous records.

Name:	Abby Fitzgerald
Age:	24
Past medical history:	Records not available but note from reception staff who know her, to tell you she has Down's syndrome and usually comes with her sister for support.
Current medication:	Nil

Notes

365

B7.2

Health disadvantages and vulnerabilities, including veterans, mental capacity, safeguarding, and communication difficulties

Case B7.2 Information for the patient

(for 2 actors if possible)

You are Abby Fitzgerald, 24. You have called the surgery today with your older sister Hayley, who wants you to talk to the doctor about not having a baby. You feel quite shy talking to the doctor because you have never met before, so your sister does most of the talking.

ICE

- Abby – You never thought about having a baby before Hayley talked about it, you feel a bit scared about the thought of having one. You're also a bit scared of an injection.
- Hayley – You have always been protective of your sister, and you are concerned she is starting to be sexually active and might get pregnant. You want to do what is best for your sister, and you hope the doctor will be able to give her the contraceptive injection.

Background

- Abby has Down's syndrome with mild–moderate learning difficulties and lives at home with her mum and sister Hayley.
- Abby attends daycare 3 times a week and does a few hours of voluntary work one day a week in a charity shop where she sorts through donated clothing.
- Abby has been friends with Callum for many years – he is a few years younger than her and also attends her daycare centre. He came over for dinner a few weeks ago and your mum found them kissing each other in Abby's bedroom.

Information divulged freely (Hayley)

Hayley does most of the talking and Abby only volunteers information if specifically asked. Hayley tells you:

- She is worried that Abby doesn't really understand that having sex can result in pregnancy, and she was hoping the doctor can talk to her about contraception.
- She doesn't think she will be able to remember to take the pill every day, and she doesn't like swallowing pills anyway.
- If the doctor mentions the implant or a coil, you are sure that Abby will not tolerate the procedure. She had the flu jab recently and tolerated it well, although she was a little scared about it beforehand.
- Abby has periods every month and is on her period at the moment. She has learnt to manage them well. She does seem to suffer with PMT and becomes quite withdrawn and tearful the week before her period.
- She takes no regular medication and is fairly well, although she does suffer with recurrent ear and sinus infections.
- She doesn't smoke and has no history of migraine / VTE / liver problems. There is no family history of cancer.
- The family trust Callum. He has autism and is very protective of Abby. There are no concerns that she is being taken advantage of.
- You have asked Abby if she has had sex and you don't think she has. You are a little embarrassed to talk about it, but when she was younger she used to masturbate in front of

other people, but you taught her that this is not appropriate behaviour. You have talked a little bit about 'where babies come from' and you know this is something she is not ready for.

Information only divulged if specifically asked (Abby)

- Abby – You have a boyfriend called Callum. You are shy and giggle to talk about it but you do kiss each other. You know that touching your private parts is something which you shouldn't do around other people. You haven't done that in front of Callum.
- You don't like taking pills. When you had an ear infection the pills you had to take made you feel sick.
- You don't want an injection or anything that hurts. If your sister reminds you about the flu injection you had recently, you remember it wasn't too bad. If the doctor is nice and explains things gently then you might feel OK about having an injection every few months. You don't want to have a baby because they cry all the time and are too loud.
- If the doctor talks about what is best for you without including you, you will feel bad and not agree with anything they suggest.
- If they talk too much about the coil/implant you will get scared. If they don't pick up on the fact you do not want this and keep talking about it you will start to cry.

B7.2

Health disadvantages and vulnerabilities, including veterans, mental capacity, safeguarding, and communication difficulties

Case B7.2 Marking scheme for the observer

patient.info/doctor/contraception-and-special-groups
patient.info/doctor/general-learning-disability

Data gathering and diagnosis

☐	☐	☐	• Elicits reasons for the call from both the patient and her sister (does not ignore Abby)
☐	☐	☐	• Finds out what the patient understands about sex and pregnancy
☐	☐	☐	• Takes a sexual and gynaecological history
☐	☐	☐	• Recognises Abby is a vulnerable adult and sensitively enquires if the family have any concerns around her relationship

Clinical management and medical complexity

☐	☐	☐	• Assesses patient's capacity to make an informed decision relating to contraception and avoids making immediate assumptions
☐	☐	☐	• Uses accessible information / visual aids (FPA produces information leaflets for patients with LD: www.fpa.org.uk/product/contraception-a-guide-for-people-with-learning-disabilities) to aid understanding, and discusses all options, not just the injection
☐	☐	☐	• Strikes a balance between empowerment and protection – LARC methods may be appropriate for some patients with LD as compliance is better, but discusses alternatives

Relating to others

☐	☐	☐	• Gives patient opportunity to make her own informed decision
☐	☐	☐	• Communicates at a slow pace and repeats information as needed to ensure understanding
☐	☐	☐	• Makes use of the patient's sister as a familiar face to support the patient during the consultation
☐	☐	☐	• Remains non-judgmental and listens to the concerns and expectations of both the patient and her sister

369

B7.3

Health disadvantages and vulnerabilities, including veterans, mental capacity, safeguarding, and communication difficulties

Case B7.3 Information for the doctor

In this case you are a GP registrar taking telephone consultations.	
Name:	Jude Damon
Age:	21
Past medical history:	Down's syndrome; severe learning difficulties; ASD surgically repaired
Current medication:	None
Blood results:	**1 year ago:** TSH 7.2, T4/T3 normal FBC normal U&Es, LFTs normal **Actions:** Repeat in one year (letter sent to patient last week requesting she book for blood tests and annual review)
Special notes:	Next of kin: Kat Damon (aunt) Patient does not have capacity to make decisions about her care (last assessed 1 year ago) Consent has been given to discuss all aspects of care with carers from the home

Notes

371

B7.3

Health disadvantages and vulnerabilities, including veterans, mental capacity, safeguarding, and communication difficulties

Case B7.3 Information for the patient

You are Svetla, the carer looking after Jude at her residential home. You have a letter from the surgery saying Jude is due some blood tests but she found it very distressing last year so you have phoned to discuss if she really needs to have them.

ICE

- You are aware the blood tests are checking for a thyroid condition but aren't really sure if this is a serious condition or not.
- You are worried the blood tests will cause Jude upset – last time she found them very painful, she screamed and cried for hours afterwards and even 2 days after she was still complaining her arm was sore.
- You hope the GP says the blood tests can be delayed or maybe are not needed at all to save the problems she had last year.

Background

- Jude has lived in the residential home for 5 years and you have looked after her all this time. She has severe learning difficulties but can communicate her needs to you. She is usually physically well.
- Her parents died 5 years ago which is why she now lives in the care home as her aunt is elderly and unable to take care of her. She does not see her aunt often but you know her aunt is keen to be kept in the loop about Jude's care.

Information divulged freely

- Jude is physically well.
- When you have asked Jude about having the blood tests taken she shakes her head and says "No".

Information only divulged if specifically asked

- Jude has had no change in weight, she is regularly weighed at the home and recently was 70 kg which is the same as 2 months ago.
- She doesn't complain of being cold. She has her bowels open regularly with no constipation. She has no complaints of dry skin, thinning hair or tiredness.
- She is eating and drinking well and has had no change in her behaviour.
- She was seen last year by a GP who visits the residential home and he asked her a lot of questions before telling the staff Jude did not have capacity to make her own decisions. You are not sure if this was in relation to having blood tests taken. She has not been seen since regarding this.
- If you ask Jude if she knows why she needs the blood tests she can't tell you. If you explain it's for a thyroid test she doesn't seem to understand this but continues to shake her head and say "No".
- If the doctor agrees to delay or cancel the blood tests you are pleased but want to know if it's dangerous to do so; you ask what harm it can do to miss this thyroid condition.

- If the doctor says the tests need to be done you do agree to bring her in but ask if there is anything you can give to help with the pain. You agree if local anaesthetic cream is offered and ask how / when to apply it before the tests.
- If the doctor requests to see Jude him / her self to assess capacity and / or do the bloods in her own environment, you agree to this.

373

B7.3

Health disadvantages and vulnerabilities, including veterans, mental capacity, safeguarding, and communication difficulties

Case B7.3 Marking scheme for the observer

patient.info/doctor/general-learning-disability
patient.info/doctor/subclinical-hypothyroidism
patient.info/doctor/telephone-consultations

Data gathering and diagnosis

☐	☐	☐	• Takes a social history including checking consent to discuss medical records
☐	☐	☐	• Enquires about what the patient understands and how she communicates with the staff normally
☐	☐	☐	• Asks about symptoms of thyroid disease and recognises last year's results were borderline

Clinical management and medical complexity

☐	☐	☐	• Is aware of the possible progression of subclinical hypothyroidism and is able to explain this to the staff member along with possible risks of untreated hypothyroidism, including worsening symptoms of hypothyroidism, high cholesterol leading to CVD and depression
☐	☐	☐	• Recognises the assessment of capacity carried out 1 year ago was not in relation to the blood tests and capacity should be reassessed in this situation
☐	☐	☐	• Is able to discuss use of local anaesthetic cream and other methods to reduce the stress caused by blood tests (such as home visit; longer appointment times; having trusted people present)
☐	☐	☐	• Appreciates the importance of having a face-to-face review with the patient for their annual review and makes arrangements for this to take place

Relating to others

☐	☐	☐	• Creates rapport with staff member
☐	☐	☐	• Is sensitive to staff member's concern about the blood tests and about the patient's previous distress, but avoids colluding with Svetla to cancel the blood tests
☐	☐	☐	• Explains clearly the reasons for the investigations and annual review and reaches a mutually acceptable plan to try to make the experience as tolerable as possible for Jude

375

B7.4

Health disadvantages and vulnerabilities, including veterans, mental capacity, safeguarding, and communication difficulties

Case B7.4 Information for the doctor

In this case you are a GP registrar taking video calls.	
Name:	Reece Hewitson (his mum Fiona will be calling on his behalf)
Age:	21
Past medical history:	Autistic spectrum disorder – non-verbal Severe learning difficulties
Current medication:	Nil

Notes

377

B7.4

Health disadvantages and vulnerabilities, including veterans, mental capacity, safeguarding, and communication difficulties

Case B7.4   Information for the patient

You are Reece's mum Fiona and have called today with concerns about some bruising on Reece's arm.

ICE

- You wonder if these bruises are caused by abuse from his carers and are obviously concerned what to do next.
- You haven't approached the care home directly because you are worried that if you are wrong, Reece may lose his place at the home.

Background

- You live at home with your husband John. Reece lives in residential care during the week but often comes home for the weekend. He has lived in his current residential home for 5 years. It is the closest home to your house which means you can see Reece on your way home from work most weekdays.
- You work as a receptionist in a private dental surgery.

Information divulged freely

- You picked up Reece from his residential home on Friday and felt over the weekend he seemed a bit distant. Although he does not speak he usually gestures if he wants food or drink and looks when you speak to him. Instead he just watched his tablet and ate very little, even of his favourite foods.
- When you helped him get undressed for his bath you noticed he had bruising on his upper arms. You are concerned they look like someone had grabbed him and squeezed him hard. These bruises were not there the previous Sunday.
- When you asked Reece about the bruises he ignored you but when you touched his arms he flinched.
- You have kept him home today and called in sick to work. You want the doctor to tell you if the bruises are from being squeezed or not and advice as to what to do next.

Information only divulged if specifically asked

- Reece was born at term with no complications. He was slow to smile and never really looked at adults or other children when he was young. When he didn't start speaking at 1 you became concerned and his behaviour became increasingly withdrawn and noticeably very different to others his age. He was referred for assessment at age 3 and received the diagnosis of ASD.
- Reece doesn't speak but is able to gesture and use non-verbal communication to make what he wants known.
- Reece goes into residential care during the week, to allow you to continue to work. You were also struggling with his behaviour as he can become aggressive towards you.
- You are aware Reece does have behavioural issues but the home have never told you he has needed restraining before. There was nothing reported to you last week about his behaviour.
- You have not previously had any concerns about the home. You are aware they do have a high staff turnover and the current manager only started a few months ago.
- You have never noted any bruising before.

- Reece does not bruise easily. There is no blood in his stool or urine. He is otherwise well.
- If the doctor suggests you speak to the manager about his bruises you would like advice on how to approach this without offending them. You also want to know what to do if they say they don't know what caused the bruising.
- If the doctor discusses a safeguarding referral or suggests informing social services you are reluctant as you don't want the home to "get in trouble". If the doctor advises that they will have to inform social services, but explains this is important to protect not just Reece but the other residents, you do understand and agree.
- If the doctor advises they will ring social services now, you agree. You ask what they advise with regards to sending Reece back to the home whilst the investigation is ongoing. You feel more comfortable if he stays with you until this is resolved.

B7.4

Health disadvantages and vulnerabilities, including veterans, mental capacity, safeguarding, and communication difficulties

Case B7.4 Marking scheme for the observer

Safeguarding training is mandatory for NHS staff and e-Learning for Healthcare offers safeguarding modules. NHS England have provided the following summary which can be used in conjunction with this case:

www.england.nhs.uk/south/wp-content/uploads/sites/6/2016/04/1085-nhs-leaflet-accesible-copy.pdf

Data gathering and diagnosis

☐	☐	☐	• Takes a history from mum of recent events including her current views on the residential care home
☐	☐	☐	• Asks about Reece's usual behaviour and identifies that mum feels there has been a recent change
☐	☐	☐	• Establishes a social history and enquires who else is involved in Reece's care
☐	☐	☐	• Considers the possibility of medical causes for easy bruising and establishes if this has happened before or if there is any bleeding from elsewhere; arranges an in-person review

Clinical management and medical complexity

☐	☐	☐	• Considers the possibility of physical abuse in this case
☐	☐	☐	• Discusses a referral to social services in order to fully investigate this incident and safeguard Reece and the other residents
☐	☐	☐	• Comes to an agreement with mum about discussing the referral with the home. Suggests mum shares her concerns with the residential home in an open manner by asking the manager if they are aware of any incidents. Offers to speak to the manager regarding the reasons for the referral
☐	☐	☐	• Considers patient safety and how the family feel about him returning to the home while this is being investigated
☐	☐	☐	• Considers the physical health of Reece and ensures he is up to date with his annual health check

Relating to others

☐	☐	☐	• Creates rapport
☐	☐	☐	• Empathises with mum over her concerns and understands she is worried about offending the residential home staff
☐	☐	☐	• Sensitively discusses social services referral even though mum is reluctant

381

B7.5

Health disadvantages and vulnerabilities, including veterans, mental capacity, safeguarding, and communication difficulties

Case B7.5 Information for the doctor

In this case you are a GP registrar in a routine morning surgery taking video calls.	
Name:	Robert Edwards (with mum Elizabeth Edwards)
Age:	42
Past medical history:	Down's syndrome, moderate learning disability
Current medication:	None
Last consultation:	
Annual review:	U&Es, LFTs, FBC, TSH normal HbA1c 44 BMI 30 BP: 136/86
Action:	see GP

Notes

383

B7.5

Health disadvantages and vulnerabilities, including veterans, mental capacity, safeguarding, and communication difficulties

Case B7.5   Information for the patient

You are Robert and Elizabeth Edwards, a 42-year old man and his 73-year old mum, who have been asked to make a GP appointment following Robert's annual review. Robert will not say much to the doctor today because he is very shy and so instead his mum will do most of the talking for him.

ICE

- You weren't told on the phone why you needed a call with the doctor but the nurse did comment at your review appointment that Robert's weight was high, so you presume the doctor wants to discuss this.
- You know that Robert has been gaining weight but you struggle to say no to him. He has a sweet tooth and loves cakes.
- Neither of you is concerned about his weight gain – he's very tall so surely he is "allowed" to weigh more?
- You expect to be given the usual lecture on his diet and told to come back next year.

Background

- You live together in a two-bedroom house – your husband died two years ago from a heart attack.
- Neither of you work but Robert volunteers in a local charity shop selling donated clothes and you are a member of the WI which involves lots of meetings and events.
- Neither of you do much exercise although Robert walks into town to get to the charity shop.
- Neither of you smoke or drink alcohol.

Information divulged freely

- Robert loves his mum's cooking and baking. He also likes fruit and vegetables but would prefer to eat cake and biscuits.
- You know you both eat too much sweet food. You often go for morning coffee with WI members where there is lots of cake. You have puddings after lunch and dinner. You like to cook and serve big portions of food.
- You were told last year about healthy eating but felt the nurse giving the advice was too judgmental and the plan she suggested sounded awful. You didn't particularly want to call today but the appointment was set up for you so you thought you should.

Information only divulged if specifically asked

- You don't know much about pre-diabetes but your friend Mitchell has diabetes and he still eats lots of cake, he tells you he just gives himself more insulin so he can eat what he wants.
- You will listen to the explanation about pre-diabetes, because you want to know what the chances are of this becoming diabetes and if it does what would the doctor do? Surely if Robert has high sugar now the doctor should be giving him insulin?
- If the doctor mentions the higher risk of heart disease associated with diabetes and being overweight you will pay attention because this is what your husband died of. You certainly take this seriously and would be keen to reduce Robert's risks of a heart attack.
- If diet is discussed in an empathetic non-judgmental way you are open to suggestions. You are accepting of advice to reduce portion size and cut down on cake or any other options

B7.5

Health disadvantages and vulnerabilities, including veterans, mental capacity, safeguarding, and communication difficulties

which you see as smaller changes, with a view to making bigger changes later on. You are also open to the idea of attending a local diabetes education class. You are not sure about Slimming World but agree to Robert being weighed regularly at the surgery to monitor his weight.

- If exercise is discussed you refuse any offers of exercise on referral – neither of you like gyms. You agree to try to walk more and perhaps try some swimming sessions at the local pool if this is suggested.
- If the doctor speaks directly to Robert he will answer with a few words; you will be pleased Robert is involved and encourage this. Robert agrees to anything the doctor suggests such as cutting down his diet, although you comment he won't be happy once he gets home and realises there will be less cake!

385

B7.5

Health disadvantages and vulnerabilities, including veterans, mental capacity, safeguarding, and communication difficulties

Case B7.5   Marking scheme for the observer

NICE CKS on Type 2 diabetes: prevention in people at high risk can be read in conjunction with this case: www.nice.org.uk/guidance/ph38/chapter/glossary

NHS guidance on diet and exercise can be found here: www.nhs.uk/live-well/

Data gathering and diagnosis

☐	☐	☐	• Identifies the reason for attendance and the patient and his mother's ideas, concerns and expectations about the appointment
☐	☐	☐	• Asks specific questions to assess the patient's diet and activity levels
☐	☐	☐	• Asks about any family history of diabetes or cardiovascular disease

Clinical management and medical complexity

☐	☐	☐	• Is able to explain pre-diabetes and that it leads to a higher risk of developing type 2 diabetes. Discusses this as an opportunity to prevent this occurring. Explains that the monitoring involves annual HbA1c tests
☐	☐	☐	• Is able to explain that diabetes will lead to a higher risk of CVD, stroke, foot problems such as ulcers, and visual loss
☐	☐	☐	• Is able to advise on healthy diet and activity levels, i.e. 30 mins of exercise 5 days a week and reducing sugary and fatty foods. Signposts to any local groups such as Slimming World, exercise on referral and Walking away from Diabetes (www.desmond.nhs.uk/about-us)

Relating to others

☐	☐	☐	• Creates rapport with the patient by including him in the consultation even though his mum takes the main role
☐	☐	☐	• Is sympathetic about their struggles to lose weight but encouraging about making small changes to their lifestyles
☐	☐	☐	• Explains the health risks of being overweight and of being diagnosed diabetic in a jargon-free patient-centred way
☐	☐	☐	• Ensures Robert is involved in the consultation and not ignored, using simple language that can be understood

387

B7.6

Health disadvantages and vulnerabilities, including veterans, mental capacity, safeguarding, and communication difficulties

Case B7.6 Information for the doctor

In this case you are a GP registrar taking telephone calls.	
Name:	Jonathan Ellis (his carer will be calling on his behalf)
Age:	42
Past medical history:	Severe learning difficulties, hypothyroidism, hypertension
Current medication:	Levothyroxine 100 mcg od, ramipril 5 mg od, amlodipine 5 mg od
Last consultation:	1 week ago: Hypertension review: BP 167/98. Refusing meds. Carer will discuss with GP.

Notes

389

B7.6

Health disadvantages and vulnerabilities, including veterans, mental capacity, safeguarding, and communication difficulties

Case B7.6 Information for the patient

You are Rose, a carer for Jonathan Ellis. You have been asked to discuss his medication with the GP. Jonny has recently been refusing to take any of his medication.

ICE

- You know he needs to take his medication but he is refusing.
- You are concerned the GP will just say to keep trying – it really is heartbreaking to have Jonny crying every morning and shouting at the carers who are trying to help.
- You would like any advice the GP can offer on how to persuade him to take the medication.

Background

- Jonny lives in residential care as both his parents have passed away. You have been his carer for over 10 years.
- He doesn't smoke or drink any alcohol.
- He is usually a happy relaxed man who loves going for walks and playing on his games console.

Information divulged freely

- Jonny used to be good at taking his medication, but about 3 months ago he had tonsillitis and after this he has refused to take any.
- When the medication is offered he turns his head away and refuses to open his mouth.
- You have tried giving him rewards when he does take them, like a little chocolate, but this didn't help.

Information only divulged if specifically asked:

- The staff have asked Jonny why he doesn't take the medication and he just points to his throat and says "ouch".
- The staff have asked Jonny if he knows why he takes his medication and he doesn't know. He gives the same answer if asked what will happen if he doesn't take them.
- The staff are aware of the reasons he is on medication – to lower his blood pressure and to replace his thyroid hormones. You know if he doesn't take his blood pressure medication he is at risk of having a stroke or heart attack.
- You have noticed he has seemed tired and has possibly put on weight, which you think is due to the missed thyroxine doses. He is otherwise eating well and drinking normally.
- If the GP would like to see Jonny to examine his throat you agree, but in the meantime ask for any suggestions for his medication.
- If the GP offers liquid medication or offers to find out if the medication is available in liquid form, you agree that might help and are happy to accept this.
- If the GP suggests mixing the medication into food you ask if this is safe, but if they say yes you are happy to try this. You do ask if it's OK to "sneak" the medication into him like this? Surely he is allowed to refuse if he doesn't want to take them? If the GP explains Jonny does not seem to understand his medication so lacks capacity to make a decision about them, you feel reassured.

Case B7.6 Marking scheme for the observer

NICE CKS Challenging behaviour and learning disabilities can be read in conjunction with this case:
www.nice.org.uk/guidance/ng11/chapter/1-Recommendations#assessment-of-behaviour-that-
challenges-2

Data gathering and diagnosis

☐	☐	☐	• Identifies the reason for the call and the history of medication refusal
☐	☐	☐	• Identifies methods the staff have already tried to persuade him to take medication and how long this has been a problem for
☐	☐	☐	• Asks about general health and considers reasons for the change in behaviour (signs of infection / pain / physical health problems; any change in environment or routine or anything else that may be upsetting him)
☐	☐	☐	• Identifies that the carers understand the reasons the medication is needed but the patient himself does not

Clinical management and medical complexity

☐	☐	☐	• Recognises a change in behaviour and offers a face-to-face review to assess Jonathan clinically
☐	☐	☐	• Picks up on the possibility of a sore throat and suggests the carers trial analgesia (liquid paracetamol) while waiting for the doctor's visit
☐	☐	☐	• Is able to suggest alternative methods of giving medication, i.e. liquid forms, and offers to prescribe appropriate medications if this is appropriate following review

Relating to others

☐	☐	☐	• Discusses the case with the carer in a professional manner, creating a good rapport
☐	☐	☐	• Considers capacity and acts in the best interests of the patient, i.e. advises that medication can be given without patient knowledge
☐	☐	☐	• Recognises the carer's anxiety and ensures they know how and when to ask for help when needed

393

B7.7

Health disadvantages and vulnerabilities, including veterans, mental capacity, safeguarding, and communication difficulties

Case B7.7 Information for the doctor

> **In this case you are a GP doing video calls. The patient will have their son Michael Harrison in attendance as well.**

Name:	Muriel Harrison
Age:	82
Reason for visit:	Confusion
Past medical history:	Angina 2006 Hypertension 2000 Lower back pain – chronic 1998
Current medication:	Ramipril 10 mg daily Aspirin 75 mg daily Co-codamol 30/500 mg prn for pain, max 8 a day

Notes

395

B7.7

Health disadvantages and vulnerabilities, including veterans, mental capacity, safeguarding, and communication difficulties

Case B7.7   Information for the patient

You are Muriel Harrison, an 82-year old lady. You don't really know why the doctor is calling – it was your son who rang to make the appointment – you feel fine. Michael says he is concerned his mum is very confused this morning. When he called her last night she said she was very tired and going to bed early. He was a bit concerned so called to see her this morning and she is totally confused.

ICE

- You feel fine and certainly do not see why the doctor is here. Your son has obviously overreacted and called them. You don't want anything done and apologise to the doctor for taking up their time.
- Michael is concerned about his mum – she has had heart problems in the past and he is worried that this is the cause of her confusion. He expects a full exam and really would prefer her to be in hospital to ensure she is safe.

Background

- Muriel lives alone after her husband died 3 years ago. She has no carers. Her son Michael lives with his wife and two children nearby. Muriel's daughter lives half an hour away.
- She does not smoke or drink.
- Michael tells the doctor she usually manages very well and still gets on the bus into town most days and walks a lot around the local area.

Information divulged freely

- Michael tells the doctor he found his mum very confused this morning with no idea what day or month it is. She keeps getting his sister's name wrong and seems to think her husband is still alive.

Information only divulged if specifically asked

- Muriel denies any symptoms the doctor asks about. She feels fine.
- Michael has noticed she has been to the toilet to pass urine several times since he arrived today; he has had to help her as she seems unsteady on her feet.
- If asked, Michael answers: "She has not had any falls. She has not mentioned any chest pain / dizziness / SOB / cough / fever / diarrhoea / abdominal pain. She has not had any recent medication changes. Her dinner was on the table uneaten from last night and she has declined breakfast." He has managed to get her to drink half a cup of tea as he noticed her urine was very dark and smelly when she went to the toilet.
- When asked about today's date, Muriel answers that it is 1990 but she does not know the date, the day or the month. She is able to identify her son but says that George (her deceased husband) is at the shops buying milk and will be back in a minute.
- Michael took a urine sample the last time Muriel was at the toilet for the doctor to test.
- If the doctor mentions hospital you say you will not go. You need to be home to look after George and you don't like hospitals. If the doctor asks, you are unable to tell them why they want you to go and you do not retain any information about the consultation. You do not understand if they mention about sepsis or a urine infection.

- Michael will discuss with the doctor: if the doctor explains your mum does not have the capacity to make this decision you agree, you feel she needs to be in hospital as she is not herself at all. You ask what to do. You are happy to try to persuade your mum if asked and will continue to speak to her about going to the hospital until the doctor asks you to stop. She will still refuse. If the doctor asks if you are able to get her to the hospital you agree you are, you ask your mum if she would come to the car with you and she agrees and you are happy to take her to the hospital.
- If the GP advises Michael they can try oral antibiotics at home you are reluctant, you and your sister both work and someone will need to stay with her at all times.
- If a home visit or in-person review is offered to discuss the matter further, Michael will accept this.

Results for the doctor

Examination provided by son who has brought round a BP machine, sats probe and thermometer from home:

- BP 105/50
- HR 100 regular
- SpO_2 98%
- Temp 37.9°C.

Case B7.7   Marking scheme for the observer

Data gathering and diagnosis

- Identifies the reason for the consultation and takes a good history of the confusion, including a systemic enquiry

- Assesses the patient's memory by asking appropriate questions

- Assesses the patient's capacity by asking her to remember, retain, weigh up and communicate the decision she is making about hospital admission

- Recognises the need for an in-person assessment

Clinical management and medical complexity

- Identifies acute confusional state with signs of sepsis (likely secondary to UTI) including tachycardia, low BP and fever

- Advises hospital admission rather than home treatment because this patient is likely to need IV antibiotics and fluids and is not safe to leave at home alone

- Identifies that the patient does not have capacity to make a decision about her treatment so acts in the best interests of the patient to take her to hospital for further treatment

- Attempts to use the family member to persuade her to attend the hospital but recognises when this is failing

Relating to others

- Creates a good rapport with patient and her son

- Involves the patient in the discussion about admission, even after they have assessed her capacity, and continues to interact with the patient

- Can discuss that her confusion is likely to resolve with treatment but considers the potential need for carers. Advises this can be monitored by the hospital team while she is an inpatient in the short term

Case B8.1 Information for the doctor

In this case you are a doctor in surgery taking telephone consultations.	
Name:	Gareth Maloney
Age:	20
Past medical history:	Tonsillectomy (2000)
Current medication:	nil Childhood immunisations up to date

Notes

Case B8.1   Information for the patient

You are Gareth Maloney, a 20 year old actor.

ICE

- You are worried you may have caught an STI and want treatment before your girlfriend notices you have symptoms.
- You have decided to pretend you have a tooth infection so you can get antibiotics which you assume will also treat the infection you have caught.

Background

- You are a 20-year old actor and have been experiencing burning on passing urine for the past week.
- Over the last 2 days you have also developed left-sided scrotal pain and slight swelling.
- You have been with your first girlfriend Sandi for 3 years, but you have started to find yourself attracted to other men. After a work night out last month you ended up having sex with your colleague Paul, and have had several more encounters with him since then.
- Your mum used to work in reception at the surgery so you are reluctant to tell the doctor about your problems as you are embarrassed. You think if you pretend to have a dental abscess then you are sure to be prescribed some antibiotics which you hope will also treat your infection.

Information divulged freely

- You tell the doctor you have called to get some 'strong' antibiotics for a tooth infection. Be fairly vague about your dental symptoms but emphasise that you are after a treatment that will kill most bugs. If the doctor is not inquisitive, and is happy to give antibiotics or directs you to a dentist, ask more about what you will be given for your teeth and if it will kill bugs elsewhere in your body too.
- If the doctor does not probe further or ask directly about other concerns then you do not divulge why you have called.
- You are usually quite fit and well with no allergies.
- You are in a 3-year relationship with Sandi, your first girlfriend from school.

Information only divulged if specifically asked

- If the doctor gets a feeling that you are hiding something and gently asks you directly if there is anything else you are concerned about, then you will admit you have had burning on passing urine for a week.
- If asked specifically about testicular pain and swelling then you will admit that you have noticed this gradually appearing over the last 2 days.
- You deny any penile discharge or testicular lumps and you feel well in yourself.
- If asked about partners, you say have not had sex with Sandi for the last 2 months as she has been working night shifts. If asked about other partners you will reluctantly admit, if you trust the doctor, that you have slept with someone from work. You will not specify that it is another man unless specifically asked. You did not use a condom.
- You will agree to examination and further testing if the doctor explains why this is necessary and you are happy to abstain from intercourse until the results are back.

- You are relieved if the doctor suggests testing for STIs and you are happy to go to a sexual health clinic.
- You are not ready to tell Sandi about Paul and if contact tracing is mentioned, you are sure that Sandi will not be affected since you have not had sex with her since meeting Paul, and you are the only partner she has ever had.

Case B8.1 **Marking scheme for the observer**

patient.info/doctor/urethritis-in-men
patient.info/doctor/epididymo-orchitis-pro

Data gathering and diagnosis

☐	☐	☐	• Identifies the patient's hidden agenda and ICE
☐	☐	☐	• Takes a sexual history in a matter-of-fact, but sensitive manner, avoiding assumptions
☐	☐	☐	• Asks questions to exclude torsion / consider testicular cancer / mumps
☐	☐	☐	• Screens for urinary / systemic symptoms

Clinical management and medical complexity

☐	☐	☐	• Considers the diagnosis of chlamydia and offers testing for this and other STIs
☐	☐	☐	• Urine testing for chlamydia has the same sensitivity as a urethral swab, and is less painful / invasive, so ideally offers an appointment for this plus urinalysis/MSU
☐	☐	☐	• Identifies the patient as high risk for STI and offers antibiotic treatment as per BASHH guidelines (doxycycline 100 mg bd 10–14 days)
☐	☐	☐	• Encourages abstinence from intercourse until diagnosis confirmed. If time allows discuss contact tracing if positive
☐	☐	☐	• Arranges appropriate follow-up in either / both sexual health clinic / GP surgery (if non-STI epididymo-orchitis then renal tract imaging advised)

Relating to others

☐	☐	☐	• Establishes rapport and gains trust of patient to enable them to divulge personal information
☐	☐	☐	• Picks up on cues from the patient to explore hidden agenda
☐	☐	☐	• Gives clear explanations of potential diagnoses and treatment options
☐	☐	☐	• Communicates risk effectively and provides options such as sexual health clinic follow-up
☐	☐	☐	• Acts in a non-judgmental manner, avoids jargon and approaches sexual history taking sensitively, avoiding unnecessary / intrusive questions and avoids making assumptions about sexual orientation / relationship status

Case B8.2 Information for the doctor

In this case you are a GP registrar taking video calls in a routine surgery.	
Name:	Rupal Qureshi
Age:	12
Past medical history:	None
Current medication:	None

Notes

Case B8.2 Information for the patient

You are Sama Qureshi, mother to Rupal, who you have called to discuss today as you are very worried your husband is sending her abroad for the "cut". Rupal is at school at the time of the call.

ICE

- You know about cutting procedures and certainly do not want your daughter to go through that.
- You are very worried the GP will say there is nothing they can do as your husband is taking her abroad.
- You want help from the GP on how to stop this happening.

Background

- You live with your husband and have been married for 24 years.
- Rupal is your only daughter and you also have a son who is 16.
- You are originally from Egypt but have been living in the UK since you were aged 10 when your family moved over here.
- You go back to Egypt most years to visit family.

Information divulged freely

- Last year when you visited Egypt the "cut" was discussed; you were clear you didn't want Rupal to have it and this led to a huge argument between you and your husband. However, once you got back home he reluctantly agreed she did not need to have it.
- This year your trip has been planned and booked for 3 weeks' time. Last night you caught your husband on the phone to his brother talking about the local man who performs the procedure and how they would be taking Rupal to visit him.

Information only divulged if specifically asked

- You are worried about asking your husband more about his arrangements. You know he is under huge social pressure from his family in Egypt to conform and you think he may even try to take Rupal away by himself if you argue with him again about it. He has the passports for the whole family in the safe at home which only he knows the code for.
- Your husband has never been physically violent towards you or your children, but you do fear a heated verbal argument if you bring this subject up with him.
- You have told your husband that you needed to speak to the GP about the headaches Rupal has been getting and you are fairly sure he doesn't suspect.
- You know the procedure does not involve anaesthetic and is very painful. You also know of women having problems in later life with pregnancy and giving birth.
- You have not undergone FGM.
- You were not aware it is illegal and ask what that means for you and your husband if she does go. Would he be arrested on his return?
- You have a sister who lives a few hours away and feel she would likely let you stay with her if the GP suggests this.

- If the GP discusses referral or discussion with social services you are reluctant; you want to know if this means your kids may be taken from you. You want to know what social services will do; can they stop your family from travelling?
- If the GP would like you to wait on the phone while they contact social services, you agree you would like this sorted as soon as possible. You do want assurances they will not call your home phone or leave any messages your husband might hear.

Case B8.2 Marking scheme for the observer

Documents related to FGM for healthcare professionals can be accessed here:
www.gov.uk/government/collections/female-genital-mutilation
www.gov.uk/government/publications/fgm-mandatory-reporting-in-healthcare
https://patient.info/doctor/female-genital-mutilation

Data gathering and diagnosis

☐	☐	☐	• Identifies the reason for calling is to discuss prevention of female genital mutilation (FGM)
☐	☐	☐	• Identifies that the patient is at risk of FGM and that a procedure is potentially being planned abroad
☐	☐	☐	• Identifies that Rupal's mother wants to prevent FGM taking place and she is worried about her husband's behaviour if she raises this issue
☐	☐	☐	• Asks about other children at home and asks if mum has been subjected to FGM herself

Clinical management and medical complexity

☐	☐	☐	• Is able to sensitively advise that FGM is a form of child abuse which is illegal in the UK, including taking a child abroad to have a procedure carried out
☐	☐	☐	• Can explain clearly that if FGM were to take place you would be duty bound to report it to the police and safeguarding services
☐	☐	☐	• Advises in this case (a young girl at risk of FGM) you will need to discuss the case with your local safeguarding lead or children's services
☐	☐	☐	• Arranges appropriate follow-up

Relating to others

☐	☐	☐	• Is able to discuss a sensitive subject in a non-judgmental empathetic manner
☐	☐	☐	• Picks up on the terminology used by the mother and is able to clarify that she is talking about FGM
☐	☐	☐	• Creates a rapport with the patient and identifies tension at home surrounding this procedure. Considers immediate safety of the family and discusses support available, including relatives they can stay with if the situation potentially becomes volatile
☐	☐	☐	• Is able to offer signposting towards information sources on FGM and support available to help the family
☐	☐	☐	• If unable to answer the questions posed by Sama, is able to speak to the local safeguarding team for advice and guidance

Case B8.3   Information for the doctor

In this case you are the duty doctor carrying out a video consultation.	
Name:	Fatima Rashid
Age:	59
Past medical history:	No PMH in records. She is a new patient to your practice.

Notes

Case B8.3 Information for the patient

You are Fatima Rashid, a 59 year-old woman who is seeing the GP via video consult today with a 3-day history of severe headache, nausea and blurred vision in the left eye. You moved to the UK from Uzbekistan 8 months ago and your knowledge of the English language is basic.

Your opening statement is: 'I need some painkillers Doctor, my head is sore'.

You are wearing sunglasses today – it feels more comfortable for your eye.

ICE

- You are a very busy housewife, looking after 3 children. You cannot cope with this headache and want some stronger painkillers. You believe your eye symptoms are due to the headache.

Background

- You started with a dull left-sided headache 3 days ago.
- This morning you woke up with sudden onset of pain and blurred vision in your left eye. You noticed it's quite red.
- You believe the blurring is due to some kind of 'pressure' from your headache.

Information divulged freely

- You are unable to do any housework due to your ongoing headache and nausea.
- You woke up with sudden pain in your left eye and everything seems blurry.
- You are angry because today is your son's birthday and there is so much you need to do.
- You have been getting occasional dull headaches for months.
- You have never had any eye injuries.
- You have distance glasses but you rarely use them.
- You never smoked and you don't drink.
- You moved to the UK because your son has been accepted to University after winning a chemistry project in your home country. You are very proud of him.
- Your husband has a furniture business with his brother, who has been living in the UK for over 10 years.

Information only divulged if specifically asked

- You had similar symptoms last year in your home country. You remember seeing an eye doctor then who prescribed some eye drops but it's been so long you can't remember what they were for. You have had no follow-up since.
- You are not sure about your family history. You grew up with your grandmother but remember your mother used to have some eye drops and heart medications.
- If the doctor offers analgesia and anti-emetics during consultation you will be very grateful and take them.
- If the doctor communicates too fast and doesn't pause to check your understanding you become upset, and answer with phrases such as 'I don't understand'.
- You are very grateful if the doctor is empathetic and uses simple and short sentences to make sure you understand all the information provided, including examination findings.

- If the doctor points out in a sensitive way that your symptoms might be due to acute glaucoma which requires immediate ophthalmology review, you will be upset and require more information on what will happen if you don't go to hospital today. If the doctor remains kind and understanding and explains possible risks of glaucoma you'll accept the reasons and agree to attend the eye clinic. You were planning to surprise your son for his birthday today and that's why you are upset but you realise you require further assessment and treatment.
- If the doctor is not sensitive and uses jargon you become very angry and walk out of the room.

Results for the doctor

Examination and image

Patient has BP machine at home and her son is present and if asked can shine a torch into patient's eyes and describe the following findings:

- Hyperaemic left eye, tender
- Photophobia
- Pupil fixed and dilated and non-reactive to light
- BP 145/80

Case B8.3 Marking scheme for the observer

patient.info/doctor/angle-closure-glaucoma
https://cks.nice.org.uk/topics/glaucoma/

Data gathering and diagnosis

☐	☐	☐	• Identifies ICE and reasons for attendance
☐	☐	☐	• Recognises red flag symptoms (reduced vision, flashing lights, redness, severe pain, photophobia, unreactive pupil)
☐	☐	☐	• Attempts remote examination. Considers arranging in-person appointment with a translator if adequate information cannot be elicited remotely
☐	☐	☐	• Suspects acute closed angle glaucoma as an emergency presentation
☐	☐	☐	• Obtains smoking, alcohol and medication history

Clinical management and medical complexity

☐	☐	☐	• Provides clear information about possible diagnoses and emphasises importance of urgent treatment. Makes it clear that the patient is at risk of losing vision if untreated
☐	☐	☐	• Offers analgesia and anti-emetics
☐	☐	☐	• Considers DVLA guidance
☐	☐	☐	• Gives clear explanation regarding prognosis of untreated glaucoma
☐	☐	☐	• Offers follow-up with an interpreter

Relating to others

☐	☐	☐	• Establishes reasons for attendance and enhances patient autonomy
☐	☐	☐	• Shows an awareness that English is not this patient's first language and speaks slowly, clearly and checks patient's understanding. Considers the use of a translating service.
☐	☐	☐	• Is patient-centred, shows empathy and interest
☐	☐	☐	• Involves patient in management plans and shares concerns

Case B8.4 Information for the doctor

In this case you are a doctor in surgery taking telephone calls.	
Name:	Samir Abbasi
Age:	55
Past medical history:	Type 2 diabetes; hypertension
Current medication:	Metformin 500 mg bd; lisinopril 10 mg od; atorvastatin 80 mg od Latest HbA1c (1 month ago) 49 mmol / mol

Notes

Case B8.4 Information for the patient

You are Samir Abbasi, a 55-year old Muslim type 2 diabetic telephoning to talk to the doctor about fasting during Ramadan.

ICE

- You fast every Ramadan but now you have diabetes you are worried that you will become unwell during this period. You want to talk to the doctor about the safest way to do this.

Background

- You were diagnosed with type 2 diabetes last year and have been taking metformin for the last 6 months without any problems. You increased the dose to twice daily a couple of months ago and the last doctor said he was happy with your control.
- You went to one of the local diabetes education classes about eating healthy foods and doing exercise, but you don't remember if they mentioned fasting and want to know if you can do it with diabetes.

Information divulged freely

- You are married and live with your wife and 2 teenage children, all of whom will be fasting during Ramadan.
- You have a desk-based job in a design studio and rarely engage in any intense physical exercise. You did buy an exercise bike when you were first diagnosed with diabetes, but it has been sitting in the garage without being used for several weeks.
- You have tried to eat better since being diagnosed, but your wife does still like to cook foods which you have now found out to be fatty.
- Your wife bought you a machine to measure your blood sugar at home, but the last doctor told you that you didn't need to check your blood sugar all the time. You have used it once or twice before when you were worried your blood sugar might be low, so you know how to use it.

Information only divulged if specifically asked

- During the holy month of Ramadan, fasting takes place from dawn until sunset for approximately 30 days. You always take part in this fasting and in previous years have 2 meals a day during this time and avoid anything else, including water or medications, during daylight hours.
- People who are sick during Ramadan are exempted from fasting, but you do not consider yourself to be unwell and would like to talk to the doctor about how you can fast without it causing problems.
- You are otherwise well at the moment. Hypertension is your only comorbidity. You have not had any episodes of hypoglycaemia since being diagnosed, but the course you went on made you well aware of the symptoms to look out for.

Case B8.4 Marking scheme for the observer

www.diabetes.org.uk/guide-to-diabetes/managing-your-diabetes/ramadan
https://cks.nice.org.uk/topics/diabetes-type-2/

Data gathering and diagnosis

☐	☐	☐	• Elicits reasons for the call and the patient's ICE
☐	☐	☐	• Shows an awareness of the risks associated with fasting (hypo / hyper-glycaemia / dehydration) and makes an assessment of level of risk this patient is at of developing problems (considers intercurrent illness / amount of physical activity involved in lifestyle / frequency of hypos…)
☐	☐	☐	• Discovers patient's social support, current medications and current understanding of his treatment

Clinical management and medical complexity

☐	☐	☐	• Reaches a shared management plan with the patient
☐	☐	☐	• Discusses risks associated with fasting and advises patient that more frequent monitoring may be needed, and what to do if blood sugars are too high or too low; ensures he is aware the fast must be broken if he has a hypo
☐	☐	☐	• Discusses meals taken during fasting to ensure patient has slow energy release foods (wheat, rice, beans) and high-fibre foods, and avoids too much in the way of fatty food
☐	☐	☐	• Discusses the role of blood glucose monitoring at home if the patient is feeling unwell and has a discussion about medication and the timings of this

Relating to others

☐	☐	☐	• Communicates risk effectively and uses safety-netting
☐	☐	☐	• Demonstrates respect and enhances patient autonomy without allowing own views to influence patient's choices
☐	☐	☐	• Has a positive attitude to reaching a solution to the patient's problems and explains things clearly to patient
☐	☐	☐	• Directs patient to resources such as https://cks.nice.org.uk/topics/diabetes-type-2 (also available in other languages)

Case B8.5   Information for the doctor

In this case you are a doctor in surgery speaking to this patient on the telephone.	
Name:	Alina Ibanescu
Age:	26
Past medical history:	Menorrhagia (Mirena coil *in situ* for 1 year)
Current medication:	nil

Notes

Case B8.5 Information for the patient

You are Alina Ibanescu, a 26-year old waitress at Pizza Express. Your first language is Romanian and your boyfriend usually helps to translate but he isn't around today. You are learning English, so you think you will be able to manage to speak to the doctor today on the telephone.

ICE

- Your feet have been hurting you for 2 weeks now, especially the right foot and you are worried that you probably have an infection and need some antibiotics. You are worried you are not going to be able to work.

Background

- You moved to the UK from Romania with your boyfriend who already had work arranged, but you have been struggling to get a job as an accountant, which is what you are qualified to do back home. You started working as a waitress about a month ago and are regularly doing 12-hour shifts.
- You are settling into life over here, and are sharing a house with 2 other Romanian couples. You do miss home, especially the food. You are disappointed you can't work in accountancy, but you know this is because your English isn't good enough yet.

Information divulged freely

- Both feet are sore, but the right is worse than the left.
- The pain is in the heel, and it's worse at the end of a long shift. Going upstairs makes it worse, and elevating your feet at the end of the day does feel better. You tried paracetamol but it didn't work.
- You haven't had any injuries and you don't go running in your free time – you haven't had 2 days off in a row since starting your new job.
- If the doctor offers an interpreter, tell them you already asked reception and they checked and there is no Romanian interpreter available. You didn't want to wait for another appointment and feel that you can manage.
- At home you would usually have bought some antibiotics by now if the pain had been going on this long, as in your experience they usually sort most problems out. This is what you want today. Doctors in this country never give antibiotics, and when your boyfriend had a sore throat recently the doctor told him he couldn't have any and he was ill all week.
- You only drink alcohol on special occasions and you smoke 10 cigarettes a day.

Information only divulged if specifically asked

- You borrowed some flat shoes from one of your flatmates for your new job; you usually wear heels, and are ashamed to admit that you can't afford to buy new ones until pay day.
- You have never had any problems with your feet before and there are no pains in any other joints. You are otherwise quite well.
- You have put on a little weight since moving to the UK. You have been eating pizzas at work and mainly McDonalds when you are off because they are cheaper and anyway you can't find the same ingredients here that you use at home.

- If the doctor dismisses your request for antibiotics without an adequate explanation, then you will be less receptive to listening to other treatment suggestions and feel resentful. If the doctor is open to listening to why you want antibiotics and what you usually do in Romania, and provides a clear reason as to why they don't think antibiotics will help you, then you will be open to other suggestions.
- If the doctor mentions painkillers you will expect a prescription for them. You pay for your own prescriptions, if the doctor asks. If the doctor explains that you can buy ibuprofen a lot cheaper from the supermarket, then you will be happy to do that, but if there isn't an adequate explanation of this you will feel resentful if you don't get a prescription.
- You do realise your shoes aren't ideal and would be happy to see a podiatrist. You have never spent as much time on your feet as you have this month, and realise that resting them a bit more would be beneficial.
- You feel bad that you have put weight on, and do want to lose it again. Maybe you can start to cook more soups and stop going to McDonalds.
- You don't like the idea of injections, and hope it will get better without that.

Case B8.5 Marking scheme for the observer

patient.info/doctor/plantar-fasciitis-pro
https://cks.nice.org.uk/plantar-fasciitis

Data gathering and diagnosis

☐	☐	☐	• Takes a history and makes a likely diagnosis of plantar fasciitis
☐	☐	☐	• Appreciates the need to confirm the diagnosis with an examination; excludes signs of infection
☐	☐	☐	• Recognises language barrier and adapts history taking accordingly (slower pace, jargon-free)
☐	☐	☐	• Bloods and imaging are of no diagnostic use, but may be useful if considering alternative diagnoses – makes arrangements for an in-person examination with an interpreter

Clinical management and medical complexity

☐	☐	☐	• Is able to approach a self-limiting condition in a positive way, without trivialising the problem
☐	☐	☐	• Addresses potential triggers to the problem: footwear / weight / time on feet in a sensitive way
☐	☐	☐	• Discusses antibiotics and gives clear reasons why prescribing them is inappropriate
☐	☐	☐	• Gives options of analgesia and stretching and suggests orthotics / night splints – considers involvement of a podiatrist
☐	☐	☐	• Offers exercise PIL: www.versusarthritis.org/media/21790/plantar-exercise-sheet.pdf
☐	☐	☐	• Gives a realistic sense of prognosis – most patients will have resolution of symptoms within a year. If asked, mentions options of corticosteroid injection, but promotes conservative therapy as first-line
☐	☐	☐	• Takes opportunity for health promotion – weight loss, healthy eating, smoking cessation

Relating to others			
☐	☐	☐	• Is alert to cues from the patient that she may not understand, and adapts to this by speaking more slowly, using simple English and offering the use of an interpreter service
☐	☐	☐	• Understands that different patients may have different health beliefs and responds to this with understanding and interest
☐	☐	☐	• Elicits social information to put patient's problem into context
			• Provides explanations that are relevant and understandable to the patient
☐	☐	☐	• Offers a follow-up appointment to examine and to have an interpreter present if appropriate

Case B9.1   Information for the doctor

You are a salaried GP in your morning surgery. The patient's husband is calling on her behalf.	
Name:	Marivelda de la Cruz
Age:	50
Past medical history:	none
Current medication:	nil

Notes

Case B9.1   Information for the patient

Your name is Alvin de la Cruz and you are calling for some advice about your wife Marivelda who has been vomiting since the early hours of the morning.

ICE

- You feel your wife has a stomach bug and are concerned about her hydration levels because she has been vomiting for 2 hours non-stop. You are hoping the doctor will reassure you about her hydration and perhaps give a prescription for some of those salts your grandson had when he was sick.

Background

- You and your wife are both 50 years old and originally from the Philippines. She works as a hairdresser and you work in a nearby office. Your wife is usually fit and well. She does not smoke or drink much and has no medical problems.

Information divulged freely

- Your wife seemed fine yesterday and went to bed as usual at 11 pm. You don't remember her getting up during the night.
- She got up and had breakfast as normal.
- You went out to get the morning paper and when you got back about half an hour later she was in the bathroom being sick.
- Since then she has vomited over 10 times.
- She has not had any diarrhoea or mentioned abdominal pain.

Information only divulged if specifically asked

- She has had no contact with anyone else with stomach problems.
- She has not complained of chest pain or acid reflux. She has not complained of shortness of breath.
- If asked if your wife can speak to the doctor herself you say 'no' – she is still in the bathroom. If asked if the phone can be taken to her or if she can come down you tell the doctor she has seemed very sleepy for the past hour or so, probably due to all the vomiting, so there would be no point the doctor speaking to her.
- If asked if your wife complained of any other symptoms, or headaches are specifically asked about, you say that she did mention she had a headache when you came back from the shop. You think she said it was down by her neck.
- If the doctor advises an ambulance you are surprised and ask for a full explanation about why, including what will happen at the hospital and what happens if this is a subarachnoid haemorrhage. You offer to drive your wife herself but are fine with an ambulance being called.

Case B9.1 **Marking scheme for the observer**

patient.info/doctor/raised-intracranial-pressure
patient.info/doctor/telephone-consultations

Data gathering and diagnosis

☐	☐	☐	• Establishes identity of the caller and makes attempts to speak directly with the patient
☐	☐	☐	• Gathers information about reason for phone call from husband including appropriate history
☐	☐	☐	• Identifies ICE from the point of view of the husband
☐	☐	☐	• Recognises the potential serious causes of vomiting in this patient and asks about additional symptoms (such as headache or altered consciousness), despite not being able to speak to or see the patient in person

Clinical management and medical complexity

☐	☐	☐	• Acts upon information gathered that this is potentially an emergency situation requiring further evaluation
☐	☐	☐	• Arranges appropriate transport and admission for this patient and explains this plan clearly to her husband along with reasons for your decision making

Relating to others

☐	☐	☐	• Explains the need for urgent assessment in a clear manner
☐	☐	☐	• Communicates effectively to the patient's husband about the plan for admission
☐	☐	☐	• Avoids jargon and develops a good rapport and a positive attitude towards helping the patient

Case B9.2   Information for the doctor

You are a doctor in surgery doing a video consultation.	
Name:	Alice Cahill
Age:	30
Past medical history:	2 months ago: Dr Scott: Dizziness, intermittent, resting ECG & bloods normal, reassured 4 months ago: Dr Scott: Dizziness continued, for resting ECG & bloods before review 6 months ago: Dr Scott: 1 week of dizziness, no red flags, likely viral, observe
Current medication:	Nil

Notes

Case B9.2 Information for the patient

You are Alice Cahill, a 30-year old lawyer who has called to request a second opinion on your dizziness, which has been ongoing for 6 months and is starting to concern you.

ICE

- You have no specific ideas about what is happening but are worried about brain tumours. You expect more tests and would be pleased if a head scan was offered.

Background

- Six months ago you started feeling dizzy when you were on the treadmill at the gym. You thought you might have an ear infection but were reassured by Dr Scott.
- Since then the dizziness has become worse and you are very worried about it.

Information divulged freely

- You are very active – you go the gym 3 times a week and usually have a long walk or cycle at the weekend. At first the dizziness occurred towards the end of a run or cycle and if you sat down for 2 minutes it cleared. However, you have now had to reduce your activity at the gym and the symptoms can take up to half an hour to resolve.
- You don't have the dizziness at any other times, just during exercise.
- You don't smoke and only drink a few glasses of wine a week.

Information only given if asked

- You do get heart palpitations with some of the more severe attacks. You don't have chest pain or feel short of breath. You have never collapsed during an episode or had a seizure. You have no problems with your ears, no ongoing upper respiratory infection and no vertigo.
- You remember your mum telling you about an uncle who died suddenly at a young age.
- If the doctor discusses the possibility of heart problems you accept an urgent cardiology referral.
- You feel angry at Dr Scott for not coming up with this – you want to know if this delay in diagnosis could lead to problems later on. You also want to know how the practice will deal with this mistake which has been made.
- You will accept a meeting with the practice manager or a discussion of complaints procedure. You will get upset if the doctor tries to defend their colleague too much.

Results for the doctor

Examination carried out by practice nurse this week

- HS normal
- PR 80 regular
- BP 120/80

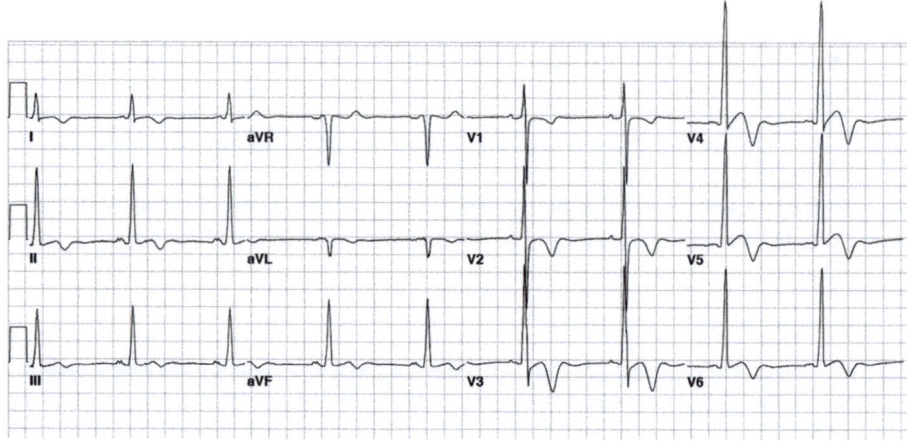

Reproduced from: http://lifeinthefastlane.com (providers of Free Open Access Meducation).

Case B9.2 **Marking scheme for the observer**

https://cks.nice.org.uk/topics/palpitations/

Data gathering and diagnosis

☐	☐	☐	• Systematically gathers information about reason for attending, to exclude other causes for the patient's presentation (specifically considering seizure activity and vertigo)
☐	☐	☐	• Recognises that a history of palpitations with adverse signs (dizziness / pre-syncope) warrants further investigation
☐	☐	☐	• Recognises abnormal ECG (T wave inversion, LVH, possible hypertrophic cardiomyopathy (https://litfl.com/hypertrophic-cardiomyopathy-hcm-ecg-library/))
☐	☐	☐	• Picks up on the family history of possible sudden cardiac death

Clinical management and medical complexity

☐	☐	☐	• Management reflects an appropriate assessment of risk – urgent or rapid access referral due to worsening of symptoms
☐	☐	☐	• Considers further primary care investigations while awaiting cardiology input (bloods/24h ECG/echo)
☐	☐	☐	• Safety-netting – advises to seek immediate medical attention if signs of haemodynamic compromise such as chest pain/SOB/syncope
☐	☐	☐	• Acknowledges her feelings about Dr Scott and is able to discuss the practice complaints procedure

Relating to others

☐	☐	☐	• Recognises the patient's agenda and deals directly with both her clinical concerns and her dissatisfaction with Dr Scott
☐	☐	☐	• Develops rapport with the patient in dealing with her complaint about the other GP. Empathises with patient whilst not commenting directly on the actions taken by the other GP.
☐	☐	☐	• Avoids jargon and has a good rapport and a positive attitude towards helping the patient

Case B9.3   Information for the doctor

You are the duty doctor calling this patient after receiving an online request from her.	
Name:	Aletha Barnard
Age:	38
Past medical history:	Nil
Last consultation:	econsult received today: "I sprained my calf a few days ago and it is swollen and sore and is not improving at all. I would like a private referral letter to see a physiotherapist please" Norethisterone 5 mg tds to delay menstruation (30-tab pack prescribed as one-off telephone consultation script prior to patient's holiday)

Notes

Case B9.3 Information for the patient

You are Aletha Barnard, a 38-year old theatrical production manager. You submitted an online consult today requesting a referral to see a physiotherapist to help with your painful right calf.

ICE

- You have a busy job in the theatre managing shows. You just returned from holiday two days ago to chaos at work and you think you sprained your calf while running around the theatre. It is getting worse rather than better and you would like a private letter from the GP to see a physiotherapist so you can sort this out sooner rather than later.
- You are not particularly concerned about this, but just want to do all you can as soon as possible to resolve the problem so it doesn't interfere with your work schedule.

Background

- You are fit and well and rarely come to see the doctor. You are single and live in a flat close to the theatre where you work long hours.
- You are originally from South Africa, and are keen to move back there, but there are few jobs back home in your chosen field. You travel back there 2–3 times per year. You have in fact just returned from a trip home for a friend's wedding.
- You smoke 10 Marlboro Lights per day and vape, and drink a couple of gin and tonics 4–5 days a week.

Information divulged freely

- You returned from a trip this weekend to a busy work schedule. You are putting together a West End show with a brand new cast so you spent all of Monday running around. You think you must have sprained your right calf because it is extremely sore and swollen. You do not recall a specific injury but it is making you limp and you really just want to see the private physiotherapist you know who helped you once with some back pain, and you require a GP referral letter to do this.
- You are ordinarily very well, you have no health problems and this is quite an inconvenience for you.

Information only divulged if specifically asked

- You have just returned from an equally busy holiday. You went to South Africa for a friend's wedding. You took two long-haul flights in the space of a week, each more than 9 hours long. You went via Dubai since that was the cheapest ticket available. Do not provide the doctor with details of your trip unless specifically asked.
- You noticed that your ankles were quite swollen on the flight, your trousers felt very tight and you had quite pronounced sock marks, especially on your right leg. You do recall having some pain in your right leg during the flight, but you considered this normal in a cramped economy seat. You tend not to move round during a flight, just have a few gins and fall asleep. You haven't really drunk much water this week either.
- You do not recall a specific injury to your leg. You have had no prior injuries and you have never had a blood clot in your legs or lungs. You think your grandma may have had a DVT when she was pregnant but are not sure.

- You have not experienced any chest pain or shortness of breath.
- You took norethisterone last week to delay your period while you were travelling. You are still taking it because work is busy and having a period now would be very inconvenient.
- You have not been sexually active for the last 6 months and are not likely to be pregnant.
- If the doctor provides you with a referral letter to see the physiotherapist you are happy. If, however, the doctor suggests you may have a blood clot in your leg, you are surprised and want to know more.
- You are curious as to what could have caused this and ask more about it.
- You are willing to have further investigations if the diagnosis is explained clearly. Work is your priority, but if an appointment for an USS can be arranged quickly and clear information on the procedure given, you are happy to follow the doctor's advice.
- If anticoagulation is discussed you are happy to accept anticoagulation now if offered. This prompts you to ask more about the treatment of a DVT and, if the diagnosis is confirmed, what will happen. If time is short, you are happy with some written information and will ask more in the hospital.

Results for the doctor

If asked, you can describe the appearance of your calf:
- Right calf measures 3 cm more than left (measured 10 cm below tibial tubercle), tender, pitting oedema apparent, nil evidence of cellulitis or superficial thrombophlebitis

Wells score calculator: www.mdcalc.com/wells-criteria-for-dvt/

Case B9.3 Marking scheme for the observer

patient.info/doctor/deep-vein-thrombosis-pro
https://cks.nice.org.uk/topics/deep-vein-thrombosis/

Data gathering and diagnosis

☐	☐	☐	• Identifies patient's idea that this is a sprain and expectation for a referral to physiotherapy, but takes a detailed history to explore the symptom further
☐	☐	☐	• Considers DVT as the most likely diagnosis and asks relevant questions about symptoms (onset, precipitating injury, other signs and symptoms such as calf swelling)
☐	☐	☐	• Enquires about risk factors for VTE (personal / family history VTE, immobilisation, recent major surgery, cancer, smoking, BMI >30
☐	☐	☐	• Attempts a remote examination by asking the patient to describe her leg; describes how to measure the swelling / look for skin changes. Recognises the limitations of remote consulting and considers converting to a video consult or arranging an in-person examination
☐	☐	☐	• Asks about symptoms of chest pain / SOB to show considering possibility of progression to PE.

Clinical management and medical complexity

☐	☐	☐	• Recognises DVT needs to be excluded as a diagnosis, uses a risk assessment tool (Wells score) to estimate clinical probability and guide management. Wells score for Aletha = 4 (immobilisation, localised tenderness, calf swelling >3 cm, pitting oedema)
☐	☐	☐	• Recognises need for USS of the right leg in view of high probability Wells score. Makes arrangements for this according to local protocols. If no scan available within 4 hours, discusses need for interim therapeutic anticoagulation; DOACs (apixiban / rivaroxaban) are first line
☐	☐	☐	• Further blood tests will be needed, especially if starting anticoagulation – shows an awareness of this and if going to hospital can be done there
☐	☐	☐	• If patient asks about definitive treatment once DVT is confirmed, can discuss anticoagulation options / provide written information about this
☐	☐	☐	• When asked what has caused this, can discuss risk factors / cumulative effect of these and address some of Aletha's modifiable risk factors (recent norethisterone use, BMI, smoking, immobilisation). Thrombophilia testing can be discussed but highlight that confirmation of the diagnosis is needed in the first instance.
☐	☐	☐	• Arranges follow-up to check progress

Relating to others			
☐	☐	☐	• Is able to communicate clearly to the patient concerns about DVT and the need for further investigation
☐	☐	☐	• Appreciates the patient's concerns and answers questions
☐	☐	☐	• Builds rapport and provides explanations the patient can understand
☐	☐	☐	• Is aware of patient's concerns and is able to calm her and guide her on management
☐	☐	☐	• Checks patient understanding and involves the patient in the decision making

Further reading

Progesterone-only pills are considered lower risk for VTE; however, there are limited data available. Bear in mind norethisterone is partly metabolised to ethinylestradiol and take care prescribing this to women to delay menstruation if they have other risk factors for VTE:

https://srh.bmj.com/content/familyplanning/47/2/102.full.pdf

Case B9.4 Information for the doctor

In this case you are a GP registrar taking telephone calls in a routine surgery	
Name:	William Stevens
Age:	45
Past medical history:	None
Current medication:	None

Notes

Case B9.4   Information for the patient

You are William Stevens, a 45-year old man, with acid reflux symptoms.

ICE

- You think you have acid reflux probably due to the extra weight you have put on.
- You are concerned about your heart because a friend of yours commented that his dad thought he had acid reflux and it was actually a heart attack.
- You expect some tests to be carried out to check your heart and a prescription for some medication to help the pain.

Background

- You live with your wife and your daughter who is 21.
- You smoke 15 cigarettes a day and have done for 25 years.
- You drink a few pints each night and at weekends have a bottle of wine each night. You are aware this is too much alcohol but are not really interested in cutting down.
- You have recently gained a lot of weight as you injured your back so stopped going to the gym.
- You work in a furniture store in the sales department so are not particularly active in your job.

Information divulged freely

- You have had problems with chest pain for the past few months. It is lower down in your chest / top of your stomach and is a dull ache.
- You feel quite sick when it comes on but have not vomited and you get the taste of acid in the back of your mouth.
- You have recently gained a lot of weight as you injured your back so stopped going to the gym.

Information only divulged if specifically asked

- The pain mainly occurs after eating and at night. It has woken you from sleep a few times.
- You have not lost weight or noticed any change in your bowel habit.
- You are worried this might be heart disease; you have not noticed the pain is related to exercise at all. You do not get short of breath with the pain and it does not radiate to your arm or jaw. You have had no palpitations.
- Your grandfather died of a heart attack when he was 78, but no one else in the family has heart problems.
- You have tried Gaviscon from the chemist and it helps but only for a few hours. You would prefer to take something which lasted all day.
- You would really like the GP to arrange some "heart tests"; if they agree to an ECG you are happy with this. If the GP feels heart disease is very unlikely and does not agree to arrange any testing you will leave unsatisfied with the outcome.
- If the GP discusses blood tests you are happy to have them done. If they discuss *H. pylori* testing you would like to ask what a positive test would mean.
- If the GP offers a prescription for lansoprazole / omeprazole you have seen a recent news update about these on This Morning. You heard they caused stomach cancer so ask the GP if this is true. You also ask what side-effects you can expect. If the GP is not reassuring about the long-term effects of these medications you will ask for an alternative.

Case B9.4 Marking scheme for the observer

https://cks.nice.org.uk/topics/dyspepsia-unidentified-cause

Data gathering and diagnosis

☐	☐	☐	• Takes a history to elicit the nature of the chest pain and associated features including risk factors for heart disease such as smoking and family history
☐	☐	☐	• Asks about red flag features of acid reflux (GI bleeding, weight loss, dysphagia, excessive vomiting, abdominal mass on examination)
☐	☐	☐	• Carries out a medication review for possible causes of dyspepsia (NSAIDs, corticosteroids, calcium channel blockers, nitrates, theophyllines, bisphosphonates)

Clinical management and medical complexity

☐	☐	☐	• Arranges appropriate investigations and is guided by patient anxiety as well as clinical need. Suggests an ECG and blood tests including FBC, HbA1c and cholesterol. Testing for *H. pylori* can be considered if there is no response to PPI
☐	☐	☐	• Discusses treatment options. Offers treatment with a PPI and is able to discuss the long-term side-effects (increased risk of fractures, increased risk of hypomagnesaemia, risk of *C. diff.* infection and possible increased risk of stomach cancer). Advises patient to take the lowest dose possible for shortest duration to reduce these risks
☐	☐	☐	• Discusses lifestyle factors for reflux such as weight loss, reducing alcohol and caffeine, smoking cessation, and eating small meals often and avoiding fatty food. Advises that lifestyle modification can be trialled first if he prefers not to take medication
☐	☐	☐	• Arranges follow-up to assess progress and review results and provides a safety net by discussing the above red flag features to be aware of and when to re-present if these occur

Relating to others

☐	☐	☐	• Creates rapport with patient by acknowledging his concerns about heart disease
☐	☐	☐	• Sensitively discusses the patient's weight and smoking / alcohol history and discusses help available locally (such as Weight Watchers and Quitsmoking helpline)
☐	☐	☐	• Considers providing written information for the patient on both dyspepsia and lifestyle modification: • patient.info/health/dyspepsia-indigestion • patient.info/health/quit-smoking-cessation/how-to-quit-smoking • patient.info/health/alcohol-and-liver-disease/alcohol-and-sensible-drinking • patient.info/health/weight-loss-weight-reduction

Case B9.5 Information for the doctor

In this case you are a GP registrar taking video calls in a routine surgery.	
Name:	Archer Irving
Age:	34
Past medical history:	None
Current medication:	None

Notes

Case B9.5 Information for the patient

You are Archer Irving, a 34-year old man, who has been getting palpitations.

ICE

- You are sure these palpitations mean you have a serious heart problem, which is really worrying you as your dad died of a heart attack last year.
- You expect some tests to be done on your heart.

Background

- You live with your boyfriend of 4 years and your dog Charlie.
- You live just around the corner from your mum who you are very close to.
- You smoke around 5 cigarettes a day and have for the past 10 years.
- You drink a few glasses of wine most nights and a few more at the weekends.
- You walk Charlie at least 3 miles each day and go the gym twice a week as well.

Information divulged freely

- For the past month you have been having palpitations where your heart feels like it's racing. This seems to happen most days and you find it very frightening.

Information only divulged if specifically asked

- You seem to get these palpitations at least once a day, more often in the evenings when you are sitting watching TV. They only last a few minutes each time.
- You don't feel faint when they start and are able to speak and walk during them, but they make you feel anxious so you tend to sit down and rest.
- You don't identify any particular triggers, they don't occur more often after exercise.
- You do often have a brief feeling of your breath being taken away, but this doesn't last. You don't get chest pain or feel light-headed and you have never passed out.
- You don't take any OTC medications.
- You drink 1 or 2 espressos a day.
- Your dad died of a heart attack last year aged 67 and he had no previous heart problems. You had a very close relationship with your dad and took his death very hard. You were off work for 2 months and went to private grief counselling. You have no other family history of heart disease or sudden death.
- If the GP offers blood tests and a heart tracing you ask what the blood tests are looking for and what the heart tracing might show. You ask if this will rule out the kind of heart disease your dad had?
- If the GP talks about wearing a monitor for 24 hours you agree that would be helpful because you get them most days so are sure monitoring over 24 hours would pick them up.
- If the GP asks you to come for a face-to-face appointment to do a physical exam you are happy to do this.
- If the GP talks about anxiety or a bereavement reaction leading to these symptoms, you accept this may be the cause, but are sure if the tests are normal you will be reassured and decline any further counselling.
- If the GP advises that lifestyle changes will help prevent the heart disease which led to your father's death you agree – you ask what services would be available on the NHS to help you stop smoking?

Results for the doctor

Examination

Provided from patient's home monitor
- BP 120/80, HR 66

Case B9.5 Marking scheme for the observer

https://cks.nice.org.uk/topics/palpitations

Data gathering and diagnosis

☐ ☐ ☐ • Takes a thorough history of the palpitations including how often they occur, for how long and any associated symptoms

☐ ☐ ☐ • Asks about adverse signs such as associated chest pain, breathlessness, syncope or dizziness

☐ ☐ ☐ • Enquires about exercise-induced palpitations and any family history of sudden death or cardiovascular disease

☐ ☐ ☐ • Arranges to perform an appropriate cardiovascular examination (BP, pulse, heart sounds, peripheral assessment)

Clinical management and medical complexity

☐ ☐ ☐ • Arranges appropriate investigations, such as FBC (to check for anaemia), U&Es (to check for electrolyte imbalances) and TSH (to rule out thyroid disease) along with a 12-lead ECG

☐ ☐ ☐ • Advises that if the investigations are negative and the symptoms continue, a 24-hour ECG could be arranged, and advises on local referral pathways

☐ ☐ ☐ • Recognises the effect the patient's bereavement may be having on their symptoms and offers appropriate support

☐ ☐ ☐ • Advises on lifestyle factors such as smoking cessation, reducing alcohol intake, increasing exercise and improving diet to prevent the development of cardiovascular disease

Relating to others

☐ ☐ ☐ • Creates rapport with the patient by empathising with their recent bereavement

☐ ☐ ☐ • Is reassuring about the current symptoms in light of the lack of red flag symptoms

☐ ☐ ☐ • Sensitively approaches the idea that stress and anxiety may be leading to the symptoms

Case B9.6   Information for the doctor

In this case you are a GP registrar taking telephone calls.	
Name:	Alison Riley
Age:	43
Past medical history:	None
Current medication:	None

Notes

Case B9.6   Information for the patient

You are Alison Riley, a 43-year old woman, with back pain.

ICE

- You think your back pain is due to spending so much time sitting at a desk at work.
- You are concerned you are making your back worse by forcing yourself to go to work each day. Your mum has chronic back pain and didn't work from age 40 due to it. She takes lots of pain pills and still complains about her back all the time.
- You expect a sick note to give your back time to rest.

Background

- You live with your husband and your French bulldog.
- You are an ex-smoker – you used to smoke 10 cigarettes a day for around 15 years.
- You only drink at special events such as weddings or Christmas.
- You have recently gained weight – since your back started hurting you stopped walking the dog and make your husband do it. You rest all weekend and in the evenings make sure you sit on the sofa which has led to you eating more.
- You work in an office, you get the bus to work and have to walk around 10 minutes from the bus stop into work. You then sit at a desk all day typing.

Information divulged freely

- You have had problems with your back for around 3 months.
- The pain is at the bottom of your back and it feels like a dull ache.

Information only divulged if specifically asked

- You have no pain radiating to your legs. You have no issues with numbness or weakness in your feet or legs. You have no changes in your bladder or bowels and you can feel your back passage normally when you are wiping yourself after going to the toilet.
- You have never had cancer or been told you have issues with your immune system. You have not lost weight or had any fevers.
- You have not injured your back.
- The back pain has made you feel low and you worry about making it worse all the time. You sleep well. Your appetite is good and your concentration is fine. You have no thoughts of self-harm or suicide.
- You are worried about this turning into the same pain as your mum's; everyone says they are fed up of hearing your mum moan about her back. She takes so many pills she often sleeps most of the day.
- You are taking occasional ibuprofen and paracetamol but are really trying not to take any tablets for this.
- If the GP advises different painkillers you are very worried about any which are addictive. If they suggest regular analgesia may be better to allow you to move about more easily you reluctantly agree, but you ask if you can't feel the pain, could you possibly push your back too far?
- If the doctor discusses investigations you are happy to have them but don't really feel you need them, you are sure this is muscular pain so don't think X-rays or blood tests will change that. However, you are happy for a face-to-face appointment for blood tests and an exam.

- If the doctor discusses your activity levels you listen and understand their suggestions. You are happy to try gentle walks with the dog and are interested in any exercises the doctor suggests. You would also appreciate a referral to the local gym in the Exercise Referral scheme if offered – you agree that speaking to a personal trainer about your back pain will make you more confident in exercising.
- If the doctor offers a physio referral you are happy to do this.
- If the doctor discusses your work you are keen for time off, because you feel that more rest will help. However, if the doctor sensitively suggests changes to your work, for example, trying to get up and walk around every half hour and getting occupational health to assess your workstation, you will agree to try this and continue going for now. If they agree to a sick note you will happily take it and want to know what to do if you need more time off.
- If the doctor discusses your weight you agree this is probably adding to the back pain and agree to reducing your sugary snacks and becoming more active.

Results for the doctor

Examination

- Patient provides height and weight details; their BMI is 28.

Case B9.6   Marking scheme for the observer

The 'STartT Back Screening Tool' can be useful to assess patients for risk of persistent back pain symptoms and guide management for both GPs and physiotherapists: www.keele.ac.uk/sbst/startbacktool/

Data gathering and diagnosis

☐	☐	☐	• Takes a history of the patient's back pain, specifically enquiring about red flag symptoms (weight loss, fever, night pain, trauma, neurological symptoms, bowel / bladder dysfunction)
☐	☐	☐	• Asks about the effects of the back pain on her occupation and personal life and asks about mood
☐	☐	☐	• Establishes what treatments she has tried already
☐	☐	☐	• Considers an in-person examination with either the GP or an in-house physiotherapist if available

Clinical management and medical complexity

☐	☐	☐	• Diagnoses mechanical low back pain and suggests no investigations are currently needed (or offers good reasoning for any investigations suggested)
☐	☐	☐	• Offers analgesia to the patient as a short-term measure to allow better mobilisation and is able to discuss the addictive nature of certain types of analgesia such as opiates
☐	☐	☐	• Signposts to physiotherapy and suggests simple exercises the patient can perform whilst awaiting this: www.versusarthritis.org/about-arthritis/exercising-with-arthritis/exercises-for-healthy-joints/exercises-for-the-back/
☐	☐	☐	• Advises the patient to keep active rather than resting; for example, suggests walking her dog short distances
☐	☐	☐	• Is able to discuss appropriate changes to her workplace and suggests liaising with occupational health at work rather than immediately agreeing to a sick note
☐	☐	☐	• Advises the patient her BMI falls into the overweight range and advises that this may be adding to her back pain. Is able to discuss simple lifestyle changes to reduce her weight and if appropriate signpost to local services such as Slimming World, Weight Watchers or Exercise Referral

Relating to others

☐	☐	☐	• Listens to patient's concerns about her back pain and acknowledges her fears of ending up like her mum
☐	☐	☐	• Sensitively discusses issues around the patient's weight and empowers the patient to engage in activities that may improve her symptoms
☐	☐	☐	• Ensures red flags are discussed with the patient and makes her aware that she should seek medical attention if she develops weakness in her legs or loss of bowel / bladder control
☐	☐	☐	• Recognises her low mood and discusses CBT. Arranges follow-up to assess progress

Case B9.7   Information for the doctor

In this case you are a GP registrar taking calls in surgery.	
Name:	Robert Fawcett
Age:	68
Past medical history:	Nil
Current medication:	Nil
Last consultation:	2 weeks ago: Face-to-face with GP: Change in bowel habit to looser stool for 3 months No PR bleeding Lost around 3 kg in weight Exam: abdo exam and PR exam normal Plan: bloods & FIT test ?referral FIT test results: **50** Hb/g (normal range 0–9) Bloods: Hb **122** (normal range 130–180), MCV **78.2** (normal range 80–100), ferritin **10** (normal range 17–291)

Notes

Case B9.7   Information for the patient

You are Robert Fawcett, a 68-year-old man who has been asked to ring to discuss your blood results.

ICE

- You are sure it is bad news as you were asked to take a call urgently about your results.
- You are very concerned about your symptoms. You have seen the adverts on the television about change in bowel habit being a symptom of bowel cancer.
- You expect the doctor to give you bad news; you feel the doctor will likely need to refer you to the cancer specialist.

Background

- You live with your wife, you have 2 grown-up children who live in the UK but not nearby.
- You retired about 6 years ago from being an HGV driver.
- You don't smoke but drink around 2–3 cans of beer each night.
- You are not very active but don't feel you have time to exercise; your weight has crept up over the years.

Information divulged freely

- You are very worried about the results; the last doctor told you he was running a "poo test" to check for cancer.
- You have noted the last 3 months your bowels have been looser, you now go 3–4 times a day when previously you would only go once a day. You haven't noted any blood in your stool. You occasionally get cramping pain before needing to open your bowels. You have not had any incontinence.
- You have lost some weight – you noted your clothes are looser. You eat the same amount and have no nausea or vomiting.

Information only divulged if specifically asked:

- Your father had bowel cancer, he had surgery and this got rid of the cancer; however, it returned several years later, by which time it had spread and he died.
- If the GP explains your FIT test is positive you ask what this means. If they explain it may mean you have bowel cancer you ask if there are any other possible causes. You will also ask why your test through the post did not show this when you sent it 2 years ago.
- If the GP explains you are anaemic you ask what the cause of this is. You are happy to take iron tablets if offered.
- You are very worried about having any further testing, you remember your Dad having a camera test and saying it was an awful experience. You would much prefer to have a scan at the hospital instead. If the GP explains more about the procedure for a colonoscopy and why it is a preferred option, you are happy to go ahead.
- If the GP mentions fast-track referrals you listen and understand the explanation of this type of appointment.

Case B9.7 Marking scheme for the observer

www.cancerresearchuk.org/health-professional/diagnosis/investigations/fit-symptomatic

Data gathering and diagnosis

☐ ☐ ☐ • Takes a history of the symptoms and recognises an appropriate exam has already been carried out

☐ ☐ ☐ • Elicits the patient's ICE early on and uses the patient's understanding to start the explanation of the results

☐ ☐ ☐ • Ensures family history is raised to put patient's fears into context

Clinical management and medical complexity

☐ ☐ ☐ • Is able to explain the results of a positive FIT test

☐ ☐ ☐ • Recognises iron-deficiency anaemia and is able to explain this to the patient

☐ ☐ ☐ • Recognises this patient meets the fast-track criteria and explains this to the patient

☐ ☐ ☐ • Is able to discuss what is involved in a colonoscopy with the patient

Relating to others

☐ ☐ ☐ • Explores the patient's concerns

☐ ☐ ☐ • Establishes good rapport

☐ ☐ ☐ • Demonstrates empathy

☐ ☐ ☐ • Checks understanding

Case B9.8 Information for the doctor

In this case you are a doctor in surgery undertaking telephone consultations.	
Name:	Fiona Haynes
Age:	46
Past medical history:	Hypothyroidism Last consultation (2 weeks ago): persistent URTI with laryngitis, not responding to OTC treatments, delayed script for amoxicillin issued. TFTs due – for routine bloods with nurse. Cervical smear overdue
Results:	BP 128/75 Pulse 80 SpO$_2$ 99% No neck lumps Chest clear ENT – NAD TFTs (taken last week) TSH 2.34 (0.4–4 mU/L) Free T$_4$ 14 (9–25 pmol/L)
Current medication:	Levothyroxine 100 µg od

Notes

Case B9.8   Information for the patient

You are Fiona Haynes, a 46-year old mother of two, who has called to speak to the doctor because of your very hoarse voice.

ICE

- You have had a hoarse voice for too long now and it is starting to interfere with your job. You will happily accept any treatment that is going to get things back to normal, but you think perhaps a stronger antibiotic will do the trick.

Background

- You work as an operator in a call centre, and colleagues and customers have been commenting on your voice being difficult to hear.
- The problem seemed to start nearly 2 months ago following a cold. You tried various remedies from the pharmacy and eventually saw the on-call doctor at the surgery a fortnight ago who gave you a delayed script for amoxicillin. You ended up taking it, but it didn't improve your hoarseness.

Information divulged freely

- You were fit and well prior to catching this cold, but have felt increasingly tired and run down over recent weeks.
- You now have no coryzal symptoms, just persistent hoarseness which you think has been there for nearly 2 months. You have no problems swallowing, but your appetite is not what it was. You don't appear to have lost any weight.

Information only divulged if specifically asked

- You used to be a heavy smoker (30 a day) and stopped 5 years ago; however, your mum died last year and you started having the odd cigarette again to help you cope, but only on your breaks at work, not around your children at home.
- You have had no problems with your breathing and have not noticed any neck lumps or haemoptysis.
- You have had a mild earache for the past few weeks in the right side but no sore throat.
- You drink roughly 2 bottles of wine per week at most, but have not had much since your birthday last month because you find it gives you bad acid reflux.
- You take your thyroid medication regularly.
- You have tried resting your voice, gargling and haven't smoked at all for the past fortnight.
- You will happily accept a different antibiotic from the doctor or medication for reflux symptoms.
- If the doctor mentions review by ENT you will be happy to attend but you have several questions about what will happen in the ENT clinic and what the diagnosis is likely to be.
- If a chest X-ray is mentioned you would like to know why.
- You have a friend who had a '2-week' referral for breast cancer and if an urgent referral such as this is mentioned you feel quite scared and worry that the doctor thinks you have cancer. You are reluctant to come out and say this, but if gently asked about any questions or concerns you will discuss this with the doctor.

Case B9.8 Marking scheme for the observer

patient.info/doctor/hoarseness-pro
www.nice.org.uk/guidance/ng12/chapter/Recommendations-organised-by-site-of-cancer#head-
and-neck-cancers

Data gathering and diagnosis			
			• Gathers information systematically to include 'red flag' features (pain, dysphagia, haemoptysis, otalgia, neck lumps, weight loss)
			• Obtains relevant social history (smoking, alcohol, voice overuse)
			• Acknowledges the need for an ENT examination and sees that this has been undertaken recently
Clinical management and medical complexity			
			• Identifies that persistent hoarseness with otalgia in a smoker requires an urgent suspected cancer pathway referral
			• Considers chest X-ray alongside the referral and the need to re-examine and assess in person
			• Simultaneously considers treatment options while awaiting ENT review, such as voice rest, steam inhalations, treatment of reflux symptoms. Discusses benefits / limitations of further antibiotic treatment
			• Promotes good health – offers smoking cessation advice and reminds patient that smear test due
Relating to others			
			• Explores ICE and the impact of the problem on the patient's work
			• Engages in honest discussion about reasons for referral, sensitively discussing the need to exclude potentially serious underlying causes to the symptoms
			• Provides explanations that the patient can understand. Deals with uncertainty and discusses possible differential diagnoses, from the serious to the benign

Case B9.9   Information for the doctor

In this case you are a GP registrar in a routine afternoon surgery undertaking video consultations.	
Name:	Eden Ullswater
Age:	51
Past medical history:	None
Current medication:	None

Notes

Case B9.9 Information for the patient

You are Eden Ullswater, a 51-year old man, who has requested a video consultation to avoid having to drive to the surgery; you have symptoms of dizziness you wish to discuss.

ICE

- You know that dizziness can be linked to your ears and wonder if you perhaps have an infection?
- You are due back at work after the weekend after taking a fortnight off to undertake some renovations on your house and you really want this to be sorted out before returning.
- You expect a prescription for some medication.

Background

- You are usually fit and well with no health complaints. You work as a psychologist and are due back at work on Monday after your time off.
- You live with your partner Helen, who is fit and well.
- You have never had anything like this before and presume it will be self-limiting, but you want a quick fix to get you back to work.

Information divulged freely

- Over the last 4–5 days you have had several episodes of dizziness which last for less than a minute each time, but leave you feeling nauseous. You have not vomited.
- You feel it is worse with sudden movements of your head – you have noticed it when turning over in bed, or when reaching up to get the teabags from the cupboard.
- Your dizziness seems unrelated to your posture or standing.
- You have not noticed any cough or cold symptoms and you have not had any fever.
- You are worried you may not be allowed to drive with these symptoms.

Information only divulged if specifically asked

- The dizziness feels similar to being drunk. The room feels like it is spinning around, as if you have just been on a merry-go-round.
- You have no earache, no discharge from your ears, no hearing loss and no tinnitus.
- You don't have a sore throat, any swallowing problems or any voice changes.
- You haven't had any headaches but you did bump your head quite hard on the doorframe at the start of the week when you were climbing up the ladder to paint the ceiling, and your head was a little sore for the rest of the day after that. You were not unconscious following this and feel it was a minor bump.
- You have not experienced any chest pain, shortness of breath or palpitations.
- You have had no weakness in any of your limbs or in your face.

Results for the doctor

Your partner is a nurse and took your vital signs this morning to provide to the doctor.
- GCS 15, afebrile 36.6°C, BP 131/80, HR 77 regular
- Helen has checked your ears and says that they appear normal
- Dix–Hallpike manoeuvre – cannot be undertaken remotely. For practice – the Dix–Hallpike test can be discussed and performed by your group to ensure you are all happy with the procedure (see over)

The Dix–Hallpike test is used to confirm posterior canal BPPV. Absolute contraindications include: recent neck trauma (fractured odontoid peg or cervical spine fracture; atlanto-axial subluxation), cervical disc prolapse, vertebrobasilar insufficiency. Caution should be taken in patients with severe rheumatoid arthritis or severe back pain, cervical stenosis, spinal cord injury, carotid stenosis or carotid sinus syncope, recent stroke, or cardiac bypass in the last 3 months. Severe orthopnoea may also restrict the test.

Remember that this test may trigger vertigo, so ensure the patient is not planning to drive themselves home.

Advise the patient what to expect and explain that transient dizziness may occur.

Prepare the couch with the headrest down so that the patient's head will overhang from the end.

Ask the patient to keep their eyes open throughout and ask them to fix on one spot such as the corner of the room.

Start with the patient sitting with their head turned 45° to the left (to test the left posterior canal). Warn them that on the count of 3 you will move them backwards, but continue to support their head, then quickly lay the patient down until the head is below the level of the couch by about 30°. Observe the eyes for nystagmus for about 30 seconds. Move the patient back up into a sitting position and observe the eyes again for nystagmus. Repeat on the opposite side.

A test is positive if a patient experiences vertigo and rotary nystagmus in posterior canal BPPV.

Case B9.9 **Marking scheme for the observer**

https://cks.nice.org.uk/benign-paroxysmal-positional-vertigo#!topicsummary

Data gathering and diagnosis

☐	☐	☐	• Takes a complete history with ENT-focused questions and confirms dizziness is related to the position of the head
☐	☐	☐	• Excludes alternative causes of the dizziness – asks about cardiac symptoms, chest pain / palpitations / posture
☐	☐	☐	• Reveals the history of recent minor head injury which may have prompted the symptoms (disruption of otolith particles from the semicircular canals)
☐	☐	☐	• Ensures the history screens for 'red flags' such as unilateral hearing loss / tinnitus, focal neurological signs, cerebellar signs, atypical nystagmus
☐	☐	☐	• Attempts a remote examination but appreciates the need for a face-to-face appointment to carry out the Dix–Hallpike test

Clinical management and medical complexity

☐	☐	☐	• Identifies BPPV as the likely diagnosis
☐	☐	☐	• Discusses treatment options to include: giving time for symptoms to self-resolve, a trial of home Brandt–Daroff exercises (https://entsurrey.com/Download/ENT-SURREY/Brandt-Daroff.pdf), a further appointment to carry out the Epley manoeuvre (www.royalberkshire.nhs.uk/media/0fslhdqf/dix-hallpike-and-epley-manoeuvres-for-bppv_pd-11_aug22.pdf)
☐	☐	☐	• Discusses timescales for improvement (symptoms are usually self-limiting over several weeks) and safety-nets for the patient to return for review, should symptoms develop or worsen
☐	☐	☐	• Picks up on the patient's desire for medication. Discusses the use of vestibular sedatives in BPPV (not usually helpful) (see NICE pathway above)

Relating to others

☐	☐	☐	• Gives a jargon-free description of BPPV that the patient can understand
☐	☐	☐	• Provides written information on both BPPV and the Epley manoeuvre (https://patient.info/health/dizziness/benign-paroxysmal-positional-vertigo)
☐	☐	☐	• Offers practical advice on how to limit symptoms (get out of bed slowly, limit head movements)
☐	☐	☐	• Advises the patient not to drive when feeling dizzy or to continue decorating at height where there is a risk of falling (experts suggest that patients with BPPV can drive once they feel safe to do so, but those with sudden and unprovoked or unprecipitated episodes of disabling dizziness should stop driving and inform the DVLA (www.gov.uk/guidance/general-information-assessing-fitness-to-drive))

Case B9.10 Information for the doctor

In this case you are a doctor in surgery video-calling a patient in response to an online consultation she submitted.

Name:	Ingrid Bauer
Age:	38
Online consultation:	"I have gritty eyes"
Past medical history:	Sterilisation
Social history:	Married, 3 children
Smokes:	5 cigarettes / day
Alcohol:	10 units / week
Current medication:	nil

Notes

Case B9.10 Information for the patient

You are Ingrid Bauer, a 38-year old woman who submitted an online consultation about your 'gritty' eyes.

ICE

- You think you should perhaps have some allergy tests and some antibiotic drops.

Background

- Your eyes are itchy and burning. You are fed up, because you have had these symptoms on and off for the past 3 months and are starting to struggle with your computer work.
- You are constantly scratching your eyes and noticed that the redness is worse towards the end of the day.
- Sometimes in the morning your eyelids are sticky with small flakes which look like dandruff.

Information divulged freely

- You work as a travel agent and use your computer daily to book holidays for your clients.
- It is important to you to look good because you are in daily contact with customers.
- You are happily married and your husband Jack suggested you see the GP because he thinks you might have some kind of allergy and that's why your eyes are itchy.
- You are not sure if Jack is right but you have never had any problems with your eyes before so you just want to make sure 'it's not a serious problem'.

Information only divulged if specifically asked

- You love your job and the people you work with, but last week your boss made fun of the appearance of your eyes. He said your eyes look 'angry' and commented that you had perhaps had too much to drink lately. You know he didn't mean it but you felt awful.
- You are not on any prescribed or OTC medications.
- You don't wear glasses or contact lenses.
- You have no allergies. You quit smoking last year and you are very proud of it.

Results for the doctor

Remote video assessment shows:

- Eye lids: pink and flaky, minimally tender on palpation, minimal crust at the base of eyelashes
- Normal conjunctiva
- Normal eye movements

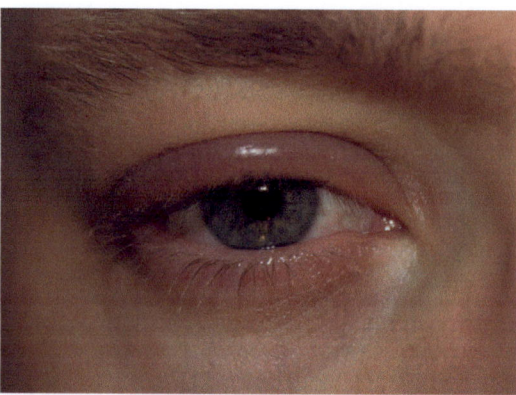

Reproduced from www.wikipedia.org under the terms of the Wikimedia Creative Commons Attribution Share-Alike Licence; author clubtable.

Case B9.10 Marking scheme for the observer

patient.info/doctor/blepharitis-pro
https://cks.nice.org.uk/topics/blepharitis/

Data gathering and diagnosis

☐ ☐ ☐ • Gathers information systematically and efficiently about reason for attending

☐ ☐ ☐ • Takes appropriate eye history, establishing the timing of symptoms, pain, trauma, contact lenses, discomfort and discharge

☐ ☐ ☐ • Attempts basic eye examination remotely and acknowledges the need for an in-person examination to check VA, pupils, lid examination, eye movements

☐ ☐ ☐ • Enquires about recent medication, eye drops, new face wash / moisturisers. Asks about pets and obtains a smoking and alcohol history

Clinical management and medical complexity

☐ ☐ ☐ • Suspects blepharitis and provides jargon-free explanation

☐ ☐ ☐ • Offers treatment options such as warm compress / lid bathing and provides an information leaflet

☐ ☐ ☐ • Offers in-person follow-up for examination and educates about prevention of further episodes

Relating to others

☐ ☐ ☐ • Establishes underlying reason for attendance

☐ ☐ ☐ • Appears alert to cues and responds to feelings and expectations

☐ ☐ ☐ • Elicits psychosocial context, is patient-centred, shows empathy

☐ ☐ ☐ • Provides reassurance and involves patient in management plan

Case B9.11   Information for the doctor

You are a GP registrar undertaking telephone consultations.	
Name:	Fiona Watson
Age:	29
Past medical history:	Anxiety
Current medication:	Propranolol 40 mg prn

Notes

Case B9.11 Information for the patient

You are Fiona Watson, a 29-year old woman who feels constantly tired. You are a single mum. Your son Josh has just turned 5. You left your partner 6 months ago and since then life has felt hectic. You are lucky that your mum lives close by and looks after Josh most evenings.

ICE

- Your main complaint is: "Doctor, I am just constantly tired".
- You work as a teaching assistant. It's been quite busy lately, you are short-staffed so staying late frequently. It's nothing new though – work's always been busy!
- You really want your bloods to be taken to check your thyroid because your mum has some thyroid issues and you've heard it could be genetic.

Background

- You are usually well. You suffer from anxiety and have had several panic attacks in the past but you are not on any regular medication. You have a supply of propranolol which you use very infrequently. You are aware of distraction strategies and breathing exercises, and you started practising yoga which really helps you relax.
- Your job has been really busy. You end up staying late to help teachers with their workload and not really seeing your son as much as you'd like. Your mum has retired and lives next to you which makes your life easier.

Information divulged freely

- You've been feeling tired for a very long time but it's been more prominent for the last 3–4 months.
- You left your partner 6 months ago; he is the father to your son. It just didn't work out for you and you simply fell out of love with him. You are now dating an old friend from secondary school and things are going well.
- Your anxiety has been more or less under control.
- Sometimes you feel you could fall asleep during the day; people at work mentioned that you look tired and pale so you've been using some make-up to cover it up.
- Your sleep is OK and you get at least 8 hours each night.

Information only divulged if specifically asked

- If asked about your mood, you are not depressed but due to tiredness you've been feeling low and have poor concentration at times, which is really frustrating.
- Your diet is not bad and you love cooking. You order take-outs every Friday. You've been avoiding red meat for about a year to try to be healthier. You have no swallowing problems, nausea or vomiting.
- You use condoms for contraception and don't want to try any other contraception options if the doctor talks about it. Your last period was 1 week ago. You have regular periods which are moderately heavy and last for about 6–7 days. You have always had heavier periods. You have no intermenstrual bleeding. Your smears are up-to-date.
- Your mum has thyroid issues, you are not sure what exactly but she had to undergo surgery for it many years ago. You definitely know it wasn't cancer, it just wasn't working quite right. She is now taking some medication for it.

- You don't smoke, and drink approximately 12 units / week. You don't take any illegal drugs.
- You have not lost any weight. You have no night sweats.
- You check your breasts regularly and have no lumps.
- Your bowels are regular with no bleeding and you have no urinary symptoms.
- If asked, you have no joint / muscle aches or stiffness and no neurological symptoms.
- You don't take any OTC medication.
- You've not been abroad recently and don't remember being bitten. No one else in your family has similar symptoms to you and you feel much the same whether you are in the house or outside.
- If the doctor suggests you might be anaemic you'd accept this but will insist on having your thyroid checked anyway.
- If offered an appointment for a set of blood tests including thyroid function, you'd be delighted. You'd expect to come and see the same doctor for a follow-up to discuss your blood results.
- You'd be happy to take on board dietary advice from your doctor.

Case B9.11 Marking scheme for the observer

https://cks.nice.org.uk/tirednessfatigue-in-adults#!topicsummary

Data gathering and diagnosis

☐	☐	☐	• Explores reason for the call and excludes tiredness red flag symptoms (night sweats / weight loss / lymphadenopathy / breast lumps / alcohol excess / bleeding, GI symptoms / dizziness / neurological symptoms)
☐	☐	☐	• Assesses mood / sleep pattern / home situation / diet / lifestyle
☐	☐	☐	• Asks if the patient is taking any OTC medications / review of current medication
☐	☐	☐	• Appreciates the need for an examination and makes arrangements for a face-to-face consultation

Clinical management and medical complexity

☐	☐	☐	• Considers iron-deficiency anaemia secondary to menorrhagia as the main differential diagnosis but remains open to alternative causes; discusses propranolol and the fact that fatigue is a known side-effect
☐	☐	☐	• Arranges face-to-face appointment for appropriate first-line investigations (FBC, LFTs, renal function tests, TFTs, haematinics – iron, B12 and folate). Also considers random glucose/HbA1c, IgA tissue transglutaminase, HIV, monospot testing and urinalysis for protein, blood and glucose
☐	☐	☐	• Discusses diet, talks about alternative iron sources
☐	☐	☐	• Arranges follow-up, safety-nets appropriately

Relating to others

☐	☐	☐	• Acknowledges patient's concern around thyroid tests and clarifies history by summarising back to the patient
☐	☐	☐	• Explores the impact of symptoms on the patient and acknowledges life stressors which may be contributing
☐	☐	☐	• Good use of pauses, empathy

Case B9.12 Information for the doctor

In this case you are a doctor in surgery undertaking telephone consultations.	
Name:	Antonia Wright
Age:	37
Past medical history:	None
Current medication:	nil

Notes

Case B9.12 Information for the patient

You are Antonia Wright, a 37-year old receptionist who is calling today to discuss some strange symptoms you have been getting in your arms and legs.

ICE

- You recently read an article in a magazine about multiple sclerosis (MS) and some of the symptoms sounded like yours. You feel certain MS is quite rare so it can't be what is wrong with you. You expect some blood tests as your grandmother had diabetes and had a similar numbness in her legs.

Background

- You want to discuss these 'episodes' you have been having for the past 5 years. They happen about once a year when suddenly you will notice you are unable to move your arm, hand or foot properly. It lasts for several hours then seems to resolve.
- The most recent episode was a week ago and the numbness in your hand lasted for a whole day. This made you worried so you made an appointment to discuss it. You feel well during these episodes and manage to go to work, look after your kids and continue your daily activities.

Information divulged freely

- You have two children aged 3 and 7. Your husband also lives at home but travels a lot for his business. You work part-time as a receptionist at a legal firm.
- You are a non-smoker and drink 2 glasses of wine per week.

Information only divulged if specifically asked

- If asked you do remember a few years ago having a day when you thought you had something in your eye as it was painful and blurred for most of the day. You had your eyes tested at the opticians a few weeks after this and everything was normal. You have never seen anyone else about these episodes.
- You will mention your concerns about MS if asked directly. If the doctor explores this further you will become very anxious and have lots of questions about what MS is, the treatment and the possible prognosis. If the doctor can answer these questions clearly you will feel calmer and happily be referred to a neurologist.

Case B9.12 Marking scheme for the observer

patient.info/doctor/multiple-sclerosis-pro
https://cks.nice.org.uk/topics/multiple-sclerosis/

Data gathering and diagnosis

☐	☐	☐	• Takes a systematic neurological history
☐	☐	☐	• Asks about other common neurological symptoms that MS can present with (visual symptoms / hearing / balance / bladder problems / pain / numbness)
☐	☐	☐	• Appreciates the need for an examination and acknowledges she is currently asymptomatic (fundoscopy, brief upper limb examination and cranial nerve assessment)

Clinical management and medical complexity

☐	☐	☐	• Refers appropriately for a neurology outpatient appointment
☐	☐	☐	• Discusses possible further investigations
☐	☐	☐	• Accepts uncertainty and communicates this effectively to the patient

Relating to others

☐	☐	☐	• Recognises the patient's concerns and answers her questions honestly
☐	☐	☐	• Elicits a social history to place her fears in context with her life
☐	☐	☐	• Is responsive to the patient's expectations (i.e. blood tests may not be particularly useful in the diagnosis of MS, but arranging them may exclude other problems and will satisfy one of her expectations)

Case B9.13   Information for the doctor

In this case you are a GP registrar in a routine surgery carrying out telephone consultations.	
Name:	Anica Moger
Age:	18
Past medical history:	Nil
Current medication:	Nil

Notes

Case B9.13 **Information for the patient**

You are Anica Moger, an 18-year old student, who has called to talk about your headaches.

ICE

- You have been having headaches almost every week for the last 2 months. You have Googled your symptoms and are worried you might have a brain tumour.
- You would like a scan of your head to find out what the problem is (but you will accept this is not needed if the doctor explains and reassures you adequately).
- You are worried this will cause you to fail your exams if the symptoms continue.

Background

- You are currently studying for your A-levels and have the first exams in a few months.
- You live with your mum and dad and hope to go to university to study Spanish if you pass your exams.
- You are fit and healthy normally and have never had any health problems before.

Information divulged freely

- You started getting headaches 2 months ago and have had them almost weekly.
- You always know when they are about to start as you get a strange feeling beforehand that you can't describe. The pain is always on the right side of your temple, is throbbing in nature and makes you feel nauseous, although you have not vomited.
- You were taking paracetamol but stopped because it didn't help. Now you go and lie in a dark room which make you feel better eventually. The headaches last around 2–3 hours.
- You feel quite stressed at the moment preparing for your exams and when you get a headache you feel guilty that it is taking time away from your revision.
- In between these episodes, you feel completely normal.
- Your mum told you that she used to suffer with migraines when she was your age, but after Googling your symptoms, what you are really worried about is a brain tumour, and you would like to have a scan of your head to rule this out before your exams start in a few months.

Information only divulged if specifically asked

- You have been drinking a lot more coffee than usual to make you more alert when you are studying. You have also been eating more chocolate as a revision treat. You don't drink alcohol and you hate cheese.
- Your last menstrual period was last week. You are not sexually active and are not using any contraception. You have not noticed that headaches are related to your periods.
- You have no visual disturbance and have not noticed any 'zig-zag' lines in your vision during these episodes. Your mum took you to get your eyes checked at Specsavers just last week and everything was fine.
- Headaches usually occur in the evening when you are studying. You have never had any in the morning and the headaches have never woken you from sleep.
- You have been systemically well in yourself and have not experienced any fever, neck stiffness or rash. You have had no head trauma and you have not lost any weight.
- You would be willing to keep a headache diary, but you would like a prescription today to make the headaches stop so you can get on with your exam preparation. After listening to what the doctor tells you, you would like to try a triptan.

Case B9.13 Marking scheme for the observer

https://cks.nice.org.uk/migraine#!scenario

Data gathering and diagnosis

☐	☐	☐	• Explores headache history to determine site, onset, severity, frequency, exacerbating / relieving factors and associated symptoms
☐	☐	☐	• Asks about headache red flag symptoms (vomiting, fever, visual disturbance, neurological symptoms, meningism) and excludes recent head trauma
☐	☐	☐	• Identifies family history of migraine
☐	☐	☐	• Asks about medication use including analgesia and contraception
☐	☐	☐	• Discusses headache triggers (stress, certain foods, menstrual cycles, sleep) and explores the effect on Anica's life
☐	☐	☐	• Acknowledges the need for a face-to-face examination because this can't be done remotely today

Clinical management and medical complexity

☐	☐	☐	• Acknowledges the patient's fears about a brain tumour and desire for a scan and offers credible reassurance that her symptoms are more in keeping with a migraine (and explains what this is)
☐	☐	☐	• Suggests keeping a symptom diary to help identify triggers and suggests cutting down on coffee and chocolate
☐	☐	☐	• Discusses options for the acute management of migraine attacks (analgesia, antiemetics and triptans discussed) and comes to a shared decision with the patient
☐	☐	☐	• Considers discussing contraception and migraines if time allows
☐	☐	☐	• Arranges suitable follow-up examination to gauge treatment effect and safety-nets by ensuring the patient is aware of when to re-present (worsening headaches that wake her, new symptoms or feeling more unwell)

Relating to others

☐	☐	☐	• Creates rapport and picks up on ICE
☐	☐	☐	• Shows empathy towards the patient's concerns and is able to reassure her that she has none of the 'red flag' features that would suggest a brain tumour and so arranges a face-to-face appointment rather than an immediate MRI
☐	☐	☐	• Empowers the patient to consider keeping a headache diary and try lifestyle measures such as avoiding trigger foods (caffeine, alcohol, chocolate), establishing regular sleeping patterns, engaging in exercise and reducing stress
☐	☐	☐	• Elicits social context and is understanding about patient's upcoming exams

Case B9.14   Information for the doctor

In this case, the patient has booked an emergency appointment this morning.

In this case you are a GP registrar in morning surgery carrying out video consultations.	
Name:	John Carruthers
Age:	56
Past medical history:	None
Current medication:	None

Notes

Case B9.14 Information for the patient

You are John Carruthers, a 56-year old man who woke up this morning with weakness in the left side of your face. Your wife wanted to call an ambulance as she thought you had had a stroke but you refused and booked a video consultation with a GP instead.

ICE

- You think your wife might be right and you have had a stroke but you were afraid of wasting the time of the ambulance crew as you feel fine otherwise.
- You are very worried that if this is a stroke you might become disabled, and the muscles in your face might never work properly again.
- You are hoping to be told you will make a full recovery from this.

Background

- You are a 56-year old man who lives with his wife. You are a retired engineer. You have three grown-up children who live away from home.
- You consider yourself very healthy. You don't smoke and rarely drink. You cycle three times a week, usually for at least two hours each time. You have a healthy diet full of fruit and vegetables.

Information divulged freely

- When you woke up and looked in the mirror this morning the left side of your face was drooping down. This was around 3 hours ago and it has not got better or worse since then.
- You have seen the advert for stroke on TV so are quick to tell the doctor you have no leg or arm weakness and your speech is normal.

Information only divulged if specifically asked

- You can't close your left eye and it is starting to feel dry and irritated. You have no loss of vision.
- You have no change to your hearing, no pain in your ear and no tinnitus.
- You have no change to your taste.
- You have no headache or jaw pain.
- You have no drooling and have had breakfast this morning but did find it difficult to eat your toast so swapped it for some porridge.
- You are extremely relieved if the doctor tells you this is not a stroke. You are keen to have Bell's palsy explained as you know your wife will ask you about it. You do also want to know if you will fully recover from this.
- If steroid tablets are offered you accept them but a friend of yours was treated with steroids for his asthma and put on a lot of weight. You want to know if there will be any side-effects like that for you.
- If antivirals are offered you will also accept these but want to know if this is an infection – do you need to avoid contact with your neighbour's young children?
- If lubricants and artificial tears are offered you are very pleased as your eye is feeling very uncomfortable.
- If referral to ENT or ophthalmology is offered you are happy to attend.

- If the doctor is not sure about the exact treatment of Bell's palsy you are happy to be called back later today with this information about prescriptions.
- If the doctor thinks this is a stroke you will be upset but accept an emergency ambulance as long as you can call your wife to let her know before you leave. You are keen to ask the doctor's opinion on prognosis though.

Results for the doctor

Remote examination

- Focused cranial nerve examination reveals weakness of the left side of the face including the forehead (7th cranial nerve weakness); see picture below, to be given to candidates.
- Can passively fully close left eye.
- Upper and lower limb power is reported as normal.
- Speech appears normal.
- No palpable neck lumps according to the patient.

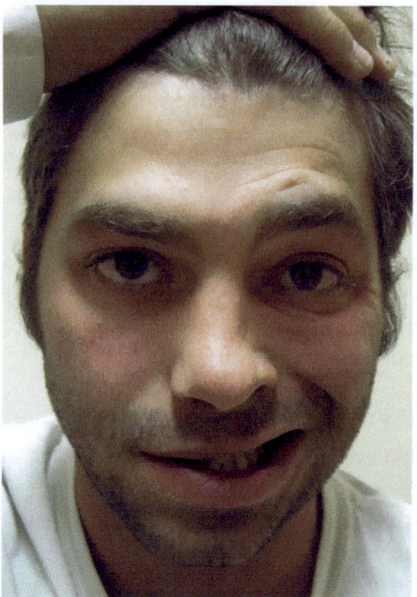

Reproduced from Wikimedia under the terms of the Creative Commons Attribution Share-Alike License, author: James Heilman, MD.

Case B9.14 Marking scheme for the observer

patient.info/doctor/facial-nerve-palsy
https://cks.nice.org.uk/topics/bells-palsy/

Data gathering and diagnosis

- Takes a full history of the facial weakness, focusing particularly on excluding a stroke and red flag features of associated limb weakness, rash in the ear and headache

- Identifies the patient's ICE, particularly his concern about stroke

- Performs an appropriate and focused neurological examination within the limitations of a remote consultation and acknowledges the need for an in-person appointment ideally

Clinical management and medical complexity

- Identifies the diagnosis of Bell's palsy

- Is able to advise on appropriate treatment including:
  - discussing use of antivirals although is aware there is little evidence supporting use of these
  - offer of steroid treatment in appropriate doses (for example 25 mg twice daily for 10 days or 60 mg daily for 5 days followed by a daily reduction in dose of 10 mg for a total treatment time of 10 days, if a reducing dose is preferred)
  - prescription of artificial tears and eye lubricants for patient's use. If the cornea remains exposed after attempting to close the eyelid, ophthalmology referral should be discussed

- ENT referral advisable if concerns of underlying cholesteatoma / parotid tumour / malignant otitis externa – nil features of this present in this case, but arranges an in-person consultation to conduct a thorough examination

- Is able to discuss prognosis and arrange appropriate follow-up

Relating to others

- Creates rapport with the patient

- Is able to explain the diagnosis and treatment of Bell's palsy without jargon

- Recognises the patient's concerns about stroke and reassures appropriately

- Allows time for the patient to ask questions and safety-nets appropriately

Case B9.15 Information for the doctor

You are a GP Registrar doing video consultations.	
Name:	Alex Wong
Age:	42
Past medical history:	None
Current medication:	Nil

Notes

Case B9.15 Information for the patient

You are Alex Wong, a 42-year old man who wants to talk about a tremor you have noticed in your hands.

ICE

- You think the tremor might be due to anxiety because there is a lot of stress in your life at the minute.
- You worry it is Parkinson's disease. Your friend's Dad has this and it started with a tremor.
- You expect to be sent for a test for Parkinson's disease.

Background

- You live alone since your wife divorced you last year. It was a difficult break-up with lots of arguments, and court proceedings are ongoing. She has since emigrated to Spain with your 10-year old son and is refusing to let you visit.
- You work in the IT department of a local financial company and work long hours.
- You drink around 1–2 bottles of beer a night and smoke 10 cigarettes a day.

Information divulged freely

- You think the tremor started around 12 months ago. It only really seems to happen at work. In the evening after you have sat down in front of the TV and had a beer it seems to stop.
- You first noticed it only on the right side but now it is affecting the left hand as well.
- You have not noticed a tremor anywhere else; your head does not tremor.
- It is present when you are holding things or doing something, when you are sitting still it is gone.
- It does not affect your sleep.
- You have been under a lot of pressure at work and at home. The more stressed you feel, the worse the tremor seems to get.
- If the doctor offers to send you for a scan or to a neurologist you will be pleased to see someone to be sure it's not Parkinson's disease.
- If the doctor explains benign essential tremor and treatment options you are happy to try some medication, although you would like reassurance that you will be referred if the medications do not work.

Information only divulged if specifically asked

- There was an incident at work last week where your boss accused you of being a drunk as your tremor was so obvious during a meeting. This is what has prompted you to call the surgery. You have been drinking more since your wife left, but you don't feel like you have an alcohol problem. You would happily listen to advice from the doctor regarding your alcohol intake but you do not feel the need to have any additional support.

Results for the doctor

Examination

- Neurological exam – normal except mild intention tremor in both arms.

Case B9.15 Marking scheme for the observer

patient.info/doctor/tremor-pro

Data gathering and diagnosis

☐ ☐ ☐ • Takes an appropriate history of the symptoms of tremor including the lack of any other neurological symptoms

☐ ☐ ☐ • Attempts to examine the tremor within the confines of a remote consultation and acknowledges the need for an in-person examination

☐ ☐ ☐ • Takes a social history and elicits the patient's personal problems and alcohol use

Clinical management and medical complexity

☐ ☐ ☐ • Explains the diagnosis of benign essential tremor and offers appropriate management (e.g. beta-blocker treatment)

☐ ☐ ☐ • Discusses alcohol intake in a sensitive manner and offers support to the patient

☐ ☐ ☐ • Arranges a follow-up appointment to examine and monitor the patient

Relating to others

☐ ☐ ☐ • Creates rapport with the patient

☐ ☐ ☐ • Empathises with the patient's difficulties at work and home and offers support

☐ ☐ ☐ • Approaches the patient's alcohol use in a sensitive, non-judgmental manner

Case B9.16 Information for the doctor

In this case you are a doctor in surgery calling a patient on your telephone consultation list.	
Name:	John Hargreaves
Age:	54
Past medical history:	Fungal nail infection; gout
Current medication:	Allopurinol 100 mg od, ibuprofen 400 mg prn / tds
Last consultation:	2 weeks ago with the advanced nurse practitioner Weight 87 kg BMI 28.8 T 36.5 BP 127/68 Chest: clear Abdomen: soft, non-tender; no organomegaly; normal bowel sounds No finger clubbing, no pedal oedema

Notes

Case B9.16 Information for the patient

You are John Hargreaves, a 54-year old man who speaking to his GP today about his chronic cough.

ICE

- You saw an NHS campaign poster at a Tube station advising to "ask your GP for a chest X-ray if you've had a cough for more than three weeks". You've had one for more than three months. You have already seen the advanced nurse practitioner, but you are suddenly concerned that you may have cancer. Your grandmother died of lung cancer.

Background

- You are a little overweight but are generally fit and well.
- You live alone but have been seeing someone for a year.
- You work as a car salesman in a Mercedes showroom.

Information divulged freely

- You have had a slight, occasional cough for several years.
- Your cough has become more noticeable to yourself and others in the last few months, but you cannot put an exact time on the worsening.
- Your cough is dry (non-productive).
- You have never felt unwell with your cough, or likened it to having a cold.
- Sometimes your throat feels a little dry and a sip of cold water usually helps.
- You don't smoke.
- You probably drink too much: sometimes you can't remember the last day you had an alcohol-free day (if specifically asked: 3–4 bottles of beer a night).
- You don't get short of breath.
- You are a little overweight and put it down to the beer. You have put a little weight on recently.
- You do not wheeze.
- You have no history of atopy (asthma / eczema / hayfever).
- You have never coughed up any blood.
- You had gout three times and now rarely need to use ibuprofen (the allopurinol keeps it at bay).
- You have not travelled anywhere exotic.

Information only divulged if specifically asked

- You have no symptoms of post-nasal drip (sensation of something trickling down the back of your throat).
- Your partner mentioned when you stay over with her, you seem to cough more at night when you are in bed.
- You have had a dog for 4 years. You don't think you are allergic to your dog.
- You occasionally notice a metallic taste in your mouth.
- You tend to eat a poor diet on the nights you spend at your own house (ultra-processed food and takeaways – anything spicy).

- You feel you make up for your diet by running for 30 minutes three times per week.
- Your grandmother had lung cancer. You don't smoke, but neither did your grandmother (so your mother tells you). You are concerned you have lung cancer.
- If asked specifically about heartburn: you don't really know what heartburn is, and don't think you've ever had it, but do complain of a discomfort in your chest at times, which is made worse by spicy foods.
- You drink around 6 coffees a day from the free dispensing machine at work. It helps drive you, and you feel it makes you more engaging in your sales pitching.
- If the doctor tells you they don't think it's cancer, you respond wondering 'why they have those big adverts about cough' and still think you should have an X-ray.
- If the doctor is understanding and explains that a routine chest X-ray should be done as part of your work-up even though they don't think it's cancer, you happily accept their plan.
- If the doctor states they think you have reflux, you explain that you don't think you suffer with heartburn.
- If the doctor explains that your alcohol intake, caffeine intake and recent weight gain could all predispose you to suffering with reflux, you understand and agree that your cough may have got worse since these lifestyle factors became more prominent in recent months.
- If the doctor suggests lifestyle changes (weight loss, reduction in alcohol and caffeine intake) you agree to make them.
- If the doctor offers you medication such as a PPI or similar, you ask if there is anything you can do other than 'take tablets' (if lifestyle measures not already addressed). If already addressed and still offers medication, you agree to have a trial.

Case B9.16 Marking scheme for the observer

patient.info/doctor/chronic-persistent-cough-in-adults
patient.info/doctor/gastro-oesophageal-reflux-disease

Data gathering and diagnosis

☐	☐	☐	• Explores ICE
☐	☐	☐	• Covers red flags (weight loss, haemoptysis, family history, smoking status, night sweats) as well as checking for infective symptoms
☐	☐	☐	• Takes thorough history to distinguish between the possible causes of chronic cough (asthma; medication-related; reflux; post-nasal drip)
☐	☐	☐	• Notes recent examination and arranges in-person follow-up if they feel a further examination is required

Clinical management and medical complexity

☐	☐	☐	• Explains the probable diagnosis of reflux-related cough
☐	☐	☐	• Arranges appropriate first-line investigations to rule out other possible causes (blood tests incl. FBC/U+Es/LFTs/CRP and routine chest X-ray)
☐	☐	☐	• Suggests lifestyle-based measures (weight loss, reduction in alcohol, caffeine, spicy foods)
☐	☐	☐	• Offers trial of medication after lifestyle measures or immediately (e.g. PPI; H2-antagonist)
☐	☐	☐	• Offers follow-up / safety-netting

Relating to others

☐	☐	☐	• Explores the patient's concerns
☐	☐	☐	• Reassures effectively
☐	☐	☐	• Establishes good rapport
☐	☐	☐	• Discusses patient's lifestyle in a non-judgmental manner
☐	☐	☐	• Demonstrates empathy
☐	☐	☐	• Checks understanding

Case B9.17 Information for the doctor

In this case you are a locum GP in the on-call surgery doing video calls.	
Name:	Victor Robinson
Age:	32
Past medical history:	None
Current medication:	None

Notes

Case B9.17   Information for the patient

You are Victor Robinson, a 32-year old man, who has called the surgery due to a flu-like illness.

ICE

- You think it is just a virus but since you are due to travel in a few days you wanted to be examined by the doctor.
- You aren't concerned about your symptoms, just worried they will stop you travelling.
- You expect to be invited in for a brief exam and to be told to "let this run its course".

Background

- You live with your partner of 5 years and your dog.
- You work as a trainer for an outdoor company who specialise in survival training. This job takes you all over the UK but usually into the Highlands of Scotland and the Lake District. You travel every month or so and are away for a week at a time. Your last trip was to Scotland around 3 weeks ago. You are due to go again in a few days.
- You don't smoke, and drink only a few glasses of wine a week when at home.
- You are very active when at home where you cycle, swim and fell walk. At work you walk long distances and swim in lakes.

Information divulged freely

- You have felt unwell for the past 3 days. You are hot and shivery with muscle aches and you feel very tired.
- You have been taking regular paracetamol, but this has not helped much.

Information only divulged if specifically asked

- You have a dull frontal headache which came on gradually. You have no visual problems.
- You have no numbness or weakness in your limbs and no speech or swallowing problems.
- You have a thermometer at home and have been getting readings around 38.5°C before you take your paracetamol.
- Your joints are painful but not swollen, red or hot.
- You have no neck stiffness, photophobia or vomiting.
- Your appetite is reduced but you are drinking plenty of water. Your urine output is normal with no other urinary symptoms.
- You have no diarrhoea or abdominal pain.
- You have no cold symptoms. Your breathing feels normal with no cough, SOB or wheeze. You have no sore throat or otalgia.
- Your partner has been well and as far as you are aware everyone in your last tour group is also well.
- You have no rashes.
- You have had no new sexual partners and no symptoms of an STI. You actually haven't even had sex in about a month because you have been away and then feeling so terrible since you got home you didn't really feel like it.
- If asked specifically you did not notice any tick bites on your last trip, but you have heard reports of people having tick bites in the areas you go to. You have not removed any ticks from your dog recently.

- If the doctor mentions Lyme disease you have heard of it but thought it was very rare. If they explain you need a blood test you agree. You want to know what the treatment is. You also ask if your partner is at risk of catching it? You also ask about your job – will you be able to go on your next trip if you have Lyme disease?
- You are happy to accept a face-to-face consultation with a view to a blood test.

Results for the doctor

Examination – details from the patient's home readings:
- Video shows patient to be alert and orientated to time and place.
- Temp 37.9°C (due paracetamol in 1 hour).
- SpO$_2$ 99%, RR 18, HR 78 regular, BP 130/80.
- No joint swelling or rashes seen.
- Moving all 4 limbs, nil neurological symptoms.

Case B9.17 Marking scheme for the observer

NICE has a helpful visual guideline for diagnosis of Lyme disease alongside its full guidance: www.nice.org.uk/guidance/ng95/chapter/Recommendations#awareness-of-lyme-disease and www.nice.org.uk/guidance/ng95/resources/visual-summary-pdf-4792272301

Data gathering and diagnosis

☐	☐	☐	• Takes a full history of a patient with fever to attempt to isolate the cause (full systems review)
☐	☐	☐	• Asks about red flag signs to exclude sepsis / meningitis, e.g. sudden onset headache, photophobia and neck stiffness
☐	☐	☐	• Asks about recent travel and takes a sexual and occupational history
☐	☐	☐	• Offers a face-to-face appointment to carry out a full examination, but recognises the results provided are normal except the pyrexia

Clinical management and medical complexity

☐	☐	☐	• Considers a differential diagnosis of Lyme disease in the context of travel history, as well as possible viral illness
☐	☐	☐	• Arranges appropriate investigations or offers to find out which tests to perform and arranges how to contact the patient
☐	☐	☐	• Offers appropriate antibiotic treatment as high clinical suspicion, or offers to discuss with microbiology team before prescribing (e.g. NICE CKS recommends doxycycline 100 mg bd for 21 days)
☐	☐	☐	• Able to advise that Lyme disease will not spread person to person so no treatment is needed for his partner, but suggests he advises his employer so the tour group can be contacted. Also advises against going on his next trip, given testing is needed and his condition may deteriorate when he is away

Relating to others

☐	☐	☐	• Creates a good rapport with patient
☐	☐	☐	• Is sympathetic to his concerns regarding his employment
☐	☐	☐	• Avoids medical jargon in explaining Lyme disease and its treatment and offers a patient leaflet for further information: patient.info/health/lyme-disease-leaflet

Case B9.18 Information for the doctor

In this case you are a doctor in surgery speaking to this patient on the telephone.	
Name:	Lewis Pinkman
Age:	21
Past medical history:	Dislocated right shoulder (5 years ago); 'Tennis elbow' right side 3 years ago; mild psoriasis
Current medication:	Nil

Notes

Case B9.18 Information for the patient

You are Lewis Pinkman, a 21-year old sports science student speaking on the telephone to the doctor about your ongoing back pain.

ICE

- You are fit and active and don't understand why you have persistent back pain. You have been doing all the exercises your physio friends have shown you and you think you must have something seriously wrong and they have advised you to see a specialist.

Background

- You are originally from Australia and came over to the UK to study sports science. You are in your final year at university.
- You play for the university lacrosse team, and as well as 2 practices each week for that you go for a run most days and work out in the gym three times a week.
- You're happy in the UK, have a good group of mates and you speak to your family back home every few weeks.

Information divulged freely

- You have had back pain for almost 4 months now, just a niggle at first, but it is definitely getting worse, and not going away with paracetamol or ibuprofen. You do play a lot of sport, but you haven't had any injuries or accidents that could be responsible for your pain.
- The pain is in your lower back, and mainly in your right buttock.
- You play lacrosse with some trainee physios and they showed you the exercises they show patients with low back pain and you have been doing these for the last 6 weeks without any improvement. You think it is time to see an orthopaedic surgeon and your mates agree.
- You don't smoke and you tend to binge drink after a big game, but generally don't drink day to day.
- You haven't had pain like this before, and no other major health problems, just sporting related injuries.
- You are feeling extremely tired at the moment which is not normal for you. You are not depressed and are generally a positive person enjoying life.

Information only divulged if specifically asked

- The pain is definitely getting worse and has woken you up in the early hours of the morning for the past fortnight. You feel quite stiff in the mornings even though you have been working out less. You actually find that going for a run or doing exercise makes the pain better.
- You have not noticed any numbness in your limbs or perianal area and have had no problems controlling your bladder. You have had no problems with your bowels either.
- You have felt feverish in bed this week and thought you might be coming down with a cold, but haven't had any coryzal symptoms. You haven't had any other symptoms of UTI or sexually transmitted disease. You haven't noticed any weight loss.
- You have had no pain in any other joints, no symptoms of peripheral enthesitis or uveitis. You have had no breathing problems or chest pains.

- If the doctor reassures you that you are young and the symptoms should settle in time, then you will feel reassured, and feel your physio friends were being a bit dramatic suggesting you need to see a specialist, and you will be happy to continue doing the back exercises.
- If the doctor agrees you need to see a specialist, then you will have questions about what they think is going on, and what sort of specialist you need to see.
- If ankylosing spondylitis (AS) is mentioned then you will get worried and want to know what it is and if it is going to stop you from doing sports. You will want to see the specialist as soon as possible.

Case B9.18 **Marking scheme for the observer**

patient.info/doctor/ankylosing-spondylitis-pro
patient.info/doctor/low-back-pain-and-sciatica – useful for listing red flag symptoms for
back pain
https://cks.nice.org.uk/topics/back-pain-low-without-radiculopathy/
https://cks.nice.org.uk/topics/axial-spondyloarthritis-including-ankylosing-spondylitis/

Data gathering and diagnosis

☐	☐	☐	• Takes a comprehensive back pain history, specifically asking about red flag features
☐	☐	☐	• Identifies the presence of red flags (morning stiffness, fever, night sweats)
☐	☐	☐	• Red flag features elicited from the history, but appreciates the need for an in-person examination
☐	☐	☐	• Considers further investigations with an awareness of their limitations (bloods – inflammatory markers (may be normal); X-ray – usually discouraged in back pain, but may show sacroiliitis)
☐	☐	☐	• Considers diagnosis of ankylosing spondylitis and enquires about related conditions in systemic enquiry

Clinical management and medical complexity

☐	☐	☐	• Recognises there is a 'red flag' diagnosis, even if unsure exactly what it may be
☐	☐	☐	• Discusses referral to rheumatology
☐	☐	☐	• Safety-nets appropriately – discusses speed of referral and when to seek medical attention in the interim if symptoms deteriorate
☐	☐	☐	• Remains positive and encourages ongoing physio and makes appropriate prescribing decisions while awaiting further review

Relating to others

☐	☐	☐	• Recognises the impact of the problem on the patient's life and is sensitive to this when discussing possible diagnoses
☐	☐	☐	• Provides explanations to the patient's questions that are clear, while accepting uncertainty
☐	☐	☐	• Is able to discuss what they know about AS and low back pain treatments in general terms

Case B9.19 Information for the doctor

In this case you are a doctor in surgery telephoning a patient who has submitted a photograph of a mole he is worried about.

Name:	Paul Stephens
Age:	61
Past medical history:	Hypertension
Current medication:	Ramipril 5 mg od; aspirin 75 mg od

Notes

Case B9.19   Information for the patient

You are Paul Stephens, a 61-year old business manager who is wanting to have a mole checked. Your wife noticed it a few months ago. You have no idea if it's been there for any longer. She is a nurse and suggested you should get it checked because it looks darker than your other moles.

ICE

- You are not particularly worried about your mole despite it being itchy and having bled on a few occasions. It's your wife who is really worried because her father had a recent diagnosis of malignant melanoma. You are hoping to be reassured that your mole is OK.

Background

- You are a very fit 61-year old. You have a history of hypertension, which is well controlled on ramipril.
- You live with your wife who works as a part-time nurse on a respiratory ward. Her dad has been diagnosed with melanoma recently. Nothing can be done for him now because it has spread into his lungs and liver. You believe your wife is understandably a little paranoid lately about moles because of this.
- You have 2 children, they are both healthy and live abroad.

Information divulged freely

- You admit your mole might have been present for many years but you are not sure because you don't generally check your back in the mirror.
- Your wife commented that she didn't like the look of your mole a few months ago and believes it's getting bigger and looks very dark.
- You are experiencing some itching and discomfort but Vaseline seems to help.
- Your mole bled a few times, but you believe it's your fault because you were scratching it.

Information only divulged if specifically asked

- You lived in New Zealand for almost 10 years during your twenties.
- You never used any sun protection.
- There is no family history of malignant melanoma.
- You had some moles removed when you lived in New Zealand. You are pretty sure they were harmless and you never required any follow-up.
- You never used sunbeds.
- If the doctor explains in a sensitive way that your mole looks very suspicious you would be surprised and demand more information.
- If the doctor remains understanding and calm and clearly identifies the reasons why this particular mole is worrying (asymmetry, irregular colour, itchy, history of bleeding, past history of living in New Zealand) you'd be cooperative and prepared to listen to the doctor's suggestions.
- If the doctor offers an urgent referral to a skin specialist you would question the urgency and reason.
- If the doctor is honest, open and supportive and shares their suspicions of a possible diagnosis of malignant melanoma, you would freeze and remain silent for a short period.

- If the doctor remains supportive and explains it is only a suspicion and that for confirmation of the diagnosis it is important to obtain a skin sample (biopsy), you'd apologise for being silent and admit you are a little bit shocked and surprised.
- If the doctor suggests a 2-week rule referral to the dermatology clinic and makes sure everything is put in place without any delays, you agree.

Results for the doctor

Examination

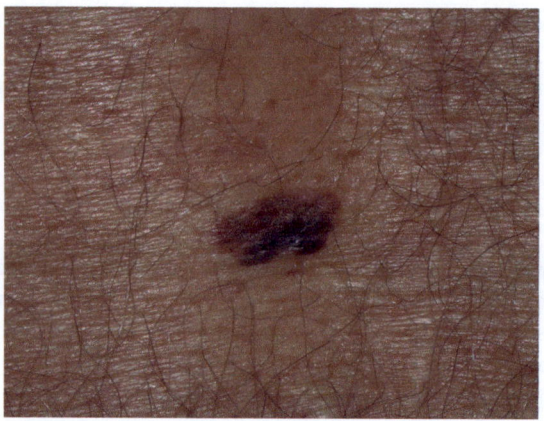

Reproduced from *Dermatology Made Easy 2e* (© Scion Publishing Ltd).

Case B9.19 **Marking scheme for the observer**

patient.info/doctor/malignant-melanoma-of-skin
www.nice.org.uk/guidance/ng14

Data gathering and diagnosis

☐	☐	☐	• Identifies ICE
☐	☐	☐	• Gathers both a personal and family skin history
☐	☐	☐	• Identifies red flags (change in size, colour, itching, bleeding…)
☐	☐	☐	• Carefully reviews the photograph of the mole. Considers ABCDE approach for examination of suspected melanoma (**A**symmetry; **B**order irregularity; **C**olour variation; **D**iameter over 6 mm; **E**volving – enlarging, changing)

Clinical management and medical complexity

☐	☐	☐	• Gives warning shot before discussing concerning features in the history and the photograph
☐	☐	☐	• Highly suspects a possible diagnosis of malignant melanoma – acknowledges the need for an in-person examination but recognises the presence of red flags requiring referral regardless of this
☐	☐	☐	• Refers appropriately to dermatology (2-week suspected cancer pathway) to confirm diagnosis
☐	☐	☐	• Offers appropriate follow-up

Relating to others

☐	☐	☐	• Involves the patient in decision making
☐	☐	☐	• Checks understanding
☐	☐	☐	• Responds to patient's agenda but remains clear abut the need for urgent referral
☐	☐	☐	• Addresses patient's concerns, builds rapport and discusses follow-up

Case B10.1   Information for the doctor

In this case you are a doctor carrying out a telephone consultation.	
Name:	Shiree Kilburn
Age:	22
Past medical history:	nil
Current medication:	nil

Notes

Case B10.1 Information for the patient

You are Shiree Kilburn, a 22-year-old care worker who has called to talk to the doctor about losing weight.

ICE

- You read an article in the *Daily Mail* about weight loss injections and you would like to have a prescription for these, or at least be prescribed some weight loss pills. You are a live-in care assistant for an elderly patient so have no time to do regular exercise and need a quick solution. You would also consider weight loss surgery.

Background

- You have worked as a resident care assistant for an elderly lady for the past 2 years. During this period you have gained at least 5 kg. As your client is sedentary, and your job is to be with her, you feel you are unable to be as active as you used to be.
- In your time off, you are too exhausted to think about exercise. You usually stay at your parents' house and tend to relax in front of the TV with a takeaway.
- You are otherwise well and take no medication.

Information divulged freely

- Your client is obese and requires assistance with all her activities of daily living and you use a hoist for all transfers. You are terrified of ending up in a similar situation to her and want to address your weight now before it becomes more of a problem.
- You used to be very active at school and played on the netball team. Since starting work you have had no time to play sports and you do miss it.

Information only divulged if specifically asked

- Your mum was recently diagnosed with diabetes and is also overweight.
- You have a very poor diet at present and generally eat crisps and chocolate when you are at work. Your mum is trying to eat better since her diagnosis, and your parents do make healthy meals for you when you are home, but you prefer to do your own thing and get a takeaway.
- You have a friend's 21st birthday party in a few months and all your old school friends will be there. You don't want to look fat in front of everyone and want to lose weight quickly. You feel an injection or pills is the way to do this. You have looked at going abroad for surgery but don't have the budget for this.
- If the doctor is sensitive, and explains the guidelines regarding weight loss medication and surgery in a non-judgmental way, you understand and are open to advice regarding diet and exercise.
- If the doctor is overly judgmental or doesn't provide enough information about why you are not being referred for an injection, surgery or pills then you become angry and feel that you are being denied a service that 'the people in the article were given on the NHS'.
- With some positive encouragement from the doctor, you would be willing to seek support improving your lifestyle.

Results for the doctor

Examination

- Shiree reports her weight and height: 76 kg and 1.62 m
- BP 123/80 on home measurement

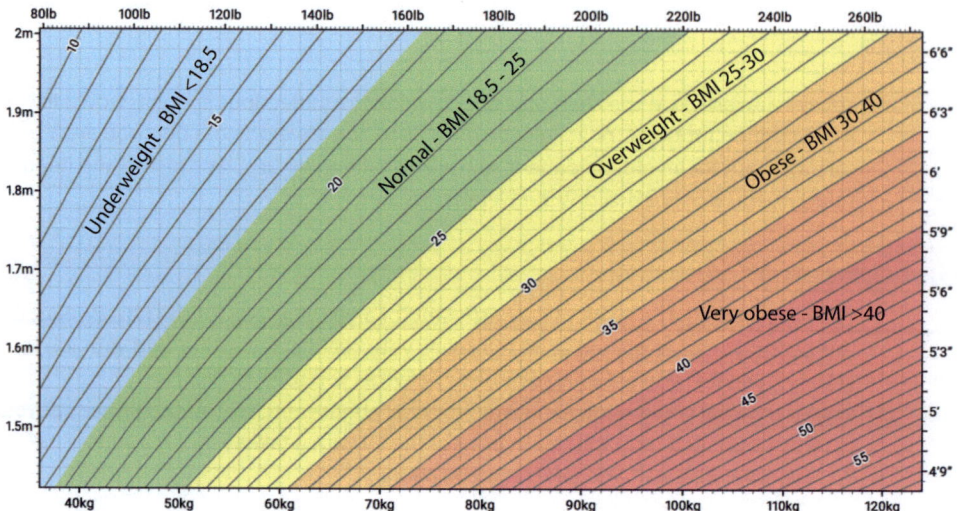

(taken from: www.bhf.org.uk/bmi/home.html)

Case B10.1 Marking scheme for the observer

patient.info/doctor/obesity-in-adults
www.nice.org.uk/guidance/ta875/chapter/1-Recommendations
patient.info/doctor/bariatric-surgery

Data gathering and diagnosis

☐ ☐ ☐	• Discovers reasons for call, ICE and builds up a picture of the patient's social circumstances
☐ ☐ ☐	• Considers any underlying contributing factors for her weight (comorbidities/ medications)
☐ ☐ ☐	• Asks about lifestyle: exercise, diet and alcohol intake
☐ ☐ ☐	• Works out BMI (using chart provided or using calculation [weight in kg / (height in m)^2]) and discusses this with patient (hers is 28.9 – in the overweight category)

Clinical management and medical complexity

☐ ☐ ☐	• Shows awareness of the NHS criteria for referral (which Shiree doesn't meet). (Semaglutide must be used in a specialist weight management service. Patients must have BMI of >35 kg/m^2 (OR BMI 30–30.4 kg/m^2 **and** a condition that can be improved with weight management, such as diabetes.)
☐ ☐ ☐	• Advises the NICE criteria for bariatric surgery specify a BMI >40 kg/m^2 or >35 kg/m^2 with significant co-morbidity. Orlistat can be considered in patients with a BMI >30 kg/m^2 or >28 kg/m^2 with significant co-morbidities
☐ ☐ ☐	• Offers appropriate alternative management options to Shiree. Is aware semaglutide can be purchased privately. Positively encourages lifestyle change (regular exercise – at least 30 minutes of moderate intensity exercise on 5 or more days a week) and healthy eating. Considers resources available locally such as the dietitian / exercise on referral schemes, weight loss apps or local weight loss groups
☐ ☐ ☐	• Discusses the longer-term, disease-preventing benefits of weight loss. Considers checking lipids, HbA1c, TFTs to assess risk factors and arranges follow-up with the patient to check weight and monitor progress, providing realistic targets for weight loss

Relating to others

☐ ☐ ☐	• Explores the patient's health beliefs and expectations and feelings about her weight, and responds to these in an understanding, non-judgmental way
☐ ☐ ☐	• Provides explanations that are understandable to the patient
☐ ☐ ☐	• Enhances patient autonomy by encouraging participation in the management of her weight and considering how the lifestyle changes discussed can be adapted to her lifestyle
☐ ☐ ☐	• Is aware of the local tier 2 lifestyle weight management programmes available (this will be area-dependent) such as a local club/course. Considers involving a social prescriber if unsure of options available

Case B10.2 Information for the doctor

In this case you are a GP Registrar in a routine clinic and the following patient is booked for a video consultation.

Name:	Pary Crick
Age:	31
Past medical history:	Asthma (recent asthma review – well controlled, never uses reliever inhaler, non-smoker, advised to return for influenza vaccination once we have it in stock)
Current medication:	Salbutamol inhaler prn, Clenil 50 bd
Allergies:	Nil

Notes

Case B10.2   Information for the patient

You are Pary Crick, a 31-year old woman, who has a video consultation with the GP today.

ICE

- You came for your asthma check recently and were told to come back when the flu vaccine was in stock this week.
- You know there is a nurse-led flu clinic you can attend, but you wanted to speak to the GP because you have some questions about the vaccine for yourself and your children.

Background

- You are a 31-year old mum of two and you work from home as an illustrator. Tamis is 5 years old and starting year 2 at school, while Ailie is 1 year old and is still at home with you. Your husband François is a paramedic.

Information divulged freely

- You are fit and well. You have asthma but it is very well controlled and your recent asthma check went well. You use Clenil twice a day and can't recall the last time you needed to use the salbutamol.
- You had the flu vaccine last year and ended up feeling ill all week. You want to ask what the point of the vaccine is if you end up getting flu? You don't really understand the difference between a cold and the flu and would appreciate an explanation.
- You heard that your kids should have it too and want to know more about how this works – they will both be terrified of needles. Also, should your husband have the vaccine too?

Information only divulged if specifically asked

- Your whole family are fit and well with no current fevers or problems of any kind. The children are up to date with their vaccinations, but you have always had bad experiences having them. If you hear the vaccination can be given to them without an injection you are very happy and keen to go ahead with this.
- You are generally in agreement with vaccinations, but hear so many reports about the flu vaccine making people ill, you are unsure what the point of it is, and want the doctor to clarify why there is such a push for people to have it this year.

Case B10.2 Marking scheme for the observer

patient.info/doctor/influenza-vaccination
The NICE CKS Guidance on seasonal influenza can be read in conjunction with this case:
https://cks.nice.org.uk/immunizations-seasonal-influenza

Data gathering and diagnosis

☐	☐	☐	• Once aware wanting to talk about the flu vaccination, takes an appropriate history regarding eligibility for vaccine on the NHS (chronic respiratory / heart / liver / kidney / neurological disease, immunosuppression, pregnancy) and any contraindications. Is aware the children's intranasal vaccination is a live attenuated virus and enquires about immunosuppression in the children
☐	☐	☐	• Enquires about any allergies (specifically asks about eggs), any previous reactions to immunisations. Enquires about pregnancy status
☐	☐	☐	• Establishes the patient is otherwise fit and well today and is able to have the vaccination

Clinical management and medical complexity

☐	☐	☐	• Can explain to the patient the groups eligible for the influenza vaccine on the NHS (see earlier links for up-to-date guidance)
☐	☐	☐	• Can advise on how the vaccination is administered to children (intranasal) and that Ailie can come to the surgery for her vaccine, while Tamas should be offered it through his school. François, as a paramedic, should be offered the vaccination by his employer. Is able to advise on where the vaccine can be obtained privately, if asked.
☐	☐	☐	• Offers advice on vaccination side-effects and safety-netting on how to seek help if concerns

Relating to others

☐	☐	☐	• Can discuss patient concerns about the vaccination in a non-judgmental, open manner
☐	☐	☐	• Can discuss the vaccination with confidence and up-to-date knowledge

Case B10.3   Information for the doctor

In this case you are a doctor in surgery taking video calls.	
Name:	Jessica White
Age:	36
Past medical history:	Two months ago • BP 120/80 • BMI 32
Current medication:	None

Notes

Case B10.3 Information for the patient

You are Jessica White, a 36-year old woman, who has called up today to discuss going on the pill.

ICE

- You want a prescription for the pill.
- You really hope the doctor does not try to persuade you to have any of those injections or coils – these make you squeamish.

Background

- You are a shop assistant and your partner is a taxi driver; you met when he took you home from a night out. You have 2 children aged 5 and 8.
- You drink 2–3 glasses of wine a week.

Information divulged freely

- You are currently in a new relationship of 4 months and have been having sex with condoms. You previously used the 'micro-something' where you had a 7-day gap and you found it great – your periods were lighter and less painful.
- Your new partner does not like wearing condoms and you are finding it expensive to buy them so that's why you decided the pill would be good. Your cycle is regular but can be heavy and painful.
- You are currently on day one of your period so are happy you are not pregnant.
- You do not suffer with migraines. You have no family history of DVT/PE, breast cancer, MI or stroke.
- You are not planning any more children but don't like the idea of having a permanent method such as sterilisation in case you change your mind.

Information only divulged if specifically asked

- You smoke 30 a day – you have tried cutting down but the shop is busy so you are very stressed. You realise you are also overweight; again you find stress makes you eat more and after a long day at work you find it's much easier to get a takeaway on the way home.
- If the GP gives you the COCP you are happy and only have a few basic questions about when to start it and the likely side-effects.
- If the GP discusses alternative methods such as the POP you are at first a bit shocked as you don't think of yourself as at risk for CVD, but if they approach it in a friendly and non-judgmental manner you accept it. You accept dietary and lifestyle advice if given in this way also. If you feel you are being judged as 'fat' and 'unhealthy' then you will simply accept the prescription and leave without any further questions.
- You are not keen on any invasive methods, but if the doctor mentions that a Mirena coil can help control heavy periods, you will accept an information leaflet about it and consider this as an option in the future.

Case B10.3 Marking scheme for the observer

patient.info/doctor/contraception-and-special-groups
www.ukmec.co.uk

Data gathering and diagnosis

☐	☐	☐	• Takes a full history of contraceptive needs
☐	☐	☐	• Identifies risk factors for cardiovascular disease
☐	☐	☐	• Appropriately considers the patient's recent BP, BMI and smoking status
☐	☐	☐	• Is aware of the UK Medical Eligibility Criteria for Contraceptive use (UKMEC) to identify potential health risks associated with certain contraceptive methods

Clinical management and medical complexity

☐	☐	☐	• Identifies age >35 plus smoking >15 cigarettes per day as an increased risk of CVD (UKMEC = 4) and discusses alternatives to the COCP such as LARC methods/POP
☐	☐	☐	• Gives lifestyle advice on smoking cessation and weight loss
☐	☐	☐	• Identifies a BMI of 30–34 as UKMEC 2
☐	☐	☐	• Recognises the patient suffers with heavy periods and mentions the place of the Mirena coil in controlling these symptoms and providing contraception

Relating to others

☐	☐	☐	• Creates rapport with the patient and discusses weight in a sensitive manner
☐	☐	☐	• If the patient opts to use the POP, doctor explains how it differs from the COCP (in particular, no 7-day gap, missed pill advice, common side-effects such as erratic bleeding)
☐	☐	☐	• Communicates risk effectively and allows the patient to come to an informed decision about the method of contraception she wishes to use, providing written information
☐	☐	☐	• Is non-judgmental, does not allow own views on contraceptive options to influence patient's decision but enhances patient's autonomy to make informed choice about what she would like to use

Further information

The UKMEC definitions

UKMEC 1 – A condition for which there is no restriction for the use of the method.

UKMEC 2 – A condition where the advantages of using the method generally outweigh the theoretical or proven risks.

UKMEC 3 – A condition where the theoretical or proven risks usually outweigh the advantages of using the method.

UKMEC 4 – A condition which represents an unacceptable health risk if the method is used.

Note: Guidance from the Faculty of Sexual and Reproductive Health supports use of Combined Hormonal Contraception up to the age of 50 years without other medical contraindications to use (UKMEC 1 under 40 years, UKMEC 2 above 40 years).

Contraception consultations are commonplace in general practice and we suggest you practise this case but change the method of contraception the patient is enquiring about, to ensure you are familiar with all of the available methods, their uses, contraindications/cautions and side-effects.

Please refer to the detailed FRSH guidance documents (www.fsrh.org/Public/Public/Standards-and-Guidance/uk-medical-eligibility-criteria-for-contraceptive-use-ukmec.aspx?hkey=82727ce6-756b-4b88-a5ab-acaf27c48669) and patient.info leaflets to aid you with the clinical knowledge.

Case B10.4 Information for the doctor

In this case you are a doctor in surgery taking telephone calls.	
Name:	Mark Evenson
Age:	34
Past medical history:	Anxiety. Stress at work 8 months ago. Appendicectomy 20 years ago
Current medication:	Citalopram 20 mg od

Notes

Age

Past medical history

Current medication

Case B10.4 Information for the patient

You are Mark Evenson, a 34-year old businessman, who has called up today to request a script for sleeping tablets because you are flying to Australia in a few weeks' time and would like to avoid jetlag.

ICE

- You expect to get a script for a sleeping pill but the main reason you called is to address your erectile dysfunction. You heard about Viagra but you believe it's for older men and are not keen to fix your problems with a tablet.

Background

- You are normally fit and well and rarely see a doctor.
- You have been with your new partner Jane for 4 months now. You are going to Australia together for your first holiday.
- You are after some sleeping tablets; you are aware they can be addictive but you just need two or three to help you with jetlag.

Information divulged freely

- You have requested zopiclone from the GP before. Last time you were flying to Africa and Thailand and on both occasions it helped you to get over jetlag.
- You have been on regular citalopram for approximately 8 months now. You were given it for anxiety and stress at work. You are much better on it, occasionally miss a pill or two by accident, and feel great in mood overall.
- You work in a busy company and everything is so much better since you employed a new partner a few months ago. You are less busy and finally don't have to work any extra hours.
- If the doctor does not directly ask about other concerns then you do not divulge why you are there and go home with a script for sleeping pills.

Information only divulged if specifically asked

- If the doctor gets a feeling that you are hiding something and gently asks you directly if there is anything else you would like to discuss, then you will admit you have had problems with erections for 4 months, since you met your partner.
- You haven't been in a relationship for 2 years. You are happy with your new partner but you are very embarrassed about what's happening in the bedroom. You have difficulties maintaining erections and you are worried that your partner will find someone else instead.
- You deny any penile discharge or testicular lumps and you feel well in yourself.
- You smoke 10–15 cigarettes a day and have approximately 3 glasses of wine per week.
- You have no significant family history.
- You have no problems with morning erections; you are able to maintain erections and achieve ejaculation when masturbating.
- You will agree to an appointment for examination and further blood testing if the doctor explains why this is necessary.
- If the doctor mentions a possible psychological cause you will be relieved but you would still agree to have further blood tests if necessary.

- If the doctor also suggests that your erectile dysfunction could be one of the side-effects of citalopram you would question if you could stop it, because in fact you don't think you need it any more.
- If the doctor offers you a script for Viagra you would be very against it and believe that this is not a solution for your problem.
- If the doctor addresses your lifestyle and smoking in a sensitive manner you would be open to this advice.

Case B10.4 Marking scheme for the observer

patient.info/doctor/erectile-dysfunction

Data gathering and diagnosis

☐	☐	☐	• Identifies the patient's hidden agenda and ICE
☐	☐	☐	• Takes a sexual history in a sensitive manner, avoiding assumptions
☐	☐	☐	• Clarifies what the patient means by erection problems (asks about morning erection / erections during masturbation)
☐	☐	☐	• Takes appropriate alcohol and smoking history and addresses lifestyle
☐	☐	☐	• Offers an in-person appointment for examination and further investigations

Clinical management and medical complexity

☐	☐	☐	• Considers possible psychogenic cause of erectile dysfunction along with possible side-effect of citalopram
☐	☐	☐	• Considers appropriate investigations (U&Es; LFTs; HbA1c; cholesterol, testosterone and would calculate the 10-year cardiovascular risk)
☐	☐	☐	• Arranges appropriate follow-up and has a clear plan on what should happen next
☐	☐	☐	• Raises Viagra as a treatment option. Discusses pros and cons of PDE5 inhibitors. Is aware a private script is no longer required
☐	☐	☐	• Addresses his request for benzodiazapines for flying – ideally do not prescribe! (NICE advises only for short-term use for a crisis in GAD, which fear of flying is not). Discusses risks associated with use (slowed reaction times, increased DVT risk, possible respiratory depression, addiction risk, illegal in some countries, should be declared to travel insurer) and suggests a fear of flying course as an alternative option (www.britishairways.com/content/information/travel-assistance/flying-with-confidence).

Relating to others

☐	☐	☐	• Picks up on cues from the patient to explore hidden agenda
☐	☐	☐	• Acts in a non-judgmental manner and maintains good rapport
☐	☐	☐	• Can discuss erectile dysfunction in a relaxed, jargon-free manner; avoids becoming embarrassed

Case B10.5 Information for the doctor

In this case you are a GP registrar in a routine morning surgery taking telephone calls.	
Name:	John Morris
Age:	55
Past medical history:	None
Current medication:	None

Notes

Case B10.5   Information for the patient

You are John Morris, a 55-year old man, who has called to talk about your hair loss.

ICE

- You know hair loss is common as you get older but you are really not happy with the appearance of your hair.
- You have just got divorced and plan to start online dating. You want to look your best and worry your hair loss makes you look older than you are. You worry because your dad is completely bald after his hair loss started at a similar age.
- You expect a referral to a dermatologist to discuss options for treating your hair loss.

Background

- You live alone after your recent divorce. You have 3 adult children who all live nearby.
- You work for a local removal firm.
- You regularly go to the gym and your work is physical. You drink 4–5 pints on a Saturday night. You don't smoke.

Information divulged freely

- Your hair has been thinning for the last 3–4 years. You hadn't been bothered by it until recently as you feel you now have a large bald patch at the back of your head.
- You have started wearing hats at work to cover it up.
- You are certain a dermatologist can help with this problem. You know there are topical medications you can use to help.

Information only divulged if specifically asked:

- You are recently divorced but are keen to start a new relationship. You have looked at some online dating websites and are feeling nervous about joining. You feel a fuller head of hair would give you more confidence and make you look younger.
- You are otherwise well. Your weight has not changed, you are not feeling tired and have no other skin / bowel / eye issues.
- You have not changed any hair / skin products recently.
- You are not using any medications.
- Your dad and grandfather both lost their hair at a similar age – your dad is now completely bald which worries you. You don't want this to get any worse.
- If the doctor advises on medication you are keen to try it, but very disappointed to hear it is only available on private prescription. You are certain a dermatologist would be willing to give you an NHS prescription and push for this. If the doctor patiently explains the consultant will not be able to do anything different, you do accept this. You would prefer to try the topical treatment than the oral medication but would like to know about the side-effects and effectiveness of both types.
- If the doctor suggests blood tests you are willing to have them done but question why.
- If the doctor suggests wigs or extensions you decline – you don't think they look attractive. If the doctor suggests referral for hair transplantation you also decline as you would prefer to use the topical medication.

Case B10.5 **Marking scheme for the observer**

NICE CKS has helpful guidelines on the management of male androgenetic alopecia (July 2018) which can be read in conjunction with this case:
https://cks.nice.org.uk/topics/male-pattern-hair-loss-male-androgenetic-alopecia

Data gathering and diagnosis			
☐	☐	☐	• Takes a full history of hair loss including pattern of loss, duration of the problem, family history and psychological effects
☐	☐	☐	• Asks specific questions to show a consideration of differential diagnoses for hair loss (hypothyroidism, iron deficiency, skin disorders, medication use, excessive dieting, recent severe infection) and if investigations / bloods are suggested, discusses why
☐	☐	☐	• Identifies the patient's expectations for a dermatology referral

Clinical management and medical complexity			
☐	☐	☐	• Is able to discuss use of topical minoxidil (unavailable as an NHS prescription but available over the counter or on a private prescription) and can discuss contraindications and side-effects (https://cks.nice.org.uk/topics/male-pattern-hair-loss-male-androgenetic-alopecia)
☐	☐	☐	• Can discuss oral finasteride and is aware it is available on private prescription only (some areas allow purchase from pharmacy under local Patient Group Directive arrangements). Can discuss contraindications and side-effects (sexual dysfunction and depression) and specifically mentions that it can decrease PSA levels and that pregnant women should avoid handling broken finasteride tablets (https://cks.nice.org.uk/topics/male-pattern-hair-loss-male-androgenetic-alopecia)
☐	☐	☐	• Discusses realistic expectation, costs and timescales of treatment (clinical results may be minimal and often require 4–6 months of treatment to begin to have an effect and would need to be continued indefinitely to maintain that benefit)
☐	☐	☐	• Mentions no treatment as an option and signposts to aesthetic options (wigs, hairpieces – men on a low income may be eligible for NHS wigs, cosmetic camouflage) or surgical hair transplantation (not available on NHS)
☐	☐	☐	• Is able to sensitively discuss referral to an NHS dermatologist for prescriptions. Awareness that NHS prescription rules still apply in secondary care. May consider a referral in the presence of underlying skin problems, an uncertain diagnosis, or if there is no response to treatment after 1 year
☐	☐	☐	• Considers health promotion by suggesting skin protection / sunscreen use on bald areas to prevent sun damage

Relating to others			
☐	☐	☐	• Creates rapport with patient
☐	☐	☐	• Is sympathetic to patient regarding the expense of private prescriptions and the reasons referral to secondary care would not change this outcome
☐	☐	☐	• Can signpost patient appropriately. If unhappy to prescribe as outside remit of NHS/GP practice, can discuss alternative providers / CQC-approved online pharmacy sites that the patient can consider
☐	☐	☐	• Elicits social context and is understanding about patient's embarrassment about his appearance
☐	☐	☐	• Considers referral to psychological support services and provides further written information for the patient (www.bad.org.uk/pils/hair-loss-male-pattern-androgenetic-alopecia)

Case B10.6 Information for the doctor

In this case you are a doctor in surgery taking telephone calls.	
Name:	Vincent Rees
Age:	43
Past medical history:	Asthma
Current medication:	Salbutamol

Notes

Case B10.6 Information for the patient

You are Vincent Rees, a 43-year old nurse who has called the GP today to request a prescription.

ICE

- You have heard about pre-exposure prophylaxis or 'PrEP' for HIV and you are hoping to find out more about this from the doctor today. You have an idea that it might not be available on the NHS yet, but you are very keen to try this and you would like to know how to get it privately if possible.
- Opening line: *"I've rung to chat about getting a prescription for PrEP"*

Background

Information divulged freely

- You are HIV negative and are keen to keep it this way. You have regular testing at the sexual health clinic and your last test was a month ago.
- You are fit and well apart from mild asthma, but you only ever use the salbutamol occasionally in the winter.
- You work as a nurse in the Emergency Department and you took post-exposure prophylaxis (PEP) a few years ago following a needlestick injury. You don't recall being bothered by the side-effects which is why you think PrEP will suit you.

Information only divulged if specifically asked

- You are not currently in a long-term relationship and have had multiple sexual partners over the past year.
- You do try to use condoms, but it is not always practical. You engage in both oral and receptive anal sex with male partners.
- You caught chlamydia 6 months ago which was fully treated but you continue to have regular check-ups at the sexual health clinic and have no concerning symptoms at present.
- You have never injected drugs or shared needles.
- You do worry about contracting HIV and feel like condoms alone do not give you enough protection. You have read about concerns from prescribers in America that patients using PrEP will stop using condoms, but you would not do this.
- If the doctor doesn't know much about PrEP but is honest about it and offers to find out more and get back to you, you are happy. However, if the doctor appears to be bluffing or if you feel you are being 'fobbed off' because it is not available on the NHS yet, you will get upset and ask for a referral to an HIV specialist. If the doctor is able to offer you an alternative solution, such as referral to a private provider you would happily accept this.

Case B10.6 Marking scheme for the observer

www.bhiva.org/PrEP-guidelines

Data gathering and diagnosis

☐	☐	☐	• Determines the reason for the patient's attendance and establishes the patient's understanding of PrEP
☐	☐	☐	• Takes a sexual history and establishes patient's risk of exposure to HIV
☐	☐	☐	• Establishes the patient's ideas, concerns and expectations
☐	☐	☐	• Asks about occupation

Clinical management and medical complexity

☐	☐	☐	• Shows an awareness of pre-exposure prophylaxis. Or, if this is new information for the candidate – they show an interest, listen to the information from the patient and make plans to learn more
☐	☐	☐	• Is able to manage uncertainty and come to a shared management plan
☐	☐	☐	• Takes the opportunity to promote safe sex and condom use
☐	☐	☐	• Signposts patient to a sexual health clinic to start the process of starting PrEP. Directs to resources such as: https://prepster.info

Relating to others

☐	☐	☐	• Takes a non-judgmental approach when discussing the patient's lifestyle
☐	☐	☐	• Is confident taking a sexual history and avoids becoming embarrassed
☐	☐	☐	• Appears comfortable in a situation where the patient is more up to date regarding a treatment than the doctor (if this is the case) and is open and honest about any lack of knowledge

Further reading

The following link provides the latest PrEP (Pre-Exposure Prophylaxis) guidelines from around the world, including UK guidance from the British HIV Association and the British Association for Sexual Health and HIV: www.prepwatch.org

Case B10.7 Information for the doctor

This is a telephone consultation.	
Name:	Donatella Carcino
Age:	80 years
Past medical history:	**2 days ago:** Home visit: Known metastatic lung cancer, refused further chemotherapy last month, gradual decline, bedbound, able to swallow meds, on 40 mg Zomorph bd, DNAR in place, patient aware symptomatic comfort care only, for review 2/7

Notes

Case B10.7 Information for the patient

You are Donatella Carcino. You are expecting the doctor to call today since Dr Shah told you on Monday that someone would call to review things. The district nurse is also present at the time of the call.

ICE

- You are very worried. You have been having difficulty swallowing your tablets for the past few days and you could not manage anything this morning. You are in pain now and worry this will only get worse the longer you are without painkillers.
- Dr Shah mentioned a machine which would give you medications and you would like to talk about this today. He left a green sheet in case prescriptions for this were needed.

Background

- You were diagnosed with lung cancer about 5 months ago which was also in your bones and liver. You did try chemotherapy for a few cycles but it made you really unwell so you decided to stop. You knew this would not give you long to live but you wanted the end of your life to be as comfortable as possible.
- You live with your husband; he knows all about your health and is aware you will likely die soon. You have told him all about your funeral plans and have updated your will.

Information divulged freely

- You have been taking morphine twice a day for a while and use the liquid stuff twice a day as well (Zomorph 40 mg bd and oramorph liquid 10 mg bd).
- You have been feeling very sick this morning.
- You are very tired and found yourself sleeping most of the day yesterday.
- You don't have any problems with noisy breathing.
- You don't feel anxious at the minute – you have come to terms with dying.
- Yesterday you struggled to swallow and did not eat anything. You drank sips of water. Today you have had no medication, food or drink. You don't feel hungry or thirsty although your mouth feels dry.
- You are still happy with your decision not to be resuscitated.
- If the doctor suggests increasing your painkillers you will be very worried. How will you swallow them as even the liquid medication is too difficult?
- If the doctor advises a syringe driver you want to know what will be in the machine, whether it will hurt being put up, what to do if you still have pain even if the machine is working. You also want to know if this means you will die soon; exactly how long would the doctor think it might be, as you want to let your daughter know who lives about a 6-hour drive away.
- The district nurse is checking about the doses of medication in the syringe driver if this is suggested.
- You will be happy to have a home review visit if this is offered.

Suggested prescription for syringe driver:

The following algorithms may help with calculations. Follow local guidelines and take care if diamorphine is being used rather than morphine, as the calculation will be different:

https://bnf.nice.org.uk/medicines-guidance/prescribing-in-palliative-care/ and
https://book.pallcare.info/index.php?tid=96

Morphine sulphate 50 mg over 24 hours via syringe driver (patient is currently taking Zomorph
40 mg bd = 80 mg modified release plus 20 mg Oramorph to equal 100 mg; dose should then be
halved to work out the SC syringe driver dose)

Also consider prescribing an antiemetic alongside the opioid analgesia and prescribe additional
stat doses morphine to be given prn (1 hourly) for breakthrough pain: 2.5 mg SC

plus
Consider prescribing other "just in case" medications alongside the analgesia and antiemetic –
such as midazolam for agitation/breathlessness; hyoscine hydrobromide or glycopyrronium for
respiratory secretions.

Case B10.7 Marking scheme for the observer

patient.info/doctor/syringe-drivers

Data gathering and diagnosis

☐	☐	☐	• Takes a focused history of the current situation
☐	☐	☐	• Identifies the swallowing difficulties and the need for an alternative to oral medication
☐	☐	☐	• Discusses pain and symptoms patient is suffering with
☐	☐	☐	• Establishes current social situation and level of support available

Clinical management and medical complexity

☐	☐	☐	• Appropriately prescribes a syringe driver (script to be written; can use *BNF* to do so)
☐	☐	☐	• Explains to the patient about use of a syringe driver and arranges a home visit
☐	☐	☐	• Recognises the patient's wishes to stay at home despite developing a symptom that would usually warrant further investigation

Relating to others

☐	☐	☐	• Shows good rapport with the patient
☐	☐	☐	• Sensitively discusses end of life care and identifies current needs
☐	☐	☐	• Is clear about the plan for starting a syringe driver and what happens next
☐	☐	☐	• Can explain pain control / syringe drivers in an understandable, jargon-free way

Case B10.8 Information for the doctor

In this case you are a doctor in surgery handling telephone consultations.	
Name:	Andre Rodrigues
Age:	21 years
Last consultation:	• BP 120/80 • Fundoscopy normal • Cranial nerves normal New patient consultation: • BMI 23 • BP 120/80 • Non-smoker • Drinks 3–4 units a week

Notes

Case B10.8 Information for the patient

You are Andre Rodrigues, a 21-year old man who has recently moved to the area. You have rung in today to sort out your repeat prescriptions (co-codamol 30/500 for your headaches).

ICE

- You really want your medication changed to something stronger as you feel it's not helping.
- You are worried about your job – you have had to take lots of sick days with your headaches. You heard a few days ago there might be redundancies coming up and feel certain you will be top of the list if you don't get these headaches sorted.
- You expect some stronger painkillers.

Background

- You have moved to the practice as you recently moved house. You work as an office manager.
- You don't smoke or drink much. You used to be very active and enjoyed cycling but have had to give that up due to your headaches. You live on your own but have a girlfriend who lives nearby.

Information divulged freely

- These headaches started about 1 year ago when you were going through a stressful period at work. After 6 months you went to your GP who told you they were 'tension headaches' and started the above medications. He also did some blood tests which he told you were normal. To try to get yourself back to work you took them most days and at first they did seem to work. After some time, your headaches started occurring more often, so now you take co-codamol every day like clockwork and they don't help at all.
- The headaches feel like someone has a band around your head. You feel fine when you wake up but then by lunch they start. There are no effects on your vision. You don't feel sick. You usually end up leaving work by 3pm and going home to bed.
- You have had the headaches every day for the past month.
- You have had a recent eye check and this was normal.
- You get no weakness or numbness with the headaches.
- Your occupational health team at work has been in touch and you are now very worried about losing your job.
- Your girlfriend has recently been complaining about the fact you can't do anything fun at the weekends because you always have these headaches.
- If the doctor discusses the fact that your medication may be causing these recurrent headaches, you are shocked at first. If you feel it is not discussed sensitively then you might feel the doctor is calling you a drug addict and this will upset you. If the topic is approached in a non-judgmental, sensitive manner then you are interested but also very worried that without the medication you will really struggle to get to work at all. You want to know how to reduce the medication and what alternatives can be used.
- If the doctor offers stronger painkillers you will happily accept.
- If the doctor offers time off work you will not accept – you feel this will make life worse. However, you would accept altered hours to allow you to go home early for a few weeks whilst you try different medication or reduce your medication.
- If you are offered a CT scan or referral to neurology then you accept although you will ask what the doctor is looking for specifically.

Case B10.8 Marking scheme for the observer

https://patient.info/health/headache-leaflet/medication-overuse-headache
https://cks.nice.org.uk/headache-medication-overuse

Data gathering and diagnosis

☐	☐	☐	• Takes an appropriate history of the headaches and use of analgesia in order to exclude red flags and recognises potential medication overuse headaches
☐	☐	☐	• Enquires about mental health; brief depression screen considered
☐	☐	☐	• Identifies difficulties at work and home in relation to the headaches
☐	☐	☐	• Considers the need for a targeted physical examination (BP/fundoscopy) and mentions a recent examination and/or makes arrangements for this to be repeated in an in-person appointment

Clinical management and medical complexity

☐	☐	☐	• Appropriately manages medication overuse headaches by advising to stop the co-codamol (see weblinks for detailed advice on assisting patient to stop)
☐	☐	☐	• Advises patient about potential worsening of the headaches and offers time off work or other appropriate suggestions to manage this (relaxation/talking therapies/headache diary)
☐	☐	☐	• Carries out safety-netting – discusses red flag symptoms and appropriate follow-up. An advice leaflet may be helpful

Relating to others

☐	☐	☐	• Establishes good rapport with the patient
☐	☐	☐	• Sensitively discusses the diagnosis with the patient
☐	☐	☐	• Is understanding of the problems the headaches are causing
☐	☐	☐	• Arranges a follow-up consultation to check in and review progress

Case B10.9 Information for the doctor

In this case you are a doctor in surgery calling this patient on the telephone. She has already been seen and examined today by a medical student at the branch surgery and you are calling her to follow up.

Name:	Jane Montgomery
Age:	34
Last consult:	Seen by medical student this morning and examination findings documented below, now wishes to speak with a doctor about her symptoms: Weight 62 kg SpO$_2$ 97% T 37.1 HR 70, regular BP 112/72 Throat – NAD, tonsils shrunken bilaterally, nil exudates, nil erythema, nasal congestion noted Chest – clear, nil focal, no wheeze Abdomen – soft, non-tender No palpable lymph nodes
Past medical history:	Medical termination 15 years ago
Current medication:	Nil

Notes

Information for the doctor

Case B10.9 Information for the patient

You are Jane Montgomery, a 34-year old woman who has already been examined today by a medical student after complaining of a dry cough, fever, and generalised aches and pains. You now want to speak to a GP.

ICE

- You feel 'rotten' and are very sleepy at work. The cough is impacting on your work as you predominantly talk to customers on the phone at a call centre. You have already been issued a warning for frequently turning up late to work, and are concerned you may get sacked. You have also missed 2 weeks rent so are concerned about both your job and your lodgings. You have called the GP to get some antibiotics.

Background

- You are normally fit and well.
- You became pregnant by accident in your late teens and had an abortion.
- You work for a mobile phone customer service centre, and have done so for 5 months. This was your first job in 2 years, having struggled to find work previously.
- You are single, and live with Wendy (in her house) as a lodger and pay her weekly rent, but missed the last 2 weeks having returned from an expensive holiday.
- You don't get along with your parents.
- You have no siblings.

Information divulged freely

- You noticed a sore throat upon return from your holiday to Spain 1 week ago.
- The sore throat lasted 2–3 days and went away.
- You then developed a dry cough and have been coughing since (approx. 4 days).
- The last few days you have felt a little 'hot-headed' and had a mild headache.
- You have had some generalised muscle aches and pains.
- You have been a little sleepy at work since your return from holiday.
- You smoke socially, no more than 20/week but smoked more on holiday.
- You tend to binge drink 2–3 times per week, but drank heavily whilst on holiday.
- Your weight is normal.
- You have no history of asthma and have never been admitted to hospital.
- Your parents are alive and well, and have no significant medical problems.

Information only divulged if specifically asked

- You have not coughed up any sputum or blood.
- You have no chest pains.
- You are not breathless.
- You do not wheeze.
- Your appetite was poor when you had the sore throat but you are eating and drinking normally now.
- You have not had any calf pain or swelling.
- You have no family history of DVTs or PEs if asked.
- You have not had any diarrhoea, nausea or vomiting.

- You have no history of atopy (asthma / eczema / hayfever).
- If the doctor asks about work, you divulge your recent stresses (fear of being sacked, as described above). You then request antibiotics to help.
- If the doctor discusses time off work, you become a little cross as taking time off work is the last thing you want to do. You just want some antibiotics to help get better.
- If the doctor uses the word 'virus' at any stage as an explanation, or if the doctor states they don't think you need antibiotics (whichever comes first), you explain that there are two other people at work with the same symptoms and they are both taking antibiotics. You mention again about fearing your boss at work, and think that if you had a pack of antibiotics to show him, he'd understand.
- If the doctor offers an appointment for a further examination and remains calm and explains why they don't think this is a bacterial infection, including an explanation of why antibiotics will not work for viral infections, you reluctantly agree and ask what they suggest instead to help you feel better.
- If the doctor explains using too much medical terminology or jargon, you become cross and say you 'have no idea what you're talking about'.
- If the doctor offers you antibiotics at any stage, you happily accept them.

Case B10.9 Marking scheme for the observer

patient.info/doctor/upper-respiratory-infections-coryza
https://cks.nice.org.uk/topics/chest-infections-adult/management/acute-bronchitis/

			Data gathering and diagnosis
☐	☐	☐	• Identifies ICE and establishes what self-care methods have been used so far, if any
☐	☐	☐	• Excludes any red flags such as haemoptysis, breathlessness, dehydration, pleurisy
☐	☐	☐	• Checks smoking history
☐	☐	☐	• Acknowledges the detailed exam carried out by the medical student, but offers further in-person assessment if patient will be further reassured by that

			Clinical management and medical complexity
☐	☐	☐	• Explains viral / bacterial / self-limiting infections coherently
☐	☐	☐	• Avoids prescribing an antibiotic and fluently explains reasoning for this in a positive manner
☐	☐	☐	• Can discuss over the counter remedies and techniques to manage self-limiting illness. Recognises the patient's fears about work and offers assistance with this.
☐	☐	☐	• Safety-netting / offers follow-up
☐	☐	☐	• Offers smoking cessation advice

			Relating to others
☐	☐	☐	• Identifies and addresses ICE
☐	☐	☐	• Remains calm and establishes rapport
☐	☐	☐	• Avoids excessive medical jargon
☐	☐	☐	• Checks understanding
☐	☐	☐	• Patient ends the call after mutually agreed plan

Case B10.10 Information for the doctor

In this case you are a doctor in surgery telephoning this patient about her online consult.	
Name:	Chloe Winter
Age:	26
Past medical history:	Asthma. Appendicectomy age 15
Online consult:	"I would like you to prescribe Roaccutane for my acne"
Current medication:	Beclometasone inhaler (Clenil 100) one puff bd; salbutamol inhaler prn

Notes

Case B10.10   Information for the patient

You are Chloe Winter, a 26-year old accountant. You have suffered from acne since the age of 16. It's never been a big problem but lately it has started affecting your forehead and chin and you are suddenly more aware of your appearance.

ICE

- You are concerned about your acne. Your close friend Emma suggested you should try Roaccutane. She tried it for her acne two years ago and it was magic because she is now completely cured.
- You expect the doctor to prescribe you Roaccutane.

Background

- You are 26 and you work as an accountant.
- You live with your partner Anna. You've been together for over two years and you've never been happier.
- You are close to your parents and you see them every second Sunday for lunch.
- Your job is OK but you've been busier lately due to maternity cover.

Information divulged freely

- You are normally fit and well and only suffer from asthma, which is well controlled with your inhalers.
- Yesterday evening you were planning to go out with your friends and while getting ready you noticed more pimples on your forehead. You couldn't cover them properly with your foundation and became quite stressed. You lost your confidence and felt embarrassed. In the end you didn't feel like going out and just wanted to hide somewhere so no one could see you.
- You are not allergic to anything.

Information only divulged if specifically asked

- Your partner mentioned a few times that she doesn't care about your acne and that she 'loves you even more' for your pimples but you think she is just trying to be nice and supportive.
- You cancelled two dinners last week because you were embarrassed to go out.
- You worry that people will judge your appearance.
- You have regular periods, have not used COCP before and have no problems with excessive hair. You do not require regular contraception and are therefore not interested if the doctor discusses COCP as a possible treatment for acne.
- You are a social smoker.
- You like an occasional wine with your dinner but you are aware of your limits.
- Sometimes you have to wash your face at work on your lunch break to get rid of the oily sensation on your forehead.
- You have used the same night cream for the last decade, and a face toner for sensitive skin in the morning. You use a basic bar of soap to wash your face 3–4 times a day.
- You've never tried any topical treatment or oral antibiotics for acne. You've never seen a GP about it because it's never bothered you until now.

- If the doctor discusses topical treatments you want to know how quickly you could see the results.
- If the doctor says GPs in the UK don't generally prescribe oral isotretinoin (Roaccutane) you initially demand referral to the specialist. If the doctor remains empathetic and explains that at this stage your acne doesn't require Roaccutane and provides reasons why, you'd feel a little better and more reassured.
- You are happy to try topical treatment first if the doctor clearly arranges follow-up to see if that works for you.
- If the doctor offers referral to a counsellor you feel like you've been listened to but you will politely decline the referral at this stage.
- If the doctor suggests you should quit smoking because it might help your skin you'd be happy to follow the advice.
- If the doctor doesn't arrange any follow-up feel free to ask for the dermatology referral anyway, for a second opinion.

Case B10.10 Marking scheme for the observer

patient.info/doctor/acne-vulgaris
https://cks.nice.org.uk/acne-vulgaris

Data gathering and diagnosis

☐	☐	☐	• Identifies patient's agenda / ICE
☐	☐	☐	• Gathers clinical information regarding severity of acne (distribution, presence of inflammatory lesions / scarring) and talks through the photograph submitted online
☐	☐	☐	• Explores psychological impact
☐	☐	☐	• Asks about PCOS symptoms (periods, hirsutism) and identifies possible triggers (recent stress at work, occasional smoking)

Clinical management and medical complexity

☐	☐	☐	• Diagnoses mild acne from the history and photograph
☐	☐	☐	• Is aware of current treatment options for mild acne (topical preparations with benzoyl peroxide or a topical retinoid / antibiotic) and discusses side-effects. Discusses next treatment steps available (oral antibiotics / COCP) if the above topical agents are not successful, and is aware of patient preferences
☐	☐	☐	• Is able to discuss criteria for oral isotretinoid and indications for dermatology referral (nodulocystic acne, scarring). Offers written information if required. Explores appropriate treatment options instead for this particular patient with mild acne
☐	☐	☐	• Takes opportunity to discuss smoking cessation
☐	☐	☐	• Is able to advise on cosmetic choices (such as avoidance of oily or creamy cosmetics and frequent usage of foundation)
☐	☐	☐	• Educates on not to over-wash face with soap (twice daily gentle wash is usually sufficient). Discusses picking and squeezing and recommends avoiding
☐	☐	☐	• Offers follow-up and realistic timeframes for improvement (6–8 weeks to see improvement, 4 months or longer for maximum response)

Relating to others			
☐	☐	☐	• Explores the patient's reasoning behind the requested management
☐	☐	☐	• Communicates severity and treatment options effectively to the patient
☐	☐	☐	• Avoids jargon and has a good rapport and a positive attitude towards helping the patient
☐	☐	☐	• Checks understanding and treatment preferences

Case B10.11 Information for the doctor

In this case you are a GP registrar in a routine surgery taking video calls.	
Name:	Lisa Holland
Age:	33
Past medical history:	Fibromyalgia Migraine Chronic back pain
Current medication:	Fentanyl patch 50 mcg/h changed every 72 h Pregabalin 100 mg bd Naproxen 500 mg tds Paracetamol 500 mg 2 qds
Last consultation:	Medicines team 5 days ago: Repeat requests for early scripts of fentanyl, asked to see GP to discuss.

Notes

Case B10.11   Information for the patient

You are Lisa Holland, a 33-year old woman. You have booked an appointment as requested about your medication. You are very polite and overly nice to the doctor, thanking them for seeing you and commenting how nice all the staff are.

ICE

- You know you have requested some early scripts recently and the medicines team were starting to make comments about this.
- You are concerned the doctor will want to stop your medication. You will struggle to manage without it as the joint pain you get is so severe.
- You expect to persuade the doctor to leave your medication as it is.

Background

- You are divorced and live with your two children who are 7 and 10. Your mum lives nearby and helps out with childcare.
- You don't smoke or drink much alcohol and have never used recreational drugs.
- You work a few mornings a week as a cleaner; you previously worked full time until the joint pains started about 5 years ago.

Information divulged freely

- You have been asked to call by the medicines team. You explain that your fentanyl patch keeps falling off in the shower or bath so you have to ask for early prescriptions. Last week when you asked they said you would have to speak to a GP.
- You apologise profusely because you feel you are wasting the GP's time. You have tried different locations for the patch and tried covering it up, but it just keeps coming off. You want the doctor to agree you can have early scripts when this happens.

Information only divulged if specifically asked

- You started having joint pains 5 years ago and after having various tests and seeing the rheumatologist, they diagnosed fibromyalgia and chronic back pain. You tried several of the suggested medications but they all had side-effects so the GP suggested morphine patches. These do work but you have had to slowly increase the dose over the years and last year the GP had to start the pregabalin as well to help with the pain.
- You have pain in all your joints with no swelling. You also have lower back pain with no sciatica. Your symptoms have not changed recently.
- You also suffer from migraine headaches, tiredness and, when your pain is at its worst, low mood. You deny being depressed at present – your sleep, appetite and concentration are all OK. You enjoy spending time with your kids and read a lot.
- On the medication you are on, you just about manage to do your cleaning job but are exhausted by the time you get home at lunchtime.
- You adamantly deny medication overuse – your patches fall off and that is the only reason for your early requests.
- When the patch falls off you do feel your pain gets worse.
- If the GP wants to change your fentanyl patches you are very reluctant, because you just manage on this prescription – if they offer a switch to oral tablets such as Longtec or MST

you will agree to try. If the risks of addiction and tolerance are sensitively explained and a slow reduction regime offered, you consider agreeing.

- If the GP suggests referral to the drug and alcohol service you decline – you are not an addict, after all these are prescribed medication not ones you buy off the street! You would prefer to see the GP regularly at the surgery. If the GP continues to ask about this you will eventually just agree to get them to stop asking, it will be clear you don't really have any intention of going. If they say they will stop your medication if you don't go, you get upset and abruptly end the call.
- If referral to a pain service is offered you are happy to go and speak to them.
- If the doctor discusses other ways to manage chronic pain you are interested to hear that exercise can help and in particular you would be interested in a local yoga class.
- If the doctor discusses the input of physiotherapists you decline – you have tried this many times in the past with no results.
- If the doctor discusses mindfulness or meditation as ways to manage your pain you are happy to try but would appreciate advice on where to find information about this.

Case B10.11 Marking scheme for the observer

The following resource can be used in conjunction with this case:
www.ouh.nhs.uk/services/referrals/pain/opioids-chronic-pain.aspx

Data gathering and diagnosis

☐	☐	☐	• Takes a pain history to include the duration of symptoms, excluding any new red flag features since patient last seen, and the effect of the pain on the patient's home and work life
☐	☐	☐	• Asks about low mood and symptoms of depression
☐	☐	☐	• Clarifies the patient's story regarding her medication and establishes what else she is taking alongside the fentanyl patches
☐	☐	☐	• Asks about past medication use, alcohol and recreational drug use

Clinical management and medical complexity

☐	☐	☐	• Identifies the difficulties with the medication and advises that although early scripts cannot be offered, an alternative solution could involve changing from patches to oral medication
☐	☐	☐	• Identifies that this patient is on high dose opiates and, given her age, would benefit from an opiate reduction regime to prevent addiction and tolerance
☐	☐	☐	• Offers the support of the drug and alcohol team but accepts the patient would prefer to see the GP regularly and makes arrangements for this
☐	☐	☐	• Advises on an appropriate starting dose for alternative opiates and knows where to seek advice regarding this conversion if unsure (see weblink above)
☐	☐	☐	• Discusses referral to a local pain service for advice on pain management and living with chronic pain
☐	☐	☐	• Offers other suggestions for living with chronic pain such as exercise, mindfulness and meditation and is able to signpost to local services or suggest online services such as Headspace (app for mindfulness)

Relating to others

☐	☐	☐	• Creates rapport with the patient by empathising with the challenges of living with chronic pain
☐	☐	☐	• Seeks to clarify the patient's story but does not make the patient feel judged or appear to disbelieve the patient's history
☐	☐	☐	• Enquires about social history and support she has at home
☐	☐	☐	• Offers leaflet on chronic pain giving advice on strategies to help: www.moodjuice.scot.nhs.uk/ChronicPain.asp

Case B11.1 Information for the doctor

In this case you are a GP Registrar in surgery and the following patient is booked for a video consultation.	
Name:	Alan Roberts
Age:	49
Past medical history:	Psoriasis
Current medication:	Nil

Notes

Case B11.1 Information for the patient

You are Alan Roberts, a 49-year old farmer. You are very upset that you may have prostate cancer and have called to discuss a PSA result that you recently obtained after a test was performed at a local community centre by a charity group.

ICE

- You have a raised PSA result and you are certain you have cancer. You want to know what happens next.

Background

- You had a PSA test yesterday in the local community centre, carried out by a prostate cancer charity group. You had seen an advert in the pub and had gone along with a few mates. The lady taking the blood had advised you to see your GP because the level was raised, but you don't know by how much.

Information divulged freely

- You have had no urinary symptoms and feel well; the only reason you had the test done was because your mates said it was a good idea.
- You were given a leaflet about the test before having it done, but no-one told you much about it. You were a bit distracted when the lady was talking about the test because you had been making plans with one of your friends to drive over to watch your football team play that evening.
- You have worked on the farm since leaving school and the work keeps you fit and well. Apart from mild psoriasis you have no other medical problems.
- You have no children.

Information only divulged if specifically asked

- You go for a run with your brother every week. The last time you did this was the evening before you had the test.
- You also had sexual intercourse with your wife the night before having the test.
- As far as you are aware, no-one in your family has had prostate cancer.
- You are a bit confused by the PSA test but are very relieved if the doctor mentions that exercise and ejaculation can cause an elevated result.
- If the doctor explains the pros and cons of the test clearly, then you decide to repeat it. If the doctor is a little vague about the test then you decide you would like to be referred to an expert to discuss things further.

Case B11.1 Marking scheme for the observer

http://patient.info/doctor/prostate-specific-antigen-psa
https://prostatecanceruk.org/risk-checker

Data gathering and diagnosis

☐	☐	☐	• Elicits patient's ICE
☐	☐	☐	• Obtains adequate history to assess if patient is symptomatic (history of LUTS)
☐	☐	☐	• Determines from the history any activities that could cause an elevation in PSA
☐	☐	☐	• Considers using a patient decision aid to assist the patient in deciding if he wants to repeat the test

Clinical management and medical complexity

☐	☐	☐	• Discusses pros and cons of PSA testing. Awareness of why there is no national screening programme for prostate cancer
☐	☐	☐	• Awareness of the factors which can cause an elevated PSA test: UTI, ejaculation or vigorous exercise in last 48 hours, recent prostate biopsy, recent DRE
☐	☐	☐	• Counsels the patient appropriately and ensures the patient is involved in decision making
☐	☐	☐	• If the patient requests referral, addresses concerns and reassures. Discusses repeat testing in the first instance

Relating to others

☐	☐	☐	• Remains non-judgmental regarding the testing process
☐	☐	☐	• Provides explanations the patient can understand and communicates risk effectively
☐	☐	☐	• Responsive to the patient's preferences and does not allow own views to inappropriately influence his decision
☐	☐	☐	• Considers providing written information to aid the patient's decision: https://patient.info/health/prostate-and-urethra-problems/prostate-specific-antigen-test-psa

Case B11.2 Information for the doctor

In this case you are a doctor in surgery doing a video consult.	
Name:	Sabine Morneau
Age:	28
Past medical history:	Takes the COCP Last consult: Contraception check – happy on COCP, not interested in LARCs, BP 110/70
Current medication:	COCP

Notes

Case B11.2 Information for the patient

You are Sabine Morneau, a 28-year old beautician who has a video call booked today to discuss a genetic condition that runs in your family.

ICE

- You want to discuss haemophilia. Your sister's son has the condition and you would like to find out more because you are planning to have children soon.
- Opening statement: 'I wanted to ask about getting testing for haemophilia'.

Background

- You were born in the south of France and moved to the UK after college to work as a nanny. You have been a beautician for several years now and are happy and settled in the UK.
- You recently got engaged to your boyfriend and have started to think about having a family together in the future.
- You really don't know much about the condition, but you know your nephew has to be very careful about sports and you want to know if it will be the same with your future children.

Information divulged freely

- You don't have any prior knowledge about genes or how conditions are inherited.
- Your nephew has had several trips to hospital when he has fallen and injured himself and you are worried about the implications of this for your children.
- You want to know what the chances are of your baby having haemophilia and if you can be tested for the gene.

Information only divulged if specifically asked

- You have discussed the condition with your fiancé in preparation for the consultation and his family have no history of haemophilia.
- You haven't started taking folic acid yet, and are happy to listen to any advice the doctor offers on pre-conceptual care.

Case B11.2 **Marking scheme for the observer**

patient.info/doctor/pre-pregnancy-counselling
patient.info/doctor/haemophilia-a-factor-viii-deficiency

			Data gathering and diagnosis
☐	☐	☐	• Determines patient's prior knowledge of the condition
☐	☐	☐	• Enquires about fiancé's family history
☐	☐	☐	• Elicits patient's reasons for enquiry and underlying concerns and expectations

			Clinical management and medical complexity
☐	☐	☐	• Explains genes and inheritance in a straightforward way. Using a family tree diagram to illustrate the point may be helpful
☐	☐	☐	• Explains that haemophilia is X-linked so if she is a carrier, her sons have a 1 in 2 chance of being affected and her daughters have a 1 in 2 chance of being carriers only
☐	☐	☐	• If unsure about testing, deals with uncertainty confidently and signposts patient to available resources
☐	☐	☐	• Takes the opportunity for health promotion, e.g. taking folic acid and vitamin D

			Relating to others
☐	☐	☐	• Answers patient's questions clearly and concisely, avoiding jargon
☐	☐	☐	• 'Chunks and checks' when talking through the condition to ensure understanding
☐	☐	☐	• Enquires sensitively if she has discussed her concerns with her fiancé and if they would wish to proceed with any invasive prenatal testing
☐	☐	☐	• Enquires what she would do with a positive result if she was to pursue testing

Case B11.3 Information for the doctor

In this case you are a doctor in surgery doing video consultations.	
Name:	Tracy Steel
Age:	35
Past medical history:	nil
Current medication:	nil

Notes

Case B11.3   Information for the patient

You are Tracy Steel, a 35-year old retail assistant, who has a video consultation booked with the doctor to discuss genetic testing.

ICE

- You want to be tested for Huntington's disease.

Background

- You were adopted as a baby and recently went to find your biological parents.
- You discovered that your biological mum died shortly after your birth as a result of Huntington's disease. You have been reading all about this disease on the internet and are very worried that you may have it too.

Information divulged freely

- You have been reading about Huntington's after recently finding out this is what killed your biological mother. You think you may have inherited the gene for this and you would like to be tested.
- You also want to arrange tests for your 5-year old daughter, Lily, so you can prepare her for the news when she is older.

Information only divulged if specifically asked

- You are aware from your reading that there is no treatment for this disease, but you are someone who likes to plan ahead and know what you are dealing with.
- You are aware that testing your daughter involves a blood test, but you have discussed this with your husband and are certain you want her tested now.
- You feel it is very important for Lily to have this test so that she can plan her life and you can plan for her future.
- If the doctor suggests Lily waits until she is older to decide for herself, you argue that children get blood tests all the time for conditions such as diabetes when they are too young to decide for themselves, so you think she should be able to have this test now too.
- If the GP explains sensitively why they will not carry out the bloods themselves in the surgery you will happily accept a referral to the genetics team to discuss things further.

Case B11.3 Marking scheme for the observer

http://patient.info/doctor/genetic-counselling-a-guide-for-gps
https://patient.info/doctor/huntingtons-disease-pro

Data gathering and diagnosis	
☐ ☐ ☐	• Discovers reason for attendance and takes history
☐ ☐ ☐	• Determines patient's prior knowledge of the condition
☐ ☐ ☐	• Elicits patient's ideas regarding testing for herself and for her daughter

Clinical management and medical complexity	
☐ ☐ ☐	• Discusses implications of testing for patient and her daughter
☐ ☐ ☐	• Refers to a clinical genetics service to explore further, with the understanding that their approach is usually only to carry out genetic testing on people over the age of 18 with informed consent
☐ ☐ ☐	• Directs patient to resources such as the Huntington's Disease Association www.hda.org.uk

Relating to others	
☐ ☐ ☐	• Responds to patient's queries with interest and understanding
☐ ☐ ☐	• Elicits patient's concerns and discusses referral options
☐ ☐ ☐	• Remains positive but realistic, and ensures the patient understands that testing for her daughter is unlikely to be agreed to by secondary care until she is 18
☐ ☐ ☐	• Is cooperative and inclusive

Case B11.4 Information for the doctor

In this case you are a doctor telephoning a patient to discuss his recent ECG.	
Name:	Dr Prakash Shah
Age:	67
Past medical history:	Bloods done last month: FBC/U&Es all normal
Last consultation:	2 days ago influenza vaccine given by nurse, BP 130/80, pulse noted to be irregular, appointment made for ECG then GP review.

Notes

Case B11.4   Information for the patient

You are Prakash Shah, a 67-year old retired ophthalmologist who is speaking to the GP today for review of your ECG which the nurse asked for because of your irregular pulse.

ICE

- You are sure this is AF and are concerned about being on warfarin since you regularly saw the complications of it in ophthalmology. You also worry about stroke as your mother was very disabled following a stroke and spent the rest of her days in a nursing home. You expect a full and honest discussion about treatment.

Background

- You attended for a flu jab a few days ago and had your blood pressure checked at the same time. The nurse noticed your irregular pulse so asked for an ECG.
- You retired as an ophthalmologist 10 years ago. Cardiology was never your forte but you have been feeling your pulse regularly and you are certain it's AF. It doesn't feel irregular constantly, however, and you think this may have been the case for months.
- Since having the ECG you have spoken to several of your colleagues about treatment and want to know about the medication that is used instead of warfarin.

Information divulged freely

- You live with your wife who is also retired. You have a son who lives in New Zealand and you try to visit every few years.
- You have had no symptoms of chest pain, palpitations or shortness of breath. You occasionally feel dizzy if you stand up too quickly or exert yourself.
- You drink a bottle of wine a week and do not smoke. You feel your diet is healthy and you walk daily and cycle 3 times a week.

Information only divulged if specifically asked

- You don't know much about the new anticoagulants except they don't need monitoring. Your main questions are about side-effects, reversal of treatment and if they are as effective as warfarin. If the GP does not know the answer you will feel frustrated. You really wanted a prescription today and are not very impressed if you feel this might not happen.
- You were not aware of the CHA_2DS_2Vasc score, or the ORBIT scoring tool. If mentioned, you are relieved to hear you are low risk.
- If given the option, you would prefer to be referred for cardioversion. You would rather avoid further medications. You are happy to discuss beta blockers although you have no symptoms and your rate is controlled.
- You are happy to accept a cardiology referral. You would prefer to start a new oral anticoagulant today, but you do not want to start warfarin.

Results for the doctor

ECG:

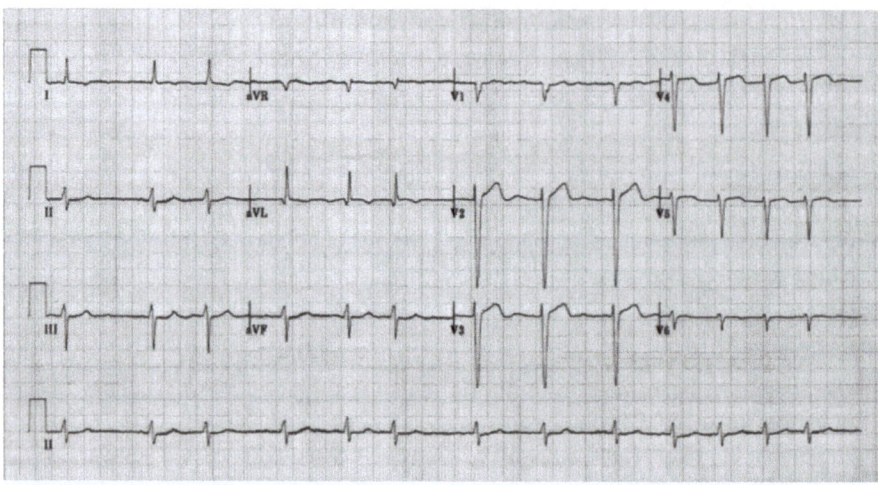

Reproduced from: litfl.com (providers of Free Open Access Meducation).

Case B11.4 Marking scheme for the observer

patient.info/doctor/atrial-fibrillation-pro
https://cks.nice.org.uk/topics/atrial-fibrillation

Data gathering and diagnosis

			• Gathers adequate information on symptoms of AF, determines onset is >48h and excludes symptoms of haemodynamic instability (tachycardia >150, low BP <90mmHg systolic, loss of consciousness, severe dizziness/syncope, chest pain, breathlessness)
			• Appropriately interprets the ECG as atrial fibrillation
			• Assesses both stroke risk and bleeding risk using CHA_2DS_2Vasc (score is 1) and the ORBIT scoring tool (score is 0) – both low risk scores
			• Elicits the patient's ideas about warfarin and treatment preferences

Clinical management and medical complexity

			• Considers the need to admit (signs of haemodynamic instability / signs of stroke or other underlying conditions); in this case the patient is stable and appropriate to manage initially in primary care
			• Discusses AF, including rate and rhythm control, with the patient. Ensures patient is aware of 'adverse symptoms' of haemodynamic compromise and when to seek help. Can discuss cardioversion and its indications if the patient asks
			• Discusses further investigations to exclude underlying causes of AF (considers the need for TFTs, electrolyte and glucose, signs of infection, echo for structural abnormalities and if cardiology input required)
			• Discusses the benefits and risks of anticoagulation (can discuss direct-acting oral anticoagulants with the patient and the monitoring needed). If unsure, deals with uncertainty and makes a plan to find out more
			• Arranges appropriate follow-up and provides written information for the patient. As this is a telephone consult, offers face-to-face if they feel further clinical assessment needed

Relating to others

			• Recognises the patient's prior knowledge and medical background; however, avoids excessive jargon and still explains the condition fully
			• Explores the patient's reasoning behind his requested management

☐	☐	☐	• Communicates effectively to the patient and ensures he knows when follow-up is planned and where to seek help if needed
☐	☐	☐	• Considers driving and DVLA requirements (www.gov.uk/guidance/general-information-assessing-fitness-to-drive). Advises patient to check their cover with their insurer
☐	☐	☐	• Considers signposting to AF support groups (https://heartrhythmalliance.org/aa/uk)

Case B11.5   Information for the doctor

In this case you are a doctor in surgery doing telephone consultations.	
Name:	Rupert Mornington
Age:	62
Past medical history:	Nil significant. Height 168 cm, weight 85 kg (BMI 30). Cholesterol/HDL ratio 5.6. QRISK2 score 14.7%
Current medication:	None

Notes

Case B11.5 Information for the patient

You are Rupert Mornington, a 62-year old man who is calling the GP today to discuss your recent cholesterol result.

ICE

- You are a little surprised you have been asked to talk about your results because they have not changed much from your check-up last year.
- You expect to be told to do more exercise and eat healthy foods like last year.

Background

Information divulged freely

- You are fit and well and have never had diabetes, heart problems, kidney disease, autoimmune disorders or treatment for high blood pressure.
- You don't smoke and never have done.
- You are not aware of any relatives who had a heart attack or angina under the age of 60.

Information only divulged if specifically asked

- You are aware that you need to lose some weight but find it difficult to fit exercise into your busy life. You do feel bad about this and remember in your 20s being very fit and playing football regularly.
- You work in the oil industry and are required to entertain clients several times a week – this involves big dinners and often a lot of alcohol (way over the recommended weekly limits). You are aware that this is likely to be a contributing factor to your weight, but it is a part of the job.
- You have never been a fan of taking medications and do not like the idea of statins. You have read the media reports and find they are often conflicting and you would welcome a balanced view from the GP regarding whether they work or not.
- If the GP is insistent that you must take a statin based on these new guidelines without an adequate explanation as to why, then you will feel patronised and refuse.
- If the GP works towards a shared management plan and acknowledges your views, you will be more inclined to consider a statin. You know that your figures haven't changed significantly from last year, but the guidelines have. You would rather spend another year working on modification of your lifestyle and may consider a statin if the situation is unchanged next year. You will happily accept the offer of some further information about statins.

Case B11.5 Marking scheme for the observer

patient.info/doctor/lipid-regulating-drugs-including-statins
patient.info/doctor/cardiovascular-risk-assessment
www.nice.org.uk/guidance/ph25

Data gathering and diagnosis

☐	☐	☐	• Assesses CVD risk and is aware of the QRISK3 tool
☐	☐	☐	• Acknowledges BP/weight as risk factors
☐	☐	☐	• Explores ICE
☐	☐	☐	• Asks about lifestyle (job, smoking, alcohol, diet)

Clinical management and medical complexity

☐	☐	☐	• Shows an awareness of the latest NICE guidelines on lipid modification (see above). In primary prevention, treatment should now be offered to patients with a 10-year CVD risk of 10% or more (previously it was 20%)
☐	☐	☐	• Is able to discuss statins with the patient including action, monitoring treatment and potential side-effects
☐	☐	☐	• Takes lifestyle factors into consideration and discusses ways in which the patient can modify his to be healthier
☐	☐	☐	• Is able to signpost the patient to any local schemes/groups that may help with weight management and alcohol (such as exercise on prescription if necessary)
☐	☐	☐	• Offers follow-up/safety-netting

Relating to others

☐	☐	☐	• Takes the patient's views into consideration when discussing treatment options
☐	☐	☐	• Adopts a flexible approach and acknowledges that guidelines change. Ensures the treatment decision is based on what is best for the patient after he has been informed of why things have changed
☐	☐	☐	• Takes a non-judgmental approach to discussing the patient's lifestyle, and remains positive about modifications that can be made

Case B11.6 Information for the doctor

In this case you are a doctor in surgery. You have the following patient waiting on line 1 wanting to discuss her recent blood test results with you.

Name:	Rosemary Jarvis
Age:	51
Past medical history:	Depression (2000) cholecystectomy (2001)
Current medication:	nil
Last consultation:	Seen by practice nurse last week, routine bloods taken
Results:	Hb 140 (120–150 g/L) MCV 85 (80–100 fL) Plt 200 (150–400 x 10⁹/L) WCC 9.0 (4.0–11.0 x 10⁹/L) Na 139 (135–145 mmol/L) K 4.0 (3.5–5.0 mmol/L) Ur **6.6** (3.0–6.5 mmol/L) Cr 83 (60–125 µmol/L) eGFR 98 (>90 ml min) TSH **9.5** (0.35–5.5 mU/L) T4 11 (8–22 pmol/L) Bili 16 (0–17 µmol/L) ALP 176 (100–300 U/L) ALT 22 (5–42 IU/L) GGT 28 (6–29 IU/L)

Notes

Case B11.6 Information for the patient

You are Rosemary Jarvis, a 51-year old full-time mum calling the doctor to find out the results of your recent blood tests.

ICE

- You called for your results this morning and were told by the receptionist that they were not normal and you had to speak to the doctor. You have been worrying about what this means all morning and just want some answers.

Background

- You are a happily married mum of three teenagers. Your husband John runs the local garage and you volunteer one day a week as an assistant at a primary school.

Information divulged freely

- The receptionist told you your blood results were abnormal and you are very worried and want to know what this means.
- You want to know as much as possible about the results.

Information only divulged if specifically asked

- You only had the bloods taken by chance. You booked in with Paula, the nurse, to have your smear done last week, and when you arrived she informed you it wasn't due for another year. You go to Pilates with Paula, so she offered to do routine blood tests for you so as not to have a wasted appointment. She said that according to your record you hadn't had any done for over 5 years.
- You generally feel quite well. You do often feel tired all the time, but you put that down to your three kids. You're not pregnant; John had a vasectomy years ago.
- You haven't had any constipation, weight gain or cold intolerance, but you have noticed that your skin gets quite dry if you don't apply moisturiser every day; but this has always been the case.
- You don't want to start medication and you are happy to have further blood tests if the doctor advises you to.
- You want to know at what stage you would have to go on medication if the results remain the same after another blood test.

Case B11.6 Marking scheme for the observer

patient.info/doctor/subclinical-hypothyroidism
https://cks.nice.org.uk/topics/hypothyroidism/management/subclinical-hypothyroidism-
  non-pregnant/

Data gathering and diagnosis

☐	☐	☐	• Establishes the reasons the blood tests were carried out and the patient's expectations of them
☐	☐	☐	• Enquires about any physical symptoms of hypothyroidism or previous ischaemic heart disease (hypothyroidism important as risk factor for cardiovascular disease – often elevated cholesterol)
☐	☐	☐	• Asks about any goitre / neck lumps; asks if patient may be pregnant because this impacts management

Clinical management and medical complexity

☐	☐	☐	• Explains clearly the nature of subclinical hypothyroidism and when it is reasonable to consider medication
☐	☐	☐	• Reasonably suggests monitoring in this case and arranges repeat TFTs, fasting lipids and thyroid autoantibody testing in approximately 6–12 weeks' time
☐	☐	☐	• If asked about when medication is started, either admits uncertainty and arranges to find out, or discusses current guidance, which suggests if TSH levels are consistently >10 and patient is symptomatic, treatment may be considered
☐	☐	☐	• Takes opportunity to discuss health promotion of cardiovascular risk factors in relation to hypothyroidism

Relating to others

☐	☐	☐	• Explores patient's concerns and elicits social information to put problem in context
☐	☐	☐	• Provides explanation that patient can understand
☐	☐	☐	• Responds to patient's questions with interest and understanding

Case B11.7   Information for the doctor

In this case you are a GP Registrar calling a patient on the telephone to discuss blood results.	
Name:	William (Bill) Norman
Age:	68
Past medical history:	Hypertension
Current medication:	Amlodipine 5 mg od

Last consultation: Spoke to locum doctor on the phone regarding results of his annual blood tests. Notes state 'Patient not known to me' – U&Es show CKD 3 on routine bloods. Patient informed and suggested book appointment to discuss further with usual GP.

Recent bloods:	All other bloods normal
Latest sample:	Na 136 (135–145 mmol/L) K 3.9 (3.5–5.0 mmol/L) Ur 4.2 (3.0–6.5 mmol/L) Cr 110 (60–125 µmol/L) eGFR **48** (>90 ml min) Urinary ACR 2.0 (<2.5 mg / mmol) Urinalysis – NAD BP 130/75 U&E results from 1 year ago: Na 140 (135–145 mmol/L) K 4.5 (3.5–5.0 mmol/L) Ur 4.9 (3.0–6.5 mmol/L) Cr 115 (60–125 µmol/L) eGFR **42** (>90 ml min)

Notes

Case B11.7   Information for the patient

You are Bill Norman, 68. You want to discuss your annual blood tests with the doctor.

ICE

- You spoke to a doctor you didn't know on the phone last week about your routine bloods and he told you that you had chronic kidney disease. You are aghast. You want to know why this has only been picked up now and the implications of it.
- Your opening line is: 'I want to talk about my severe kidney disease'.

Background

- You are a retired gardener and are enjoying your retirement with your wife Edie.
- You have always considered yourself quite fit and well. Although you are not outdoors as much as when you were working, you still potter around the garden most days and are a keen fell walker.

Information divulged freely

- You are very concerned that you have a chronic disease. You understand that chronic means very severe. You are confused about how it could have reached this stage without being picked up earlier. Why wasn't it spotted at stage 1 or 2? You will continue to talk about the disease as severe unless the doctor asks why you think this, and you will explain the locum doctor on the telephone said it was chronic. If the doctor gives an understandable explanation of what chronic actually means, you will feel slightly reassured.
- You have had high blood pressure for over 10 years but don't see it as a problem; you take your medicine every day and it has always been controlled at your yearly checks. You feel fit and well and wonder why you have no symptoms if the disease is so bad.

Information only divulged if specifically asked

- If the doctor mentions that your bloods results are unchanged from the results you had a year ago you will feel quite indignant that you were not told about your kidney failure last year, and will demand an explanation for this. If the doctor gives an understandable explanation of CKD and the implications of the results then you will feel reassured. If not you will continue asking questions about the implications to your kidneys and ask to be referred to 'someone who knows what they are talking about' before the problem gets worse.
- You don't smoke and drink 4 pints of beer every week.

Case B11.7 Marking scheme for the observer

patient.info/doctor/chronic-kidney-disease-pro
https://cks.nice.org.uk/chronic-kidney-disease-not-diabetic

Data gathering and diagnosis

☐	☐	☐	• Establishes the patient's concerns about the results and takes account of the previous results and history provided
☐	☐	☐	• Makes note of the presence of hypertension, but is reassured that the other bloods exclude diabetes, anaemia, significant renal disease and uses this information to be able to reassure the patient
☐	☐	☐	• Interprets the results correctly (CKD Stage 3a) and establishes that the patient is symptom-free and not on any nephrotoxic medication
☐	☐	☐	• Reviews previous results to assess the degree of deterioration (if any)

Clinical management and medical complexity

☐	☐	☐	• Provides a clear explanation of CKD stage 3, common causes, reassurance that it rarely progresses to the need for dialysis and offers a patient information leaflet
☐	☐	☐	• Explains the need for monitoring and for good control of blood pressure
☐	☐	☐	• Discusses the link between CKD and developing cardiovascular disease. Latest NICE guidelines advocate starting atorvastatin 20 mg and an antiplatelet drug in CKD3 patients; explores this with patient
☐	☐	☐	• Discusses avoidance of nephrotoxins (NSAIDs, radiocontrast agents)
☐	☐	☐	• Discusses eligibility for annual influenza / anti-pneumococcal vaccination

Relating to others

☐	☐	☐	• Responds to the patient's concerns and expectations and provides understandable answers to the questions asked
☐	☐	☐	• Establishes the patient's understanding of the word 'chronic' and provides reassurance
☐	☐	☐	• Works in partnership to develop a shared management plan
☐	☐	☐	• Avoids jargon

Case B11.8 Information for the doctor

> **You are a GP Registrar in your afternoon surgery telephoning a patient to discuss his recent blood results.**

Name:	Diego Urbano
Age:	31
Past medical history:	None
Current medication:	Nil
Previous consultation:	Seen by Dr Veneto last week c/o total body pain. Nil specific injury/triggers. Systemically well, nil other symptoms or concerning features. Normal examination. For routine bloods and review.
Blood results:	Hb 138 (120–150 g/L) MCV 90 (80–100 fL) Plt 340 (150–400 × 10^9/L) WCC 8.1 (4.0–11.0 × 10^9/L) Na 139 (135–145 mmol/L) K 3.7 (3.5–5.0 mmol/L) Ur 5.6 (3.0–6.5 mmol/L) Cr 110 (60–125 µmol/L) eGFR 94 (>90 ml/min) 25-hydroxyvitamin D **31** nmol/L (>75 nmol/L optimal) LFTs, calcium, PTH, ferritin, CK and TFTs – normal

Notes

Case B11.8 Information for the patient

You are Diego Urbano, a 31-year old waiter, who wants to talk about your recent blood results.

ICE

- You have been feeling generally 'achey' for weeks and hope the blood results will give you an explanation for this problem.

Background

- You are originally from Colombia and moved to the UK last year to work as a waiter at a high-class hotel.
- You have always been fit and well.
- You don't smoke and drink the occasional beer after a shift at work.

Information divulged freely

- You came to see another doctor at the surgery over a week ago because you have been feeling generally 'achey' for weeks, maybe months. The doctor examined you and found nothing wrong, and arranged for you to have some bloods taken.
- You work hard, that's the nature of the job, and your role does involve lifting heavy trays, but you have not had any specific injuries that would be responsible for the muscle pains you have been experiencing.
- You have never felt 'achey' like this before. At home you used to enjoy going running and you have been diligent about trying to stretch after your shifts, but this has made no difference. You occasionally take paracetamol which does help.
- You are relieved if the doctor suggests your symptoms may be caused by a lack of vitamin D and you are interested to hear more about why this has happened – is it because of your diet? You would like an explanation about what you need to do to correct this.
- If asked to take a supplement you would like the doctor to write down exactly what you need because your English isn't perfect and you don't want to get it wrong. If you could have an NHS prescription for the supplement you would be even happier. You want to know how long you need to take it for.
- You wonder if your girlfriend should get tested too because she also spends a lot of time indoors – what does the doctor advise?

Information only divulged if specifically asked

- You work long hours at the hotel because you are looking for a promotion. You often work until the early hours of the morning and then have to be up early for the breakfast shift. You tend to catch up on sleep during your afternoon break. If specifically asked you will realise that you don't spend much time outdoors at all – it is way too cold in the UK! On your days off you tend to sleep, and occasionally use the hotel gym.
- Your diet has also suffered since moving to the UK. Staff meals at the hotel are poor and you tend to be picky. Often you will get a pizza or eat crisps and unhealthy snacks between shifts.
- You have never broken any bones or taken any medications in the past – you have always been healthy.
- You have no problems with your bowels and have not noticed loose stools.

Case B11.8 Marking scheme for the observer

https://patient.info/doctor/vitamin-d-deficiency-including-osteomalacia-and-rickets-pro
https://cks.nice.org.uk/topics/vitamin-d-deficiency-in-adults/

Data gathering and diagnosis

☐	☐	☐	• Re-explores the patient's history and considers vitamin D deficiency as a potential cause of the patient's non-specific symptoms (excludes other plausible explanations)
☐	☐	☐	• Assesses for risk factors that may warrant high strength replacement (fragility fractures, medications, conditions associated with malabsorption)
☐	☐	☐	• Asks about lifestyle factors which put the patient at risk of deficiency

Clinical management and medical complexity

☐	☐	☐	• Can discuss vitamin D and bone health, and offer advice on safe sun exposure
☐	☐	☐	• Can name some foods containing vitamin D (oily fish, egg yolk, fortified cereals) but is aware that sun exposure is main source compared to dietary intake
☐	☐	☐	• Recognises vitamin D insufficiency and advises an oral replacement and maintenance
☐	☐	☐	• Is aware that vitamin D testing is not recommended in asymptomatic population-risk individuals – offers his girlfriend lifestyle advice and suggests over-the-counter supplements

Relating to others

☐	☐	☐	• Builds rapport with the patient and shows understanding towards his busy work schedule
☐	☐	☐	• Is mindful that English is not the patient's first language and keeps the explanations clear and jargon-free
☐	☐	☐	• Considers use of NHS resources and can advise the patient (and his girlfriend) in a tactful manner on obtaining over-the-counter maintenance supplements
☐	☐	☐	• Offers a follow-up appointment in a reasonable amount of time if the symptoms have not improved

Case B11.9 Information for the doctor

You are a GP registrar telephoning your next patient to discuss the results of his recent tests.	
Name:	Calum Richards
Age:	54
Past medical history:	Anxiety / depression GORD
Current medication:	Citalopram 20 mg od Lansoprazole 30 mg od

Spirometry report attached:

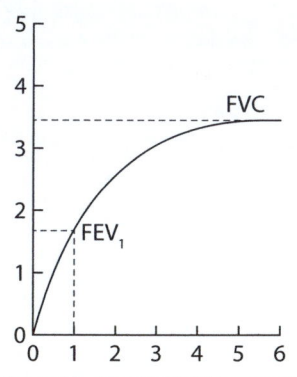

Name: *Calum Richards*   **Age**: *54*   **Height**: *174cm*

	Best	Predicted	% Predicted
FEV₁:	1.89	3.64	51.9%
FVC:	3.51	4.65	75.5%
FEV₁/FVC:	53.8%		

Good technique; repeatable values. Results demonstrate predominantly obstructive picture. Some coughing afterwards.

Last examination during spirometry:	SpO₂ 96% RA RR 16/min BP 129/73 HR 74 Chest: reduced air entry throughout, no wheeze, nil focal
Previous consultation:	4 weeks ago: c / o increasing SOB on exertion for over a year, feeling worse after flu over Xmas and not right since. Does cough but still smoking – cessation advice given. Note CXR last month reported clear. Not losing weight. Can walk around ½ mile on the flat at own pace but previously 1–2. Still working as normal. O/E: reduced air entry throughout. SpO₂ 97% RA, BP 112/71, HR 82, HS normal. Plan: spirometry and review with results.

Case B11.9 Information for the patient

You are Calum Richards, a 54-year old man, who would like to discuss the results of your recent breathing tests. You don't think you did these very well at the time, so expect them to be terrible. Your GP ordered the tests after you complained of slowly worsening exertional breathlessness which has been present for at least a year, but perhaps longer.

ICE

- You presume the results of the breathing tests will be poor due to your perceived bad technique when performing them.
- You think that your breathlessness may be due to your cigarette smoking but are afraid to admit it. Your father died from emphysema aged 69 and you don't want to go through the same thing.
- You expect that you will be told to stop smoking and that this will make you better, but you aren't willing to do so.

Background

- You have suffered with both anxiety and depression since the death of your long-term partner, Elsie, who tragically died in a car accident 7 years ago. This is well managed, however, with citalopram.
- You suffer with occasional heartburn, particularly after spicy foods, but again, this is well managed with medication.
- You live with your labrador, Jessie. You take her for walks twice each day, but have been slowing down recently owing to breathlessness. Your mother is still alive and well, and lives locally.
- You work as an estate agent.

Information divulged freely

- You have noticed that you cannot walk as far as you could last year, and are needing to stop for around 5 minutes if you walk for about half a mile.
- You suffered with what you believe to be the flu a few months ago over Xmas, and had a nasty cough for several weeks. At the time, this was productive of green / yellow sputum.
- You noticed your breathing was worse around this time, and saw your GP who organised a chest X-ray – which you have been told was clear.
- Your breathing has improved now, but not quite to the level you were used to before you were ill.
- You cut down to 10 cigarettes / day when you were unwell recently, but prior to this you had smoked around 20/day since you were in your teens (around 40 years smoking in total).
- You have a cough most days and this is productive when you get up in the morning but dry thereafter. Your sputum is usually grey in colour. You have had this for as long as you can remember and think it is a "smoker's cough".

Information only divulged if specifically asked

- If asked about family history, your father had emphysema. If specifically asked about your father's smoking habits, your father was a heavy smoker (at least 30/day).
- There is no family history of asthma, eczema or hay fever.

- There is no family history of cancer that you are aware of.
- You tried smoking marijuana in your 20s a couple of times but did not smoke this regularly.
- If you are encouraged to stop smoking, you will tell the GP that you have done it all your life and enjoy it, and have no intention of stopping at the moment. If the GP offers you written information or another appointment to discuss this another time, you will accept this.
- You do not drink any alcohol.
- You have not coughed up any blood.
- You have not lost any weight.
- Your mood is good.
- Your reflux is controlled.
- You never suffer with chest pains.
- You have noticed that you wheeze a little if you get a cough or a cold, which happens around twice a year, particularly over winter.
- Your breathing does not get better or worse throughout the day.
- You do not wake up in the night breathless.
- You have not been exposed to any inhaled dusts or chemicals that you can recall.
- Your ankles do not swell up.
- If the GP gives you a diagnosis of chronic obstructive pulmonary disease (COPD), you have never heard of this and do not understand what it means.
- If it is further explained that this diagnosis encompasses emphysema (which your father had), you will be concerned that you will die like him, in your 60s, and be more open to the suggestion of stopping smoking (if brought up).

Case B11.9 Marking scheme for the observer

https://cks.nice.org.uk/topics/chronic-obstructive-pulmonary-disease/
https://goldcopd.org

Data gathering and diagnosis

- Checks patient's current wellbeing and screens for any new symptoms since last review

- Assesses smoking history and current smoking status

- Checks relevant family history (particularly COPD, asthma, lung cancer)

- Explores red flags, such as exertional chest pain, weight loss and haemoptysis

- Interprets spirometry report in the context of the patient's symptoms

Clinical management and medical complexity

- Explains that the results of the spirometry report (in the context of this case) would be consistent with a diagnosis of COPD, and explains the diagnosis to the patient in a jargon-free way

- Encourages smoking cessation, provides information / smoking support, or offers follow-up to discuss another time if the patient is resistant to discussing it today (www.nhs.uk/smokefree/help-and-advice/support)

- Offers a prescription for an inhaler; a short-acting beta-2 agonist (SABA) or a short-acting muscarinic antagonist (SAMA) prn would be an appropriate first step in this case

- Offers to discuss inhaler technique with the patient, either during the consultation, or arranges to do so at another time, such as with a practice nurse or pharmacist

- Does *not* offer a referral for a hospital assessment at this stage as the diagnosis has just been made and a treatment has not yet been trialled. Considers appropriate GP follow-up to assess the effects of the inhaler and to consider further pharmacological treatment according to response

Relating to others

- Acknowledges patient's concern about dying from the same condition as his father

- Emphasises the huge importance of smoking cessation

- Checks current mood given prior history of anxiety / depression

- Appropriate use of pauses, empathy

Case B11.10 Information for the doctor

In this case you are a GP registrar taking telephone calls after a routine surgery.	
Name:	Christian Johnson
Age:	25
Past medical history:	None
Current medication:	None
Last consultation:	
3 weeks ago:	4/12 Hx of intermittent diarrhoea with urgency. No PR bleeding. No weight loss. No nausea. FH ulcerative colitis. Needs bloods and faecal calprotectin. ?IBD.
Results:	FBC: Hb **113** (120–150 g/L) MCV **79** (80–100 fL) Ferritin **15** (normal range 17–291) CRP normal Faecal calprotectin **453** (normal range <50)
Action:	to discuss with GP.

Notes

Case B11.10 Information for the patient

You are Christian Johnson, a 25-year old man, who was asked to call in about his blood results.

ICE

- You are certain this call is bad news. Your cousin had ulcerative colitis and died of colorectal cancer at 34 so you have been very worried about getting a similar diagnosis.
- You don't know much about inflammatory bowel disease, but know your cousin was sent for lots of "camera tests" when he was alive and at one point they talked about doing surgery to have a stoma bag put on his stomach.
- You expect to be sent for a camera test and want to be sent for it as soon as possible, ideally within the week.

Background

- You are a student living with 3 housemates.
- You are studying geography with a plan to become a teacher.
- You smoke occasionally when you are on a night out.
- You drink around 4 nights a week; two of these are usually "heavy" nights and the others are a few beers at the local pub.

Information divulged freely

- The GP receptionist called you 3 days ago about the results and this was the earliest call back appointment she could give you. You have been worried sick since then about these results.
- You know the tests were for bowel problems but the last doctor didn't really explain what all the tests were for.

Information only divulged if specifically asked

- Your cousin was diagnosed with ulcerative colitis at 16 and always seemed to be in hospital. He also refused the surgery offered to him. By the time he was diagnosed with cancer it had spread to his bones and he died around 8 months later.
- You have had symptoms for the past 4 months but have been so worried about the cause you decided to ignore it. When you have diarrhoea it happens around 5–6 times a day but with no bleeding, there is sometimes mucus and you have to rush to get to the toilet. Your appetite is reduced when your bowels are bad but you don't think you've lost any weight. You get abdominal cramps when you have diarrhoea too. You feel tired all the time despite sleeping well.
- You want to know more about the test results – does this mean you definitely have ulcerative colitis? If the doctor mentions you are anaemic you want to know what to do about this.
- You want to know what the next step is and how quickly this can be arranged. You will be outraged if the doctor suggests any longer than a week wait – surely this is an urgent matter? You want to know if the doctor can speak to the consultant about the camera test and ask them to do it earlier. If the doctor is reluctant you will ask about a private referral – how much would this cost?
- You want to know more about inflammatory bowel disease: what is the treatment and does everyone get cancer like your cousin?

Case B11.10 Marking scheme for the observer

Data gathering and diagnosis

☐	☐	☐	• Identifies the reason for the telephone consultation and briefly re-explores the history of the presenting complaint and ensures no worsening of symptoms since last being seen
☐	☐	☐	• Asks about the patient's knowledge of the tests being performed before explaining them, i.e. do they know which tests were done and why?
☐	☐	☐	• Identifies the patient's concerns regarding his family history and takes this into account when explaining the test results

Clinical management and medical complexity

☐	☐	☐	• Explains that the faecal calprotectin test is used to identify inflammation in the bowel and that the patient has a strongly positive test which could be consistent with inflammatory bowel disease
☐	☐	☐	• Explains that the patient also has iron-deficiency anaemia which is likely due to inflammation in the bowel. Offers a prescription for iron tablets whilst further tests are awaited and advises how / when the prescription will be prepared
☐	☐	☐	• Can explain more about the nature of inflammatory bowel disease, expected symptoms and possible treatments (medication and / or surgery depending on the severity of symptoms). Offers a leaflet: patient.info/health/inflammatory-bowel-disease
☐	☐	☐	• Explains the need for referral to gastroenterology for colonoscopy and is able to discuss what this will entail
☐	☐	☐	• Does not falsely reassure or overestimate the risk of colorectal cancer in IBD. If unsure, defers to the gastroenterology team to explain the risks. Is aware that regular colonoscopies are usually carried out in diagnosed patients in order to pick any cancer up at the earliest opportunity

Relating to others

☐	☐	☐	• Creates rapport with the patient by acknowledging his concerns about bowel symptoms in light of his family history and death of a relative at an early age
☐	☐	☐	• Explains faecal calprotectin, IBD and cancer risk in a clear jargon-free manner
☐	☐	☐	• Sympathises with the patient's wish for an urgent test and tries to reassure him about the speed of the referral
☐	☐	☐	• Asks the patient to return if the symptoms get worse while waiting to see the gastroenterologists

Case B12.1   Information for the doctor

In this case you are a doctor in surgery taking video calls.	
Name:	Britanny Lear
Age:	35
Past medical history:	None
Current medication:	Cerazette 75 mg od

Notes

Case B12.1 Information for the patient

You are Britanny Lear, a 35-year old woman. You have called up today to discuss a termination of pregnancy. However, your opening statement is "This is completely confidential right – you can't tell anyone what I say today?"

ICE

- You want to request a termination of pregnancy but are very worried about the paperwork involved. Your husband's sister works as a secretary in the neighbouring practice and you know she has lots of friends in this surgery. You really do not want this consultation to be recorded in the notes at all.
- You hope the doctor will agree not to record the consultation and will give you the name of a private clinic where you can go.

Background

- You are a 35-year old shop assistant who is married to a local politician. You already have two children who are 7 and 5. You don't smoke and rarely drink.

Information divulged freely

- You are on the mini pill but are not very good at taking it every day. You think you are about 8 weeks pregnant.
- You have had no abdominal pain or abnormal bleeding. You have been experiencing morning sickness and breast tenderness.
- This was an unplanned pregnancy and you really don't feel you can manage another child now.

Information only divulged if specifically asked

- If specifically asked why you do not want the consultation recorded, you will tell the doctor you don't want your husband finding out. If asked why and you feel comfortable telling the doctor then you admit the baby is not his – you know he would work out he was staying down in London on the date of conception. You have been having an affair with the man who owns the shop you work in.
- You want no record of the conversation and will get quite upset if the doctor says they have to, even if reassurance is given that the notes are kept confidential. You are sure the secretaries will talk. You will, however, accept a priority '0' or 'hidden' consultation when it is explained that this will hide the record of the consultation, only if this is fully explained and reasons for recording your information are pointed out e.g. if you were to become unwell after the procedure.
- You are aware of how the procedure is performed and have decided you will tell your husband you are going to stay with your sister for a few days. You have told your sister all about the pregnancy so you know she will lie for you.

Case B12.1   Marking scheme for the observer

patient.info/doctor/termination-of-pregnancy
www.gmc-uk.org/guidance/ethical_guidance/confidentiality.asp

Data gathering and diagnosis

☐	☐	☐	• Takes an appropriate history, including possible length of pregnancy and last menstrual period; works out gestation
☐	☐	☐	• Enquires about abdominal pain / PV bleeding (nil acute concern of ectopic)
☐	☐	☐	• Asks sensitively about reasons for requesting a termination and establishes the patient's view that being pregnant will have a detrimental effect on her mental health

Clinical management and medical complexity

☐	☐	☐	• Is aware of options for recording sensitive information in the notes. Some computer systems give the option of recording a 'priority 0' consultation where the notes are hidden from general viewing
☐	☐	☐	• Can advise about the procedure for medical terminations even if is an objector to referring
☐	☐	☐	• Discusses the availability of LARC / alternative forms of contraception which may suit the patient better in the longer term
☐	☐	☐	• Discusses local options for referral and assists the patient to arrange this

Relating to others

☐	☐	☐	• Identifies and discusses the patient's concerns about confidentiality early on with no false reassurance given about the potential need to break confidentiality in some situations
☐	☐	☐	• Is non-judgmental about the lifestyle of the patient and does not allow own views to inappropriately influence dialogue
☐	☐	☐	• Gives explanation of the importance of recording information in the notes
☐	☐	☐	• Empathises with the patient

Case B12.2 Information for the doctor

In this case you are a doctor in surgery taking telephone calls.	
Name:	Kathleen Roberts
Age:	70
Past medical history:	1 week ago: Discussed in gynae MDT: metastatic endometrial cancer with liver and bony metastases, for chemotherapy
Current medication:	Nil

Notes

Case B12.2   Information for the patient

You are Kathleen Roberts, a 70-year old lady who has called the surgery today to discuss your plans for your future health.

ICE

- You would like to put things in place for your future health.
- You don't want people jumping on your chest if you have died to try to bring you back. You also don't want to spend your last days in a hospital but want to be at home with your family.
- You don't want to tell your husband any of this and want the GP to reassure you they won't. You are worried they might make you tell him.

Background

- You live at home with your husband of 50 years.
- You have 2 sons and 5 grandchildren.
- You don't smoke or drink alcohol.

Information divulged freely

- You had some funny bleeding from down below about 4 weeks ago and were sent to the fast track clinic. They did a scan and a biopsy but told you it was probably cancer. A week or so after that they rang you with biopsy results to confirm this. Then they did a scan which showed it had spread to your liver and bones. They have told you they will carry out chemotherapy shortly to try to stop the spread. They have told you this is not curative.
- You know you will die of this cancer and nothing is going to stop that, so you have decided you don't want any chemotherapy; it will only make you unwell for what is left of your life.
- You want to make plans for your death. You went to the solicitor yesterday and sorted out your will.
- You want to die at home if possible; if not, a hospice but certainly not a hospital.
- You do not want to be resuscitated if you die – you do not want to end up on a life support machine.
- You have called to ask the GP how to go about making all this official. Is there paperwork they can give you to fill in?

Information only divulged if specifically asked

- You have not told your husband any of this.
- None of the rest of your family know either. You have confided in two close friends, one of whom had breast cancer last year.
- You really don't want to tell your family. You feel this will make it all seem real. You also know they will worry a lot about it and you really don't want to upset them.
- If the GP encourages you to talk to them you want to know what will happen if you say no – will he/she phone them and tell them anyway? You also want to know how long you have got left, as there is no point worrying your family if you might have years left.
- If the GP is sensitive and understanding about the worry it might cause your family you will ask if you could bring your husband here and then you could tell him together. Then he can ask all his questions of the GP straight away which you think will help.

- If the GP is not sensitive or encouraging then you will refuse to tell your family; you will 'cross that bridge when you come to it'.
- If the GP discusses DNAR (Do not attempt resuscitation) documents you are happy to call in to collect these and then take away to read and sign.
- If they discuss advance directives you want to know how to write one and if your family will then have to do as it says.

Case B12.2 **Marking scheme for the observer**

patient.info/doctor/advance-care-planning

Data gathering and diagnosis

☐	☐	☐	• Takes a history of the reason for the call and identifies the palliative nature of the cancer diagnosis
☐	☐	☐	• Identifies the fact the family are unaware of the diagnosis
☐	☐	☐	• Gathers information on the patient's wishes for end of life care

Clinical management and medical complexity

☐	☐	☐	• Listens to everything the patient has to say, and can talk generally about end of life decisions, but remains cautious about prognosticating and giving advice on the condition until all the facts are available (discusses the need to speak with the gynae team)
☐	☐	☐	• Is able to advise the patient on DNAR and advance directive decisions
☐	☐	☐	• Encourages family participation in these decisions
☐	☐	☐	• Is able to direct patient to online resources and support groups that can help her at this difficult time

Relating to others

☐	☐	☐	• Discusses end of life care in a sensitive manner
☐	☐	☐	• Empathises with patient's desire not to worry her family
☐	☐	☐	• Encourages her, without being too forceful, to tell the family

Case B12.3 Information for the doctor

In this case you are a GP registrar triaging telephone calls in the local Out of Hours service. Triage note reads: "Daughter Rose called to report expected death, district nurse cannot verify as patient not seen recently by GP".

Name:	Margaret Thackeray
Age:	99
Past medical history:	Full record unavailable
Current medication:	Full notes unavailable

Notes

Case B12.3   Information for the patient

You are Rose Wade, the daughter of Margaret Thackeray who has just passed away this evening.

ICE

- You would like the doctor to come and visit to explain what you need to do now your mum has died. You would like to ask a lot of your main questions over the phone now.
- Your mum's main wish was to donate her body to medical science to help future doctors learn, and you want to make sure that everyone involved is aware of her wishes.
- You know you need a death certificate from the doctor and would like to get this as soon as possible so you can make further arrangements.

Background

- You and your husband Stan have been looking after your mum at your home since she was discharged from hospital last month. She hated hospital and was very clear that she didn't want to go back in there and told you if anything else happened to her she wanted to stay at home.
- She seemed to get worse over the weekend. You called the GP on Friday night to let them know she had had a fall going to the bathroom late afternoon. You found her sitting on the floor and she had bumped her head. She hadn't been knocked out and you were able to get her up and mobilising normally. She then started burning up with a fever and became more chesty. You spoke to the doctor about mum's wishes to stay at home and the doctor said to call the OOH service if you were worried over the weekend.
- You have been keeping a close eye on her all weekend and she has been weak and spent all the time in bed, but has been comfortable and you didn't think you needed to call the doctor out. When you checked on her just now she had stopped breathing.

Information divulged freely

- You have never seen a dead body before, so you do want the doctor to come and check mum for you, but she has stopped breathing and is starting to feel cold.
- Mum had several hospital admissions over the last year and her death is not unexpected.
- She has had a 'Do Not Attempt Resuscitation' order in place for several years. The hospital doctors discussed this with you all again during her last admission and it was kept in place.
- Your mum wanted to donate her body to medical science and registered with the local university. You have all the paperwork and want to make sure your mum's wishes are carried out. It says you need a death certificate before you can contact them and you want to ask if the doctor can give you this when they visit.
- You want to know what will happen to your mum's body and whether you need to contact someone to move her to the university.

Information only divulged if specifically asked

- Your mum had a fall about 6 months ago and broke her hip. She was in hospital for some time, but when she came home she was able to get around the house with her Zimmer frame and was having carers every morning to help her get dressed.

- She was admitted to hospital last month with a chest infection and has been living with you since discharge. She has been frail since then, but was still able to mobilise to the toilet and was managing with the carers once a day.
- She had cold symptoms all last week but on Friday seemed to get worse. She felt feverish and was a bit chesty. She didn't want you to get a doctor out because she really wanted to avoid hospital, but you did speak to the GP just before they went home on Friday to let them know she wasn't well and that she had had a fall.
- The chestiness continued and she spent all weekend in bed, not eating much but quite peaceful, just sleeping a lot until tonight when she stopped breathing.
- She hasn't been seen by a doctor since she was discharged from hospital over a month ago.
- If the doctor says the death needs to be reported to the coroner you want to know more about what this will involve. If a post-mortem is mentioned you will be quite upset – will this mean that mum will not be able to donate her body to the university as she requested?

Case B12.3 Marking scheme for the observer

The following links may help you with this case:

Confirmation and certification of death: www.england.nhs.uk/coronavirus/documents/
death-certification-processes-information-for-medical-practitioners-after-the-coronavirus-
act-2020-expires

Reporting deaths to the coroner: www.gov.uk/after-a-death/when-a-death-is-reported-to-a-coroner

Data gathering and diagnosis

☐	☐	☐	• Opens the consultation confirming you are speaking to the patient's daughter and with an acknowledgement that Margaret has died. Listens to the daughter's story
☐	☐	☐	• Establishes the events leading to her death and who was present. Asks when she was last seen by a doctor
☐	☐	☐	• Confirms the presence of a DNAR order and asks about any end of life care discussions that have taken place
☐	☐	☐	• Picks up on the recent fall and is aware that deaths related to falls/fractures need to be reported to the coroner. A full list of deaths which must be reported can be found here: www.manchester.gov.uk/info/626/coroners/5532/when_death_occurs/2
☐	☐	☐	• Attempts to establish the cause of death

Clinical management and medical complexity

☐	☐	☐	• Recognises this as a death that should be reported to the coroner (recent fall) and can explain to the patient what this entails. The patient has also not been seen by a doctor within 28 days
☐	☐	☐	• Discusses certification of death with Rose and explains that, as the OOH doctor, you cannot issue this and it is typically done by the patient's own GP. As the death will be reported to the coroner, they will decide if a certificate can be issued or if further investigation (such as a post-mortem examination) is needed
☐	☐	☐	• Acknowledges the wishes of the patient to donate her body to medical science. Picks up on Rose's comments about paperwork and, if asked, suggests going through it all during the visit

☐ ☐ ☐		• Can signpost Rose regarding what they need to do next and the practical arrangements around death. Typically a funeral director can be contacted to move the body; however, in this case advise that the family should wait until you have spoken to the coroner's office before moving Margaret. A patient leaflet may help: www.mariecurie.org.uk/help/support/bereaved-family-friends/practical-legal/medical-certificate or www.kctrust.co.uk/what-to-do-when-someone-dies
☐ ☐ ☐		• Arranges to visit the family to confirm death and discuss their questions further in person (check the protocol in your local area)
Relating to others		
☐ ☐ ☐		• Shows empathy towards Rose and her loss
☐ ☐ ☐		• Listens and responds appropriately to Rose's reactions
☐ ☐ ☐		• Gives Rose time to ask questions and is prepared to repeat answers, acknowledging that there is potentially a lot of information and emotion for Rose to deal with
☐ ☐ ☐		• Avoids jargon when explaining the death administration process and keeps things as straightforward as possible

Changing regulations

www.gov.uk/government/collections/death-certification-reform-and-the-introduction-of-medical-examiners

www.gov.uk/government/publications/medical-certificate-of-cause-of-death-draft-regulations

The Draft Regulations for England and Wales have been published at the links above, and are expected to come into force in September 2024.

Medical Certificate of Cause of Death (MCCD)

Under the new regulations, any medical practitioner who has "attended" the deceased during the deceased's lifetime will be eligible to complete the MCCD and confirm a cause of death to the best of their knowledge. (Prior to this there was a requirement to have attended the deceased during their final illness.)

The requirement is to have "attended" the patient can be taken to mean "provided healthcare for", which could include remote management.

Case B12.4 Information for the doctor

You are a salaried GP. The receptionist was asked to book a double appointment for you with Dorothy Lane, a 68-year old patient that you have never met before. The receptionist has warned you to check previous records and a personal inbox message from Dr Smith, a GP partner who was on call last night and got a worrying fax report from the radiology department. You are speaking to Dorothy via a video call because she cannot make it into the practice today.

Name:	Dorothy Lane
Age:	68
Past medical history:	Hypertension GORD
Current medication:	Ramipril 5 mg once a day Omeprazole 20 mg od
Previous consultation:	1 week ago: c/o constant cough for many months, no SOB, thinks her cough is getting worse. Coughing up purulent sputum, some streaks of blood last week, one episode – no haemoptysis since. Smoker since the age of 15. Has had 10 cigarettes/day for the last decade (cut down from 30/day). Smoking cessation briefly discussed, not interested. Denies weight loss. Good appetite. No fever. Retired, lives alone. O/E: apyrexial, chest clear, good A/E, no added sounds. SpO$_2$ 96% RA, BP 151/76, HR 80, HS normal. Plan: urgent CXR and review with results.
CXR report:	Moderate hyper-expansion noted. There is a well-circumscribed lesion in the left upper lobe, approximately 2.5 × 3.5 cm with adjacent atelectasis. No obvious hilar lymphadenopathy. No obvious bony lesions. Cardiac size and borders appear normal. Chest otherwise clear. Conclusion: appearances highly suspicious of primary lung malignancy. Please arrange urgent CT chest and suggest urgent respiratory review. *report faxed and phoned through to GP*
Inbox message from Dr Smith:	Hi, so sorry to hand over this difficult task but I will be away for a week and Dorothy's usual GP (Dr Malik) is still on long-term sick leave as you know. See CXR result – Dorothy is a heavy smoker so it's not good news. I've already referred on the 2 week wait pathway and asked our receptionist to book a double app. with Dorothy so you should hopefully have enough time to discuss her X-ray report and next steps. I met her last week, lovely lady. I made sure you are not on call so you shouldn't be interrupted but please remind them not to put any calls through just in case. Thanks again. John.

Case B12.4 Information for the patient

You are Dorothy Lane, a 68-year old woman, who wants to discuss the results of your chest X-ray. The receptionist was very vague on the phone yesterday, she just mentioned the doctor had asked for a longer appointment to discuss your X-ray results. You didn't sleep very well last night; the need for a double appointment makes you think the results are more likely to be abnormal.

ICE

- You suspect the results of the chest X-ray to be abnormal because you were given a double appointment. Your gut feeling almost never lets you down and you are concerned.
- You've been anxious for a while and delayed coming to see a doctor because deep down you know it's not just a simple cough. You've been smoking all your life. Your father died of lung cancer in his 60s and he was coughing up blood for a long time prior to any investigations. When you noticed some blood in your sputum last week it prompted you to book an appointment.
- You expect to be told you have cancer. You hope the doctor is straight and honest with you.
- You need to sort out your Will as soon as possible if it's cancer.

Background

- You've had a cough for many months. It's always been a little bit phlegmy but last week your sputum had some blood in it. It was just a small amount but it made you worry and think about your father.
- You suffer with occasional heartburn, particularly after a glass of port in the evenings, but omeprazole usually works.
- You live alone. Your husband Rob died in a car accident 10 years ago. You miss him very much and have not had a partner since. Your close friends Mary and her husband Keith are your next door neighbours. You do most things together: volunteering in a local charity shop twice a week, going for walks, playing cards.
- You have two children. Your daughter Michelle lives in France with her husband Pierre. They own a little restaurant and you see them every 3 months. Your son Connor is a journalist and travels a lot; you don't see him very often, but whenever he is back in the UK he spends a long weekend with you.
- You are retired and used to work in a local library.

Information divulged freely

- Your cough is getting on your nerves but it's been a while since it started. It has probably been present for around 5 months but you are not sure, your life has been a little busy lately. You went to France to visit your daughter recently; you are volunteering for a charity and spending a lot of time outdoors with your neighbours.
- Last week you coughed up some blood – it happened three times in two days. You immediately called the doctor who arranged for a chest X-ray.
- Your breathing is OK, you don't think you are breathless or wheezy.
- You are embarrassed to talk about your smoking, but you've been a smoker since you were 15 years old. You remember stealing cigarettes from your dad – he was a heavy smoker. Your children don't smoke and you are proud of them for not doing so.

- Since your husband died you significantly reduced the number of cigarettes you smoke. You admit Rob never liked your awful habit and kept telling you to quit. You cut down to 10 cigarettes / day from 30 which you think is pretty good for you.
- You are not interested to stop smoking: "I know the damage has been done, I just want to enjoy the rest of my life now. I am sure I'll meet Rob again soon, I can just tell".

Information only divulged if specifically asked

- If asked about family history, your father died of lung cancer. He was coughing up blood for months and had some tests really late, he ended up dying in hospital, you remember he was very unwell.
- You drink a few glasses of port almost every evening.
- You have not lost any weight.
- Your mood is good.
- You never suffer with chest pains.
- You have not been exposed to any inhaled dusts or chemicals that you can recall.
- You know it's bad news. You think you have lung cancer.
- If the GP is vague and takes too long to discuss your X-ray result you'll get a little bit impatient and ask him to finally get on with it and tell you the truth. If the doctor keeps referring to a 'mass' or a 'lesion' you will directly ask if he means cancer. You just need to know this so you can start planning your Will.
- If the GP suggests that it may be something else, such as infection, you will be relieved that you don't have cancer!
- If the GP is honest and open with you and mentions that there is a strong possibility that you might have lung cancer, you'll start crying but in a way you are relieved and are grateful that the doctor is straight with you. You'll start talking about planning and organising your Will. You will need a moment to cry and will be grateful to be given some space to digest this information.
- If the doctor tells you that you'll still need a CT and an urgent outpatient appointment (2 week rule referral) to the respiratory department you will specifically ask if it could still be something less serious. If the doctor is not ruling it out but explains the reasons why the findings remain worrying, and that the confirmation of diagnosis is very important, you'd be on board with a referral.
- You are grateful if the doctor asks if you have someone around who can make you a cup of tea and talk through this news with you. You thought you were prepared for bad news and are surprised that you are feeling a little bit shaky.
- If the doctor offers you a follow-up appointment / help to contact relatives / see you with your friends – you will decline at this stage but you will make sure they accompany you to the hospital appointment.

Case B12.4 Marking scheme for the observer

You can find some useful information below regarding consultation skills on breaking bad news: https://patient.info/doctor/breaking-bad-news and www.gponline.com/consultation-skills-best-break-bad-news/article/776491
https://cks.nice.org.uk/lung-and-pleural-cancers-recognition-and-referral

Data gathering and diagnosis

☐	☐	☐	• Ensures privacy, knows all the facts prior to the consultation
☐	☐	☐	• Checks with the patient reasons for CXR, explores what they already know
☐	☐	☐	• Gives a clear explanation step by step, allows the patient to control the amount of information they receive
☐	☐	☐	• Listens to patient's concerns, covers ICE
☐	☐	☐	• Remembers to check patient's understanding and repeats information if needed

Clinical management and medical complexity

☐	☐	☐	• Fires a warning shot suggesting that some unpleasant news may follow, for instance: "Unfortunately, I have some difficult news I have to tell you" or "The results are a little bit more serious than we had hoped"
☐	☐	☐	• Breaks bad news in stages, avoids overloading or telling news all in one go
☐	☐	☐	• Explains what further investigations / tests are required and the next steps
☐	☐	☐	• Checks at the end if the patient has any questions about any of the information given
☐	☐	☐	• Offers follow-up (ensures the patient has support at home, offers to see again with relatives / friends)

Relating to others

☐	☐	☐	• Establishes rapport with patient
☐	☐	☐	• Remains calm when speaking with the patient
☐	☐	☐	• Shows empathy and understanding
☐	☐	☐	• Uses pauses, allows time and space for answers
☐	☐	☐	• Body language and tone of voice appropriate for situation

Case B12.5 Information for the doctor

You are GP in surgery calling Oliver's mum.	
Name:	Oliver Haddon
Age:	4 months
Past medical history:	None
Current medication:	None
Last consultation:	**Yesterday – out of hours:** OOH consultation resulting in emergency hospital admission
	Yesterday morning – telephone triage: Dr Roberts: bad night, now sleepy, cough continues, further reassurance given
	2 days ago: Dr Roberts: cough 2/7, feeds reduced, felt hot, exam – chest clear, note new young mother ++anxiety, reassure and advise

Notes

Case B12.5   Information for the patient

You are Julie Haddon, age 20, and you want to discuss the recent treatment of your son Oliver by Dr Roberts.

ICE

- You want to discuss the circumstances leading to Oliver's hospital admission.
- You are worried this may happen to other patients if Dr Roberts is allowed to continue poorly examining his patients.

Background

- You live with your boyfriend. You are not at work as you are on maternity leave but usually work on the checkouts in Asda. Your boyfriend is on long-term sick leave with back pain so he is also at home. You don't smoke and haven't been drinking since you found out you were pregnant. You do have social support from your mum and sister in the local area.

Information divulged freely

- You called to discuss your consultation with Dr Roberts, which happened 2 days ago. You brought your son to discuss a recent cough and fever. You were very worried as he was taking much less milk than usual and had fewer wet nappies. You felt Dr Roberts was very dismissive and made reference to your age when considering why you were so worried.
- Following the consultation, Oliver worsened overnight so you called the surgery the next morning to speak to Dr Roberts who again was very dismissive and told you *"Well, what did you expect? These things take time."* At this point Oliver had been very sleepy all morning and you were worried this meant he was getting worse. Unhappy with Dr Roberts' advice, you attended the OOH GP who thoroughly examined Oliver and found he has a chest infection and was dehydrated. He admitted him to the ward where he is now. He is having IV antibiotics and fluids.
- You want to tell this whole story first and if the doctor tries to interrupt, you will get upset and ask to finish the story first.
- You feel Dr Roberts did not do his job properly and want to know why. You also want to know if this GP would have done anything differently.
- You have not made an appointment to discuss this with Dr Roberts as you feel too angry and think you would start shouting. If an appointment with him is offered you will not accept.
- You mainly want your concerns noted today. If a written complaint is discussed you would like to go ahead.
- If the doctor tries to defend Dr Roberts you will get very upset. They were not present during the consultation so you don't feel it is their place to comment.

Case B12.5 Marking scheme for the observer

www.themdu.com/learn-and-develop/course-listing/complaints-local-resolution

			Data gathering and diagnosis
☐	☐	☐	• Listens to mum tell the story without interruption
☐	☐	☐	• Identifies the patient's ideas, concerns & expectations
☐	☐	☐	• Elicits social history
			Clinical management and medical complexity
☐	☐	☐	• Is aware of the complaints procedure in their practice
☐	☐	☐	• Can discuss the next steps with the patient regarding taking the complaint forward / resolving her concerns
☐	☐	☐	• Recognises the impact this has had on the patient, offers support and follow-up
			Relating to others
☐	☐	☐	• Shows good rapport with the patient
☐	☐	☐	• Makes early apology for her anger and upset
☐	☐	☐	• Does not try to defend or blame colleague – listens and advises patient only
☐	☐	☐	• Obtains the story by allowing the patient to talk with minimal interruptions

Case B12.6   Information for the doctor

In this case you are a doctor in surgery calling this patient on the telephone.	
Name:	Eva Abraham
Age:	35
Past medical history:	PCOS diagnosed 2 years ago
Current medication:	Cerazette

Notes

Case B12.6 Information for the patient

You are Eva Abraham, a 28-year old woman. You want to discuss a sick note.

ICE

- You have called to request a sick note and fully expect to be given one. You have several friends on the sick and they never have problems getting notes.

Background

- You are a 28-year old shop assistant. You don't smoke. You drink one bottle of wine a week. You are overweight and are aware you need to lose weight but feel you don't have any time to exercise. You live with your boyfriend.

Information divulged freely

- You want a sick note for work due to your polycystic ovarian syndrome. This gives you hair on your face and chest which you find very embarrassing and you feel you are unable to work due to this.
- You work as a sales assistant in a nearby clothes store. No-one at work has ever mentioned your hair problem to you before.
- You have recently been diagnosed with PCOS after coming to speak to the GP about this and your irregular periods. You are aware the excess hair growth is part of this.
- You currently wax the hair on your upper lip but it grows back quickly. You have not tried anything for the hair on your chest.
- Your boyfriend is not bothered about the excess hair.

Information only divulged if specifically asked

- If a sick note is refused you will get very upset. How are you meant to work with the public when you are too embarrassed to show your face in the shop?
- If other options are offered for the hair growth you turn down electrolysis and laser treatment as they are far too expensive as they are not available on the NHS. You have tried the hair removal creams and shaving as well as waxing but they don't seem to last any time at all either.
- If your weight is discussed you are aware you need to lose weight but feel you have no time to exercise. You eat as healthily as you can, given your budget.
- You tried different pills in the past including Dianette but it gave you mood swings and you refuse to try it again.
- If a referral to dermatology or endocrinology is offered you accept but want a note until you have an appointment.
- As far as you know there is no occupational health department at work but your boss is horrible and you feel you certainly can't talk to her about this problem to ask about different duties. If a sick note with amended duties is offered you will want more information about what this is and are not sure your work will accept it, but will be happy after an explanation to take it.
- If a sick note is offered you will be very pleased and end the consultation with a big thank you.

Case B12.6 Marking scheme for the observer

patient.info/doctor/sickness-certification-in-primary-care
patient.info/doctor/long-term-sickness-and-incapacity
www.gov.uk/government/collections/fit-note

Data gathering and diagnosis

☐	☐	☐	• Takes an appropriate history, including occupational history
☐	☐	☐	• Establishes which other methods have been tried to reduce hair growth
☐	☐	☐	• Elicits impact of the problem on the patient's life

Clinical management and medical complexity

☐	☐	☐	• Discusses options for removal of excess hair growth, including knowledge of which procedures are freely available on the NHS
☐	☐	☐	• Establishes how the problem affects patient while at work and offers practical solutions to minimise her distress to allow her to continue work (make-up, clothing to cover up)
☐	☐	☐	• Recognises weight reduction could improve symptoms and gives appropriate advice
☐	☐	☐	• Recognises that providing a fit note may be 'easy' but will not be addressing the patient's main problem and may have potential detrimental consequences (encouraging patient to adopt the sick role) and makes an effort to explain this to the patient and look for alternative solutions
☐	☐	☐	• In this case – avoids writing a note. If patient is insistent, explains self-certification process (first 7 days) but encourages the patient to consider alternatives to the sick role

Relating to others

☐	☐	☐	• Develops rapport with the patient
☐	☐	☐	• Recognises the patient is struggling with work and allows her to discuss concerns about her employer, and identify options for support and help at work
☐	☐	☐	• Reaches an appropriate plan where the patient and doctor are in agreement

Case B12.7 Information for the doctor

In this case you are a doctor in surgery undertaking telephone consultations.	
Name:	Karen Hall
Age:	59
Past medical history:	Chronic neck pain 6 years ago Termination of pregnancy 35 years ago
Current medication:	Co-codamol 30/500 Gabapentin 300 mg TDS

Notes

Case B12.7 Information for the patient

You are Karen Hall, a 55-year old woman. You are extremely angry. You asked for copies of your medical records for an insurance claim you are making. The records say you had a termination, which is not true.

ICE

- You are very angry about this mistake in your records. You are 'pro-life' and would never consider a termination under any circumstances.
- You are worried that people seeing this record would judge your behaviour.
- You expect a full apology and the information to be removed.

Background

- You are a 55-year old woman who lives with her husband. You have a 29-year old son who lives in Glasgow. You worked at a factory nearby until 5 years ago when a 'slip and trip' on a wet floor left you with chronic neck pain. You smoke 3 cigarettes a day and drink 2 bottles of wine a week.

Information divulged freely

- You have recently been involved in making a claim against your old employer for loss of earnings. This led to your request for your medical records – fortunately you asked to see them first before they were sent away.
- You were not pregnant in 1990 – your only pregnancy was with your son.
- When you first speak, your statements include *"You have some explaining to do"*, *"You people think you can write what you like on people's records and it doesn't matter"* and *"What if my son or husband had seen these records?"*
- You want to tell your full story with no interruptions.
- If you are given time to tell your story and an early apology is made, you will calm down and be willing to discuss the issue.
- You want the information removed from your records and also you would like an explanation of how it came to be in your records – is it a patient with a similar name?
- You will be very pleased if told this issue will be discussed as a significant event and feedback given to you.

Case B12.7 **Marking scheme for the observer**

https://patient.info/doctor/data-security-and-caldicott-guardianship
www.gponline.com/medico-legal-alterations-medical-records/article/985144

Data gathering and diagnosis			
☐	☐	☐	• Takes a full history of what happened
☐	☐	☐	• Gives patient time to speak and fully express her concerns uninterrupted
☐	☐	☐	• Establishes the patient's wishes and how she would like to proceed with this situation
Clinical management and medical complexity			
☐	☐	☐	• Demonstrates awareness of the practice complaints policy
☐	☐	☐	• Demonstrates awareness of the practice policy to deal with significant events
☐	☐	☐	• Demonstrates awareness of information governance and medical record keeping / changes to patient notes
Relating to others			
☐	☐	☐	• Gives patient time to tell their story
☐	☐	☐	• Gives an early apology
☐	☐	☐	• Enables patient to feel at the end of the consultation that the GP took their concerns seriously and will fully investigate this incident

Case B12.8 Information for the doctor

You are a locum GP doing telephone consultations.	
Name:	Pritiya Mahadik
Age:	53
Past medical history:	Osteoarthritis left hip Recent consultation 2 weeks ago: urinary incontinence – urge, no prolapse, no stress incontinence, urinalysis negative. Would like treatment, try oxybutynin 5 mg & report 2/52
Current medication:	Paracetamol 1 g qds Oxycontin 5 mg bd

Notes

Case B12.8   Information for the patient

You are Pritiya Mahadik, a 53-year old lady. You want to discuss the new medication the doctor gave you for your urinary problems because you were asked for a review after 2 weeks.

ICE

- You want to report on this new medication – it has not helped your bladder in the slightest but oddly you have noticed your hip has been much better since taking it.
- You have no concerns today.
- You would like an alternative medication for your bladder but as this does seem to be helping your hip maybe you could also continue these?

Background

- You are a 53-year old woman who came in 2 weeks ago with urinary incontinence. You could not reach the toilet in time and had had a few accidents.
- You are working as an office manager so this waterworks problem is quite troublesome and embarrassing.
- You live with your husband and have two children away at university.
- You don't smoke and you drink around 12 units a week.

Information divulged freely

- You have been taking these tablets twice a day for two weeks now and they are not helping your bladder at all. Your urge incontinence is just as bad.
- However, your hip is very much better. Previously you were getting pain after around 100 metres walking and after climbing the stairs at work. Now you are pain free!
- A week ago you decided to read the leaflet that came with your medication and it said they are in fact a pain killer so that makes sense. You know doctors often use medication for other reasons than on the leaflet so that did not concern you.
- You are not getting any other side-effects from the medication.
- If the doctor advises you there has been a prescribing error you are very upset; how could this happen? What if you had had a terrible reaction? When you find out you were given an opiate-based medication you are even more upset; you could have become addicted to it!
- If the doctor apologises and explains how this type of error can occur (i.e. the medications have similar names), you will accept the apology and don't think you want to take the complaint further.
- If they offer to prescribe the correct medication for your bladder you are more cautious this time and want to know more about it and its side-effects.
- If they want to stop the oxycontin you are reluctant – it really has helped your hip! If offered an alternative or review of your pain relief you will accept this. If they are happy to continue your oxycontin you think you would like to.

Case B12.8 Marking scheme for the observer

patient.info/doctor/urinary-incontinence-pro
Dealing with complaints (MPS):
www.medicalprotection.org/docs/default-source/pdfs/Booklet-PDFs/eng-med-complaints-
    booklet.pdf?sfvrsn=4

Data gathering and diagnosis

☐	☐	☐	• Identifies the reason for the consultation
☐	☐	☐	• Identifies the medication error which occurred
☐	☐	☐	• Re-explores the patient's urinary symptoms rather than relying on the prior consultation

Clinical management and medical complexity

☐	☐	☐	• Is able to discuss the appropriate management of urinary incontinence
☐	☐	☐	• Is able to discuss analgesia for this patient, including appropriate alternatives to opiate-based medication
☐	☐	☐	• Is aware of the complaints procedure in the surgery or offers to find out

Relating to others

☐	☐	☐	• Creates a rapport with the patient
☐	☐	☐	• Apologises for the medication error and explains how it has occurred
☐	☐	☐	• Discusses appropriate complaints procedure with the patient
☐	☐	☐	• Comes to a shared management plan with the patient regarding both her problems

Case B12.9 Information for the doctor

In this case you are a GP registrar in a routine surgery undertaking telephone consultations.	
Name:	Noah Carruthers (dad James will be attending on his behalf)
Age:	5
Past medical history:	None
Current medication:	None
Last consultation:	5 days ago in surgery (Dr Roberts): Seen with dad, 3 days hx sore throat, appetite OK, no fever, been off school, lethargic, dry cough. Exam: HR 90, temp 36.6°C, throat – red swollen tonsils, no exudate, no LN present. Centor score 0. Advised likely viral. Analgesia and see if concerns. 4 days ago in OOH surgery (Dr Williams): Seen with dad – saw own GP yesterday with sore throat but dad unhappy no abx given, patient no better. Exam: HR 88, temp 36.5°C, throat – red swollen tonsils, no exudate. Discussion with dad – he requests abx script given signs, prompt to viral but given second presentation and level of parental anxiety abx given.

Notes

Case B12.9 Information for the patient

You are James Carruthers, a 30-year old man, father to Noah Carruthers. You have called today to make a complaint about another GP in the surgery. You start the consultation extremely angry.

ICE

- You want to complain about Dr Roberts. He refused to give your child antibiotics when he obviously needed them. Noah spent the next day in pain before you took him to the out-of-hours GP to get a prescription.
- You are concerned this will happen again the next time Noah is sick and needs antibiotics and you want to make it clear you should be able to request them next time.
- You expect an apology and reassurance that next time you will be able to ask for antibiotics and have them given.

Background

- You live with Noah by yourself, you are divorced from your wife and she lives with her new husband and stepchildren around an hour away. She sees Noah every other week for the weekend.
- You don't smoke or drink much alcohol.
- You work as an electrician and Noah attends the local primary school. Your mum lives nearby and she helps a lot with childcare; she does most of the school runs too.

Information divulged freely

- You are extremely unhappy with the consultation with Dr Roberts last week. You felt he was dismissive of Noah and his symptoms. You asked at the time if he could have antibiotics but Dr Roberts said no. The next day Noah was still in pain and had to be off school again. This meant cancelled work for you as your mum is away on holiday. The out-of-hours doctor clearly agreed with you that Noah needed the antibiotics. Since he started them he has been much better and went back to school 2 days ago.
- You feel all doctors are scared to prescribe antibiotics now and are sure all the hype about resistance is just another tabloid drama. Surely children are more at risk of getting nasty infections and they should be given antibiotics more readily.
- After you have said all this you do calm down and apologise, saying: "It's not your fault doc, I'm sure you would have given him antibiotics wouldn't you?".

Information only divulged if specifically asked

- If the doctor discusses Dr Roberts' consultation with you, you are interested to hear their opinion. You want to know why he didn't give the antibiotics. You ask what the Centor score is and what this score means. If the GP explains the low score makes bacterial tonsillitis unlikely you don't accept this – surely all children are different. After all the out-of-hours doctor agreed with you didn't she?
- If the out-of-hours consultation is discussed with you, you are surprised to hear this GP also felt the throat infection was viral, but now you start thinking back to the consultation maybe she didn't say Noah needed the antibiotics. You admit you were very abrupt with her and asked several times for antibiotics.

- You want to know why Noah seemed much better after the antibiotics were started if this was a virus; you seem unconvinced by the explanation that the virus would have improved on its own; this seems like a big coincidence to you.
- If the GP advises that avoidance of antibiotics in viral illnesses is important to prevent spread of resistance you laugh – you are sure this is made out to be worse than it is. However, you do admit to hearing about MRSA and *C. diff*. Surely giving one child antibiotics would not change this though, it's the hospital specialists that should be stopping their prescriptions.
- If the GP takes you through the important points in the consultations (low Centor score, likely viral symptoms, OOH GP giving script due to parental concern) you do feel you understand the events better and calm down.
- You ask what will happen next time, because you still feel parents should be able to insist their child gets antibiotics when they need them. If the GP offers strategies such as delayed scripts, review appointment at the surgery or swabs in cases of throat infection, you agree to this and feel fully satisfied with the consultation. You decline any offer to take the complaint further. If the GP advises that you are unable to request scripts and does not offer any suggestions for the next occasion, you do want to complain and take details of the complaints process.

Case B12.9   Marking scheme for the observer

Advice on how to stay calm when dealing with angry patients can be read in conjunction with this case: www.gponline.com/consultation-skills-staying-calm-angry-patients/article/1051676

Data gathering and diagnosis

			• Actively listens without interrupting whilst the patient speaks about their complaint and the events which occurred and gives time for him to vent
			• Acknowledges dad's concerns and reasons for his anger
			• Establishes the patient's understanding of the use of antibiotics in viral illness and antibiotic resistance

Clinical management and medical complexity

			• Reflects and legitimises the patient's anger, e.g. "I can understand why you are unhappy that Noah continued to be in pain and you had to take extra time off work"
			• Takes the patient through the details of both consultations explaining why both doctors agreed Noah's illness was likely a viral illness
			• Is able to discuss the Centor scoring criteria as a tool to guide antibiotic use (www.nice.org.uk/guidance/ng84/chapter/terms-used-in-the-guideline)
			• Advises that antibiotics in viral illnesses will be ineffective, will lead to side-effects and antibiotic resistance in the general population. Considers providing an information leaflet: https://antibioticguardian.com/keep-antibiotics-working
			• Focuses on Noah's presentation and suggests the approach you would have taken at the time would be to discuss medications that would help him feel better (such as analgesia for the sore throat), a discussion on typical timescales for resolution and when he should seek further medical review. Is able to offer strategies for any further illness such as 48 hour review appointments, delayed prescriptions for antibiotics or, in case of sore throat, a swab could be considered to rule out bacterial infection
			• Can provide details of the local complaints procedure if needed

			Relating to others
☐	☐	☐	• Remains calm, composed and speaks slowly and clearly, avoiding any raised voices
☐	☐	☐	• Listens quietly and encourages the patient to tell his story
☐	☐	☐	• Chunks and checks any information given for understanding
			• Phrases such as "I'm sorry you are feeling so angry about this" or "Thank you for sharing how you feel about this so we can come to an understanding" may be useful
☐	☐	☐	• Is able to discuss antibiotics and their use in a jargon-free manner

Case B12.10 Information for the doctor

In this case you are a GP registrar taking video calls in a routine surgery.	
Name:	Charlotte Richards
Age:	22
Past medical history:	None
Current medication:	None

Notes

Case B12.10   Information for the patient

You are Charlotte Richards, a 22-year old woman, who wants to talk to the GP about your cousin's recent death.

ICE

- You have been told by your aunt that your cousin died due to heart problems and they advised you to go to your GP for testing.
- You are worried that you may suddenly die too. You have been struggling to sleep due to the worry about your heart.
- You expect to be sent for some further tests.

Background

- You are a student at a local college studying to be a social worker. You live with your two friends near the college campus. You also work in a local restaurant a few nights a week as a waitress.
- You don't smoke cigarettes but occasionally smoke cannabis, probably around once a month.
- You go out a few times a week and have 3–4 glasses of wine.
- You go to the gym a few times a week.

Information divulged freely

- Your cousin died about 3 months ago – he suddenly collapsed whilst out running. There has been a post-mortem and an inquest and your family have just been told he had hypertrophic obstructive cardiomyopathy (HOCM).
- Your aunt told you the whole family have been advised to "have tests".

Information only divulged if specifically asked

- You have no symptoms. You have not experienced any shortness of breath, chest pain, palpitation or syncope.
- You have no other family history of sudden death. Your parents are both alive and well and you have a brother who is also well.
- You have been very anxious waiting for this appointment and you have stopped going to the gym in case it leads to heart problems. Your sleep has been disturbed and you are distracted in your classes. You are feeling upset about what happened to your cousin, but you have no symptoms of depression and don't feel you need any help with your bereavement.
- You have looked up the condition on the internet and know it involves the heart muscles being thicker than they should be. You are keen to obtain as much information as possible but didn't want to look too much up on the internet in case the information was all wrong.
- Your questions regarding the condition are:
  ° You were told the condition is genetic, what does this mean?
  ° What are the chances you have HOCM too?
  ° What are the chances of any children you have having HOCM?
  ° What tests are needed to see if you have HOCM?
  ° Whilst waiting for the tests would the GP suggest you stop exercising?

Results for the doctor

Examination

Provided from patient's home monitor
- BP 120/80, HR 68

Case B12.10 Marking scheme for the observer

Data gathering and diagnosis

☐ ☐ ☐ • Takes a family history of an inherited condition

☐ ☐ ☐ • Asks about cardiovascular symptoms – chest pain, breathlessness, palpitations and syncope

☐ ☐ ☐ • Identifies the recent bereavement and screens for depression

Clinical management and medical complexity

☐ ☐ ☐ • Arranges appropriate investigations including a 12-lead ECG and cardiology referral for echo. Discusses typical timescales to be seen

☐ ☐ ☐ • Is able to explain what HOCM is and discuss its genetics in a jargon-free way (autosomal dominant inheritance, see: www.genomicseducation.hee.nhs. uk/education/videos/autosomal-dominant-inheritance)

☐ ☐ ☐ • Discusses her concerns about her children inheriting the condition (children of affected parents have a 50% chance of inheriting the disease and early screening is advisable)

☐ ☐ ☐ • Discusses exercise and signposts to guidance: www.cardiomyopathy.org/ physical-health/exercise

Relating to others

☐ ☐ ☐ • Chunks and checks the information given about genetics and HOCM and provides a leaflet (patient.info/health/hypertrophic-cardiomyopathy-leaflet)

☐ ☐ ☐ • Assesses the patient's level of prior knowledge before starting their explanation and also identifies that the patient would like to be well informed about the condition

☐ ☐ ☐ • Creates rapport with the patient using good non-verbal communication

☐ ☐ ☐ • Recognises that the patient has had a recent bereavement and offers support with this

APPENDIX

Case list by subject

Subject	Relevant case(s)	Page reference
Abdominal pain	B2.5, B3.3, B5.9, B6.1, B9.4	135, 195, 321, 327, 447
Acne	B10.10	597
Advance care planning	B4.7, B12.2	261, 675
Alcohol misuse	B5.6, B5.9	303, 321
Allergy	B1.4	93
Alopecia	B3.7, B10.5	219, 567
Antibiotic prescribing	B10.9, B12.9	591, 717
ASD	B7.4	375
Atrial fibrillation	B11.4	627
Atrophic vaginitis	B2.6	141
Back pain	B9.6, B9.18	459, 531
Behavioural change (LD patient)	B7.6	387
Bisphosphonates	B4.2	231
Blepharitis	B9.10	483
BPH	B2.9	159
BPPV	B9.9	477
BRCA gene	B2.3	123
Breaking bad news	B12.4	687
Cannabis use	B5.4	291
Capacity assessment	B4.1, B6.2, B7.3	225, 333, 369
Cardiovascular risk assessment	B11.5	633
Cellulitis	B6.4	345
Cervical screening	B2.10	165
Chronic pain	B10.11	603
CKD	B11.7	645
Complaint	B12.5, B12.7, B12.9	693, 705, 717
Confusion / agitation	B4.6, B5.3, B7.7	255, 285, 393
Conjunctivitis	B1.6	105
Constipation	B1.1	75
Contraception	B1.5, B2.7, B2.12, B7.2, B10.3	99, 147, 177, 363, 555

Subject	Relevant case(s)	Page reference
COPD	B11.9	657
Cough	B9.16, B10.9	519, 591
Death administration	B12.3	681
Depression	B5.1, B5.4	273, 291
Dermatitis	B3.6	213
Diabetes	B7.5, B8.4	381, 417
Difficult consultations	B1.5, B4.1, B4.6, B5.4, B5.8, B6.1, B6.2, B6.3, B7.1, B7.2, B8.3, B9.2, B10.7, B11.2, B11.3, B12.1	99, 225, 255, 291, 315, 327, 333, 339, 357, 363, 411, 435, 579, 615, 621, 669
Dizziness	B6.3, B9.2, B9.9	339, 435, 477
DNACPR discussion	B12.2	675
Down's syndrome	B2.2, B7.3	117, 369
Dyspareunia	B2.5, B2.6	135, 141
Dyspepsia	B9.4	447
Eating disorder	B5.5	297
ECG interpretation	B6.3, B9.2, B11.4	339, 435, 627
Ectopic pregnancy	B6.1	327
Eczema	B1.4	93
End of life care	B4.6, B4.7, B10.7, B12.2, B12.3	255, 261, 579, 675, 681
End of life prescribing	B4.7, B10.7	261, 579
Endometriosis	B2.5	135
Erectile dysfunction	B10.4	561
Facial nerve palsy	B9.14	507
Falls	B4.5, B5.3	249, 285
Familial hypercholesterolaemia	B3.1	183
Fear of flying	B10.4	561
Fertility	B2.2, B2.11, B11.2	117, 171, 615
FGM	B8.2	405
Genetic testing	B2.2, B2.3, B3.1, B11.2, B11.3	117, 123, 183, 615, 621
Glaucoma	B8.3	411
GORD	B3.3, B9.16	195, 519
Gout	B6.5	351
Haematuria	B2.8	153
Haemophilia	B11.2	615
Headache	B8.3, B9.13, B10.3	411, 501, 555
Heart failure	B3.2	189
Hoarseness	B9.8	471
HOCM	B12.10	723
HPV vaccination	B2.10	165

Subject	Relevant case(s)	Page reference
HRT	B2.4	129
Huntington's disease	B11.3	621
Hypothyroidism	B7.3, B11.6	369, 639
Infertility	B2.5	135
Inflammatory bowel disease	B11.10	663
Influenza vaccination	B10.2	549
Insomnia	B5.7	309
Intermenstrual bleeding	B2.10	165
Iron-deficiency anaemia	B4.3, B9.7	237, 465
Learning disability health check	B7.3, B7.5	369, 381
Lung cancer	B12.4	687
LUTS	B2.9	159
Lyme disease	B9.17	525
Maldescended testes	B1.3	87
Medication error	B12.8	711
Medication overuse	B5.8, B10.8	315, 585
Melanoma	B9.19	537
Memory problems	B4.4, B5.3	243, 285
Menopause	B2.4	129
Miscarriage	B2.11	171
Multiple sclerosis	B9.12	495
Osteoporosis	B4.2	231
Palpitations	B9.2, B9.5	435, 453
Perinatal mental health	B5.2	279
Plantar fasciitis	B8.5	423
Pre-exposure prophylaxis (PrEP)	B10.6	573
PSA testing	B2.9, B11.1	159, 609
Safeguarding	B1.5, B7.1, B7.4, B8.2	99, 357, 375, 405
Sepsis	B6.4	345
Shortness of breath	B3.2, B6.2	189, 333
Sickness certification	B12.6	699
Snoring	B3.4	201
Social care	B4.1	225
Spirometry	B11.9	657
STI	B8.1	399
Suicidal ideation	B5.1	273
Suspected cancer referral	B4.3	237
Termination of pregnancy request	B12.1	669

Subject	Relevant case(s)	Page reference
Third party consultation	B1.1, B1.2, B4.1, B4.6, B5.3, B7.1, B7.2, B7.3, B7.5, B7.6, B9.1	75, 81, 225, 255, 285, 357, 363, 369, 381, 387, 429
TIA	B4.8	267
Tinnitus	B3.5	207
Tiredness	B9.11	489
Travel advice	B2.1	111
Tremor	B9.15	513
Upper respiratory tract infection	B10.9	591
Vaccination	B10.2	549
Vasectomy request	B2.7	147
Venous thromboembolism	B6.2, B9.3	333, 441
Visual disturbance	B8.3	411
Vitamin D deficiency	B11.8	651
Vomiting	B9.1	429
Weight loss	B10.1	543